Pediatric Psychogastroenterology

Bringing together international experts in psychological and behavioral treatments for pediatric gastrointestinal symptoms, this book provides detailed, evidence-based protocols targeting gastrointestinal distress and associated mental health concerns for patients and their families.

The first consolidated resource on the topic, *Pediatric Psychogastroenterology*, gives mental health professionals access to the most up-to-date clinical knowledge and practice. Taking a holistic approach, it guides the reader on the treatment and care of pediatric gastrointestinal (GI) patients, as well as how to work with and support children's parents and families. The book is structured around symptom presentation and common challenges, enabling the reader to focus quickly on the area of need. Each chapter includes clinical pearls of wisdom and 62 developmentally appropriate worksheets for patients and their families to facilitate treatment, available for download.

This practical, authoritative guide is an essential resource for mental health professionals who work directly with pediatric cohorts, as well as postgraduate students in health psychology, behavioral medicine, or social work.

Miranda A.L. van Tilburg is Research Director at Cape Fear Valley Health in Fayetteville, NC, USA. She also holds professor positions at the University of North Carolina, Marshall University, University of Washington, and Campbell University. Dr van Tilburg is an expert in psychogastroenterology.

Bonney Reed is Pediatric Psychologist and Associate Professor of Pediatrics at Emory University School of Medicine and Children's Healthcare of Atlanta, USA. In working with patients and conducting clinical research, she aims to use psychological principles to improve disease outcomes and quality of life in patients affected by GI conditions.

Simon R. Knowles is Associate Professor and Clinical Psychologist based at the Swinburne University of Technology, Melbourne, Australia. His clinical and research interests relate to the biological and psychological interactions of GI conditions and the brain–gut axis.

Pediatric Psychogastroenterology

A Handbook for Mental Health Professionals

Edited by Miranda A.L. van Tilburg,
Bonney Reed and Simon R. Knowles

Routledge
Taylor & Francis Group
LONDON AND NEW YORK

Designed cover image: © Shutterstock

First published 2024
by Routledge
4 Park Square, Milton Park, Abingdon, Oxon OX14 4RN

and by Routledge
605 Third Avenue, New York, NY 10158

Routledge is an imprint of the Taylor & Francis Group, an informa business

ISBN: 9781032312347 (hbk)
ISBN: 9781032312330 (pbk)
ISBN: 9781003308683 (ebk)

DOI: 10.4324/9781003308683

Typeset in Times New Roman
by Deanta Global Publishing Services, Chennai, India

Access the Support Material: routledge.com/9781032312330

Miranda: This book is dedicated to the countless children, past and future, whose lives I've had the honor to briefly visit. I learned so much from your grace, grit, and generosity.

Bonney: I dedicate this book to my mentors in pediatric psychogastroenterology and to my patients.

Simon: I dedicate this book to my parents, Robert and Irene Knowles, who like all wonderful parents provided a loving and caring environment in which to learn and grow.

Contents

List of tables *x*
List of figures *xi*
List of boxes *xii*
List of acronyms *xiii*
List of contributors *xv*
Acknowledgments *xxi*
List of editors *xxiii*
Foreword *xxiv*
Preface *xxvi*

PART 1
Introduction to pediatric gastrointestinal physiology and conditions, the brain-gut axis, and working within health care teams **1**

1 Gastrointestinal anatomy and physiology 3
JORDAN M. SHAPIRO

2 Stress, psychological factors, and the brain–gut axis 22
JULIE SNYDER CHRISTIANA AND SAMUEL NURKO

3 Common gastrointestinal conditions in pediatrics 35
ASHISH CHOGLE

4 Medical procedures/testing in pediatric gastroenterology 53
SHAUNTE MCKAY AND JOSE GARZA

5 Helping youth manage medical procedures 67
DELANE LINKIEWICH, OLIVIA DOBSON, AND C. MEGHAN MCMURTRY

6 Case conceptualization and assessment 77
MICHELE H. MADDUX AND AMANDA D. DEACY

7 Collaborative, multidisciplinary treatment 87
JENNIFER VERRILL SCHURMAN AND CRAIG A. FRIESEN

8 Working with parents and primary caregivers 101
KARI FREEMAN BABER AND KELLY A. O'NEIL RODRIGUEZ

9 Caring for youth and families with complex medical and psychosocial concerns 114
BRADLEY JERSON AND AMY E. HALE

PART 2
Psychological approaches in pediatric psychogastroenterology 129

10 Feeding difficulties: Introduction 131
HAYLEY H. ESTREM, JACLYN PEDERSON, AND KAITLIN B. PROCTOR

11 Feeding difficulties: Food refusal 142
MEGHAN A. WALL, ANDREA BEGOTKA, AND CINDY KIM

12 Feeding difficulties: Food selectivity 152
KAITLYN MOSHER, ROBERT DEMPSTER, VALENTINA POSTORINO, AND T. LINDSEY BURRELL

13 Feeding difficulties: Difficulty swallowing and the fear of aversive consequences 164
NANCY L. ZUCKER, ILANA B. PILATO, AND SARAH LEMAY-RUSSELL

14 Nausea and vomiting 177
SALLY TARBELL

15 Pain disorders: Introduction, assessment, and psychophysiology 189
LIZ FEBO-RODRIGUEZ AND MIGUEL SAPS

16 Pain disorder interventions: Cognitive behavior therapy and acceptance and commitment therapy 198
TASHA MURPHY, MIRANDA A.L. VAN TILBURG, AND RONA L. LEVY

17 Pain disorder interventions: Hypnotherapy 211
ARINE M. VLIEGER

18 Constipation and soiling: Infant/toddler 219
CHRISTINA LOW KAPALU AND JOHN M. ROSEN

19 Constipation and soiling: Children and adolescents 228
JACLYN A. SHEPARD AND ALEX C. NYQUIST

PART 3
Transition and future challenges in pediatric Psychogastroenterology 237

20 Chronic illness adjustment and transition 239
SARA L. LAMPERT-OKIN, MEGHAN M. HOWE, ANGELA YU, KIM GRZESEK, AND RACHEL NEFF GREENLEY

21 Supervision and future challenges in pediatric psychogastroenterology 252
BONNEY REED, SIMON R. KNOWLES, AND MIRANDA A.L. VAN TILBURG

Index *259*

Tables

2.1 Developmentally appropriate metaphors to explain the brain–gut connection, nervous system hypersensitivity, and the concept of chronic GI symptoms 29
3.1 Common GI conditions in youth 36
3.2 Commonly used medications for GI conditions in youth 37
4.1 Common indications for laboratory testing 55
4.2 Summary of common imaging descriptions 57
4.3 Common motility testing indications 62
5.1 Assessment of pain and fear (all measures are freely accessible) 70
6.1 Language adaptations by age and developmental level 79
7.1 Sample roles by patient population (assessment phase) 90
7.2 Role definition and communication strategies for integration of psychology into GI care 92
7.3 Key strategies to enhance communication and collaboration in multidisciplinary care 93
7.4 Recommended talking points with administrative leaders 96
11.1 Summary of contributing factors associated with food refusal 144
11.2 Summary of common psychological and behavioral issues and suggested assessment questions/comments and interventions 149
14.1 Rome IV diagnostic criteria for pediatric nausea and vomiting disorders 178
15.1 FAPD subtypes 191
15.2 Pharmacologic management of abdominal pain 194
17.1 Stages of hypnosis in gut-directed hypnotherapy 212
19.1 Summary table of behavioral issues and suggested interventions 232
20.1 Evidence-based interventions to enhance psychosocial functioning, adherence, and transition readiness 242

Figures

1.1	The anatomy of the GI tract	4
1.2	Layers of the GI tract	5
1.3	Esophageal phase of swallowing	9
1.4	The role of the lower esophageal sphincter in gastroesophageal reflux disease	10
1.5	Anatomy of the stomach	10
1.6	Sites of absorption of macronutrients and micronutrients along the GI tract	13
1.7	Pancreatobiliary system	14
1.8	Functions of the liver	15
1.9	The anatomy of the anorectal canal	17
2.1	The brain–gut axis	24
3.1	Classification of esophageal atresia	38
4.1	Child performing breath test	56
4.2	Child on tilt table drinking contrast for upper GI X-ray	58
4.3	Child receiving colonoscopy	63
5.1	A longitudinal view of medical procedures	69
7.1	Process map with key elements to consider within each phase	88
10.1	History of PFD and ARFID	134
10.2	Patient ages per diagnostic code use	135
11.1	Bite-size fading	146
12.1	Picky eating and selective eating	153
12.2	Parent–child feeding interaction	155
12.3	Treatment goals for food selectivity	156
13.1	An example of a maladaptive fear gradient following a choking incident	166
13.2	Cycle of somatic avoidance resulting from fear generalization	167
13.3	Throat sensation characters	172
16.1	Impact of child and parent catastrophizing on child and health outcomes	200
16.2	Tension–pain cycle	203
18.1	A vicious cycle: constipation	220

Boxes

3.1	Red flags suggestive of organic conditions	42
8.1	Supporting a 9-year-old in daily medication adherence	104
8.2	Addressing parental overprotection	108
9.1	Discussing refractory symptoms amid reassuring test results	115
9.2	The chicken or the egg? GI symptoms and anxiety disorders	118
9.3	Navigating trauma disclosures	119
9.4	Responding to commonly expressed treatment concerns	120
9.5	Systemic barriers in action	124
9.6	Tips for enhancing treatment collaboration with a school and/or coach	125
10.1	Visualizing antecedent-based challenges	139
14.1	Recommended assessment for NVD	179
14.2	Case example of CVS treatment	184
15.1	Can everyone feel pain?	193
17.1	How to discuss hypnotherapy with youth and parents	215
18.1	Red flags indicating the need for further evaluation	221
18.2	Is toilet training a contributor to constipation?	223
18.3	"Help! I'll fall in the toilet"	225
19.1	Examples of school accommodations	231

Acronyms

ACE	Adverse childhood experience
ACT	Acceptance and commitment therapy
AN	Anorexia nervosa
ANS	Autonomic nervous system
ARFID	Avoidant/restrictive food intake disorder
ASD	Autism spectrum disorder
BGA	Brain–gut axis
BMP	Basic metabolic panel
CBT	Cognitive behavior therapy
CHS	Cannabinoid hyperemesis syndrome
CNS	Central nervous system
CRP	C-reactive protein
CVS	Cyclic vomiting syndrome
DGBI	Disorders of gut–brain interaction (formally known as functional gastrointestinal disorders; FGIDs)
EBT	Evidence-based treatment
EndoFLIP	Endoluminal functional lumen imaging probe
ENS	Enteric nervous system
ESR	Erythrocyte sedimentation rate
FAP	Functional abdominal pain
FGIDs	Functional gastrointestinal disorders (now referred to as disorders of gut–brain interaction; DGBI)
FN	Functional nausea
FOAC	Fear of aversive consequences
FV	Functional vomiting
GI	Gastrointestinal
H. pylori	*Helicobacter pylori* bacteria
HPA axis	Hypothalamic–pituitary–adrenal axis
IBD	Inflammatory bowel disease
IBS	Irritable bowel syndrome
IV	Intravenous
LGBTQIA+	Lesbian, gay, bisexual, transgender, queer, intersex, asexual, +
NFI	Nonretentive fecal incontinence

NG Nasogastric
NVD Nausea and vomiting disorders
OR Observer report
OT Occupational therapist
PFD Pediatric feeding disorder
PFPT Pelvic floor physical therapy
POTS Postural orthostatic tachycardia syndrome
SAM axis Sympathetic-adreno-medullar axis
SDOH Social determinants of health
SLP Speech-language pathologist
SR Self-report
TAs Topical anesthetics
TF-CBT Trauma-focused cognitive behavior therapy

Contributors

Kari Freeman Baber, PhD

Clinical Assistant Professor of Psychiatry, Perelman School of Medicine, University of Pennsylvania & Psychologist, Department of Child and Adolescent Psychiatry & Behavioral Sciences and Department of Pediatrics/Gastroenterology, Hepatology & Nutrition, Children's Hospital of Philadelphia
Philadelphia, Pennsylvania, USA.

Andrea Begotka, PhD

Assistant Professor, Pediatric Psychologist, Medical College of Wisconsin
Milwaukee, Wisconsin, USA.

T. Lindsey Burrell, PhD

Adjunct Assistant Professor, Departments of Pediatrics, Emory University School of Medicine & Clinical Psychologist
Atlanta, Georgia, USA.

Ashish Chogle, MD, MPH

Associate Professor, Division of Pediatric Gastroenterology, CHOC Children's, University of California-Irvine
Irvine, California, USA.

Julie Snyder Christiana, Psy.D

Assistant Professor of Psychology, Harvard Medical School
Pediatric Psychologist, Boston Children's Hospital
Boston, Massachusetts, USA.

Amanda D. Deacy, PhD

Associate Professor, Department of Pediatrics, University of Missouri, Kansas City (UMKC) School of Medicine & Psychologist, Division of Gastroenterology, Hepatology, and Nutrition, Children's Mercy Kansas City
Kansas City, Missouri, USA.

Robert Dempster, PhD

Clinical Assistant Professor, Department of Pediatrics, The Ohio State University
Program Director, Comprehensive Pediatric Feeding and Swallowing Program, Nationwide Children's Hospital
Columbus, Ohio, USA.

Olivia Dobson, MA

PhD student, University of Guelph
Guelph, Ontario, Canada.

Hayley H. Estrem, PhD, RN

Assistant Professor, University of North Carolina Wilmington
Wilmington, North Carolina, USA.

Liz Febo-Rodriguez, MD

Assistant Professor & Pediatric Gastroenterologist, The University of Texas Medical Branch
Galveston, Texas, USA.

Craig A. Friesen, MD

Pediatric Gastroenterologist & Professor of Pediatrics, University of Missouri Kansas City School of Medicine
Associate Division Director for GI Research, Children's Mercy Kansas City
Kansas City, Missouri, USA.

Jose Garza, MD

Pediatric Gastroenterology Physician, GI Care for Kids
Atlanta, Georgia, USA.

Rachel Neff Greenley, PhD

Psychologist, Rosalind Franklin University of Medicine and Science
North Chicago, Illinois, USA.

Kim Grzesek, BS

Clinical Psychology Doctoral Student, Rosalind Franklin University of Medicine and Science
North Chicago, Illinois, USA.

Amy E. Hale, PhD

Assistant Professor of Psychology, Harvard Medical School
Pediatric Psychologist, Division of Gastroenterology, Hepatology & Nutrition, Boston Children's Hospital
Boston, Massachusetts, USA.

Meghan M. Howe, BA

Clinical Psychology Doctoral Student, Rosalind Franklin University of Medicine and Science
North Chicago, Illinois, USA.

Bradley Jerson, PhD

Assistant Professor of Pediatrics, University of Connecticut School of Medicine
Pediatric Psychologist, Division of Digestive Diseases, Hepatology, & Nutrition, Connecticut Children's Medical Center
Farmington, Connecticut, USA.

Christina Low Kapalu, PhD

Associate Professor & Pediatric Psychologist, Children's Mercy Kansas City, University of Missouri
Kansas City, Missouri, USA.

Cindy Kim, PhD, ABPP

Pediatric Psychologist, CHOC Children's Hospital of Orange
Orange, California, USA.

Simon R. Knowles, PhD

Associate Professor & Clinical Psychologist, Swinburne University of Technology
Melbourne, Victoria, Australia.

Sara L. Lampert-Okin, MS, LPC

Licensed Professional Counselor & Clinical Psychology Doctoral Student, Rosalind Franklin University of Medicine and Science
North Chicago, Illinois, USA.

Sarah LeMay-Russell, PhD

Clinical Associate & Clinical Psychologist, Duke University Medical Center
Durham, North Carolina, USA.

Rona L. Levy, MSW, PhD, MPH

Professor and Associate Dean for Research, University of Washington
Seattle, Washington, USA.

Delane Linkiewich, MA

PhD student, University of Guelph
Guelph, Ontario, Canada.

Michele H. Maddux, PhD

Associate Professor, Department of Pediatrics, University of Missouri, Kansas City (UMKC) School of Medicine
Licensed Psychologist, Division of Gastroenterology, Hepatology, and Nutrition, Children's Mercy Kansas City
Kansas City, Missouri, USA.

Shaunte McKay, MD

Pediatric Gastroenterology Fellow Physician, Ann & Robert H. Lurie Children's Hospital of Chicago
Chicago, Illinois, USA.

C. Meghan McMurtry, PhD, C. Psych

Associate Professor, University of Guelph, McMaster Children's Hospital
Hamilton, Ontario, Canada.

Kaitlyn Mosher, PhD

Clinical Assistant Professor, Department of Pediatrics, The Ohio State University & Clinical Psychologist, Department of Pediatric Psychology and Neuropsychology, Nationwide Children's Hospital
Columbus, Ohio, USA.

Tasha Murphy, PhD

Senior Research Scientist, University of Washington
Seattle, Washington, USA.

Samuel Nurko, MD

Professor of Pediatrics, Harvard Medical School
Director, Center for Motility and Functional Gastrointestinal Disorders, Boston Children's Hospital
Boston, Massachusetts, USA.

Alex C. Nyquist, PhD

Assistant Professor of Pediatrics, Cincinnati Children's Hospital Medical Center
Clinical Child & Adolescent Psychologist
Cincinnati, Ohio, USA.

Jaclyn Pederson, MHI

CEO, Feeding Matters
Phoenix, Arizona, USA.

Ilana B. Pilato, PhD

Medical Instructor & Clinical Psychologist, Duke University Medical Center
Durham, North Carolina, USA.

Valentina Postorino, PhD

Departments of Pediatrics and Psychiatry, University of Colorado, Anschutz Medical Campus, JFK Partners
Aurora, Colorado, USA.

Kaitlin B. Proctor, PhD

Assistant Professor, Division of Autism & Related Disorders, Department of Pediatrics, Emory University
Atlanta, Georgia, USA.

Bonney Reed, PhD, ABPP

Associate Professor of Pediatrics, Emory University School of Medicine
Clinical Psychologist, Children's Healthcare of Atlanta
Atlanta, Georgia, USA.

Kelly A. O'Neil Rodriguez, PhD

Assistant Professor of Clinical Psychiatry, Perelman School of Medicine, University of Pennsylvania & Psychologist, Department of Child and Adolescent Psychiatry & Behavioral Sciences and Department of Pediatrics/Gastroenterology, Hepatology & Nutrition, Children's Hospital of Philadelphia
Philadelphia, Pennsylvania, USA.

John M. Rosen, MD

Professor & Pediatric Gastroenterologist, Children's Mercy Kansas City, University of Missouri
Kansas City, Missouri, USA.

Miguel Saps, MD

Professor & Pediatric Gastroenterologist, Miller School of Medicine
Miami, Florida, USA.

Jennifer Verrill Schurman, PhD, ABPP, BCB

Clinical Psychologist & Professor of Pediatrics, University of Missouri Kansas City School of Medicine & Section Chief of GI Psychology, Children's Mercy Kansas City
Kansas City, Missouri, USA.

Jordan M. Shapiro, MD, MS

Assistant Professor of Gastroenterology, Baylor College of Medicine
Staff Gastroenterologist, Baylor College of Medicine/ Baylor St. Luke's Medical Center
Houston, Texas, USA.

Jaclyn A. Shepard, Psy.D

Associate Professor of Psychiatry and Neurobehavioral Sciences, University of Virginia School of Medicine & Clinical Psychologist
Charlottesville, Virginia, USA.

Sally Tarbell, PhD

Professor (retired)
Pediatric Psychologist, Northwestern Feinberg School of Medicine
Chicago, Illinois, USA.

Miranda A.L. van Tilburg, PhD

Research Director Cape Fear Valley Medical Center, Professor of Medicine, Marshall University, Adjunct Professor of Medicine, University of North Carolina, Affiliate Professor of Social Work, University of Washington
Chapel Hill, North Carolina, USA.

Arine M. Vlieger, MD, PhD

General Pediatrician, St Antonius Hospital Nieuwegein
Nieuwegein, The Netherlands.

Meghan A. Wall, PhD, BCBA

Assistant Professor, Pediatric Psychologist, Medical College of Wisconsin
Milwaukee, Wisconsin, USA.

Angela Yu, BS

Medical student, Rosalind Franklin University of Medicine and Science
North Chicago, Illinois, USA.

Nancy L. Zucker, PhD

Professor & Clinical Psychologist, Duke University Medical Center
Durham, North Carolina, USA.

Acknowledgments

Simon: I wish to thank the patients I have had the honor to work with; your valuable time and determination to make your life better despite having significant gastrointestinal difficulties are inspiring. Thank you to the allied and medical health professionals and researchers who continue to have a significant impact on my work with patients and research in psychogastroenterology. Finally, I wish to thank my coeditors, Bonney Reed and Miranda van Tilburg, who are leaders in psychogastroenterology, and despite significant workloads, agreed to take on this daunting project with me.

Bonney: I would like to thank my graduate school mentor, Professor Ronald L. Blount, who first introduced me to GI psychology and my long-time collaborators and supporters including Dr Jeffery D. Lewis. Only through the support of mentors have I been able to develop a career in psychogastroenterology. I would also like to acknowledge my GI psychology trainees who have made my career in psychogastroenterology possible and rewarding, including Dr Grace Cushman, Dr Sharon Shih, and Dr Kelly Rea. My husband's steadfast support throughout the writing and editing of this book, much of which occurred in the evenings, cannot go unacknowledged. Finally, I would like to thank my coeditors, Simon Knowles and Miranda van Tilburg, both are distinguished experts in the field of psychogastroenterology, from whom I have learned so much.

Miranda: I would like to honor the scientists and clinicians who laid the foundations of Psychogastroenterology before such a field was even named. A special thanks to the scientific mentors in my life: Dr Ad Vingerhoets, Dr Richard Surwit, Dr Bill Whitehead, and Dr Rona Levy. Thanks for allowing me to stand on your shoulders. I could not have done this without the amazing pediatric gastroenterologists who accepted me in their midst, at a time when psychologists were not commonly employed in the field. I especially want to thank Dr Denesh Chitkara who ushered me in, Dr Nader Youssef who has always been an intellectual sparring partner, and Dr Miguel Saps who has been there in every step of the way. We are better when we work together. Finally, I am privileged to have worked with an amazing editorial team. Bonney Reed and Simon Knowles, I am glad we shared this journey.

The editors would also like to acknowledge and thank:

- Mr Maxwell Rapach for his expert research assistant and editing support.
- Mr James Overs for his expert research assistant and editing support.
- Dr Edward Giles (Consultant Pediatric Gastroenterologist at Monash Children's Hospital, Melbourne, Australia) for his assistance in reviewing and revising Handout 4.1.
- Professor Carlo DiLorenzo for his very kind Foreword.
- Finally, we would like to thank all the contributors who provided chapters for this handbook. Each of you is a highly respected clinical expert in your field and consequently providing your valuable time to provide a chapter was very much appreciated. This handbook was an enormous challenge made much easier by your professionalism and dedication to this project, and your willingness to make changes to your chapters even right up to the end of the editorial process. Thank you.

List of editors

Dr Miranda A.L. van Tilburg is a Research Director at Cape Fear Valley Health in Fayetteville NC. She also holds professor positions at the University of North Carolina, Marshall University, University of Washington, and Campbell University. Dr van Tilburg is an expert in psychogastroenterology. She develops and tests brain–gut treatments such as cognitive behavioral therapy and hypnotherapy, for gastrointestinal diseases particularly for children. Dr van Tilburg has over 200 publications in her name and has received >$10M in grant funding. She has advised the FDA, EMA, NIH, and Center for Medicaid/Medicare. Dr van Tilburg was appointed to the Rome committee, which establishes diagnostic criteria for pediatric disorders of gut–brain interaction. She is a previously elected council member of the American Neurogastroenterology and Motility Association and a current elected ethics chair of the North American Society for Pediatric Gastroenterology, Hepatology, and Nutrition.

Dr Bonney Reed is a Pediatric Psychologist and Associate Professor of Pediatrics at Emory University School of Medicine and Children's Healthcare of Atlanta. In working with patients and conducting clinical research, she aims to use psychological principles to improve disease outcomes and quality of life in patients affected by GI conditions. She carries an active caseload of patients, regularly publishes clinical research in peer-reviewed journals, and trains future GI mental health professionals.

Dr Simon R. Knowles is Associate Professor and Clinical Psychologist based at Swinburne University of Technology, Melbourne. His clinical and research interests relate to the biological and psychological interactions of GI conditions and the brain–gut axis. Associate Professor Knowles has published over 100 peer-reviewed articles, 3 books, including *Psychogastroenterology for Adults: A Handbook for Mental Health Professionals* in 2019, and attained over $5.8(AUD) million in research funding. He has developed multiple online resources and optimal health programs for gastrointestinal conditions, which have been used by over 600,000 users to date.

Foreword

Optimal functioning of the gastrointestinal (GI) tract is central to youth's ability to grow, learn, and be happy. Yet, diseases and disorders affecting the GI tract impact one in four youth. These may not only impact biological factors such as appetite or defecation but also are known to negatively influence children's psychosocial development. Many children with GI symptoms are at risk for significant school absence with negative consequences on academic and social development. Long-term negative outcomes range from job insecurity to imprisonment. The relationship between psychosocial factors and gastrointestinal health is complex and as a child grows into adulthood, changes in social, psychological, and biological development can impact the many facets of the brain–gut axis.

Despite the long recognition of the importance of the brain–gut axis in the development and impact of many GI disorders and the more recent appreciation of the benefit of multiple psychological and behavioral treatments, the true integration of mental health professionals in the treatment of youth with GI diseases is relatively new. Increasingly, the value of a multidisciplinary collaboration to help youth with GI symptoms is recognized and GI practices are looking for ways to incorporate mental health professionals in their care delivery. Also, pediatric populations present with diverse developmental and emotional needs, requiring a greater range of therapeutic approaches. In response to such needs, pediatric GI psychology has now become a highly focused field that requires specialized training. Simply treating general mental health aspects is no longer deemed sufficient or appropriate for youth with complex GI problems.

A shortage of adequately trained pediatric GI mental healthcare providers has left GI practices with difficulties in hiring providers with the needed expertise. Until recently, most pediatric GI mental health providers did not have access to training, other than in a few specialized academic centers, often concentrated in large urban areas, hence excluding access to GI mental health to many youth, particularly those in rural areas. The current book is the first to provide comprehensive information needed for any mental health professional entering the field or established providers looking for an update on recent practices and approaches. Drawing on the latest research and clinician experience, the authors offer practical advice and evidence-based strategies for addressing psychosocial issues in youth with GI conditions, aiming to improve overall health and well-being.

The book includes background information on GI physiology, diseases, and medical assessment/treatment for those new to the field. It provides an in-depth description of mental health assessment and treatment of the most common GI symptoms such as abdominal pain, constipation, nausea, and feeding issues. In addition, the book has a very original format with learning points, "pearls of wisdom", practical scenarios, and suggested readings. This book is a pleasure to read and will be an invaluable resource for any mental healthcare provider encountering youth with GI issues.

Carlo Di Lorenzo, MD
Chief, Division of Pediatric Gastroenterology
Nationwide Children's Hospital
Professor of Pediatrics
The Ohio State University

Preface

Pediatric gastrointestinal (GI) conditions are common, and concerns around abdominal pain, digestion, stooling, and feeding are several of the most common reasons parents seek pediatric healthcare. Pediatric GI problems are heterogeneous and may include aberrations in meeting feeding and toileting developmental milestones, disorders of gut-brain interaction (DGBI) such as irritable bowel syndrome, and pediatric onset of chronic illnesses such as Crohn's disease. Particularly DGBI are common: In the Unites States of America 1 out of 4 infants, toddlers, and children fulfilled criteria for a DGBI. Worldwide, 13.3% of children suffer from functional abdominal pain [1], likely one of the most common GI conditions. Another common condition seen in GI practices is inflammatory bowel disease. Although this condition affects only 0.08% in the US, every single one of these patients needs regular care of a pediatric gastroenterologist. In addition, the rate of pediatric IBD has increased 133% from 2007 to 2016 with no definitive explanation [2]. Diagnosis with a pediatric GI disorder places youth and their family at risk of impaired quality of life [3], missed school/work [4], psychological distress [5], and increased healthcare costs [6].

As anyone can attest, our brain and gut are intimately connected. Who does not recognize butterflies in one's stomach or stomach cramps before an important event? The role of psychosocial factors in pediatric GI symptoms is well established. A sizeable literature describes associations between GI symptoms and many psychosocial factors such as child's and parent's thoughts, emotions, coping strategies and a history of negative life events [7]. Thankfully, it is increasingly recognized that comprehensive treatment for pediatric GI conditions includes addressing both biological as well as psychological and social factors impacting disease outcomes. It is no longer evidence-based or acceptable to treat a pediatric GI condition without addressing the social and psychological factors that may be influencing symptoms directly through an association with their onset and maintenance or contributing to a patient's distress through maladaptive coping [8]. This increased recognition has given rise to a new field of psychogastroenterology.

Psychogastroenterology can be defined as "the application of psychological science and practice to gastrointestinal health and illness" [9]. It examines how psychosocial factors can influence GI symptoms, develops and tests psychological treatments for GI disorders, and examines the crucial role mental health clinicians play in multidisciplinary teams. Although wide evidence exists for the efficacy and safety of psychological treatments in GI disorders, these are not available to most patients due to lack of GI-trained mental health care providers, low referral rates in the absence of clear psychological distress, and poor insurance coverage for these treatments. The aim of this book is to develop a compendium of expert opinion on the practice of pediatric psychogastroenterology. The book aims to serve as a resource for students/trainees, established mental health practitioners who are new to treating youth with GI disorders, other clinicians interested in psychological treatments of GI disorders, and established GI mental health providers who desire a state-of-the-art reference book for their practice. Through education and dissemination, we hope to make psychological treatments available to any pediatric patients in need of psychogastroenterology approaches.

Psychogastroenterology: Development and history

Pediatric psychogastroenterology has a long history. The earliest published literature stems from the 1950s at a time when Sigmund Freud's theory on psychosexual development was widely accepted. Bodily symptoms were often interpreted as repression of unconscious threatening thoughts or emotions. To discover the state of unconsciousness, clinicians interpreted the patients' symptoms, behaviors, and language, assigning meaning largely outside of the patients' own experiences We now know Freud was spectacularly wrong, therefore the examples below will feel outdated.

(1) **Constipation:** In 1947 Editha Sterba published a case report of "psychogenic constipation" in a two year old child [10]. Psychogenic constipation was seen as a normal developmental stage of the child's libido during potty training. Children were thought to derive anal pleasure from bowel movements and constipation was seen as anal eroticism and/or penis envy. Repeated use of enemas to aid in bowel movements elevated anal libido and thus constipation. These ideas remained popular even in the mid seventies. For example, Dr Glenn [11] published a case report of a young girl with constipation arguing the girl's symptoms were due to penis envy, pseudo pregnancy, and a masochistic father. This despite evidence in 1966 that 'psychogenic' constipation can be treated with an enema in 40 out of 56 young patients [12].

(2) **Inflammatory bowel disease:** In 1958 a report in the Royal Society of Medicine [13] describes young patients with colitis as dependent upon their parents, having difficulty expressing emotions, and preoccupation with cleanliness. Although not specifically discussed, the names of these psychosocial factors clearly are in line with the psychoanalytic framework of Freud in which parental sexual jealousy, suppressed emotions, and anal (erotic) fixations were thought to explain symptoms. Psychogenic causes of IBD where commonly accepted at that time [14].

(3) **Abdominal pain:** Although published in 1957 the study by Dr Apley and Naish [15] on recurrent abdominal pain feels refreshingly modern. The authors relied on empirical techniques rather than psychoanalytic insights. The authors studied 1000 school children and found those with recurrent abdominal pain, compared to those who with abdominal pain, show increased anxiety/timidness as well as increased excitability and fussiness. The authors relied on reports of mothers and school personnel, rather than psychiatrists' interpretations of the patient. In addition, their use of concepts such as anxiety and excitability are more aligned with current conceptualizations rather than their psychoanalytic zeitgeist. Thus, contrary to their compatriots the authors did not interpret psychological factors as evidence of repressed feelings being expressed in a physical way. However, not much later

> the idea that abdominal pain is entirely caused by emotional issues becomes very well entrenched (for example see the 1970 article by unlisted authors in the British Journal of Medicine) [16].

Despite these early empirical studies, it was decades before well-designed empirical studies of psychosocial factors in GI disease become common place. We have to place these studies in the light of the reigning models explaining health and disease. The biomedical model proposes that psychosocial factors can play a role in disease in two ways. Psychological factors can be *a consequence* of medically explained diseases. It may influence such things as health care seeking. For example, Engstrom observed in 1999 that the well-being of children with IBD depends on psychological and social complications from the disease [17]. The biomedical model also predicts that symptoms that are medically unexplained are caused by psychological factors. If it is not in the body, it must be in the brain. Many case control studies seem to support this assumption: Anxiety rates were much higher in patients with DGBI than in healthy controls [7]. Yet, Drs Walker and Greene observed no difference in anxiety or depression between children with medically explained and unexplained GI diseases [18].

The biopsychosocial model (see Chapter 2), proposed in 1977, introduced the idea that psychosocial aspects play a role in all diseases. But it would take several decades for these ideas to be widely accepted in medicine. We can see this from the timeline of studies (see Figure 0.1) that shows a clear focus of early psychosocially oriented studies on DGBI, disorders that do not have a clear medical explanation. While early studies in IBD, an inflammatory disease with a clear medical explanation, focused primarily on the consequence of living with a chronic disorder. For example, the first trial of cognitive behavioral therapy (CBT) for IBD in 2004 was aimed at treating comorbid depression. Over time, more blurring of the lines between 'medically explained' and 'medically unexplained' occurred, particularly with the recognition of IBS-IBD overlap. We now know that DGBI have important biological factors in their pathophysiology, and IBD has important psychosocial aspects affecting disease outcomes.

Although DGBI, particularly IBS/functional abdominal pain, and IBD are still primary targets for most studies, over time more studies have included other disorders or symptoms such as constipation, nausea, vomiting, feeding issues etc. (see Figure 0.1). These are important developments making psychogastroenterology far more inclusive and offering much needed psychological care to children across GI conditions. Furthermore, the type of psychosocial factors examined have become more diverse (see Figure 0.1). Where the early literature focused primarily on general anxiety and depression, as either causes of or reactions to GI symptoms, a shift can be observed towards examining more GI focused concepts such as GI specific anxiety, somatization, pain catastrophizing etc. which are stronger predictors of outcomes. Social aspects are also increasingly studied, and the strongest evidence comes from the social learning literature, showing parents protectiveness increases the pain and disability of their children. In 2017 this culminated in a novel trial showing that intervening only with parents can reduce disability in children with DGBI [19].

As evidence for the use of CBT and hypnosis across various pediatric GI disorders was building (see Figure 0.1), this has increased the number of mental health care providers embedded in pediatric GI clinics. The number of clinicians trained has exponentially increased, but is still too small to be able to offer care to all patients. Particularly patients living in rural areas with limited access to mental health care providers. Yet official training does not yet exist for pediatric psychogastroenterology. Mental health care providers often learn from mentorship of others in the field.

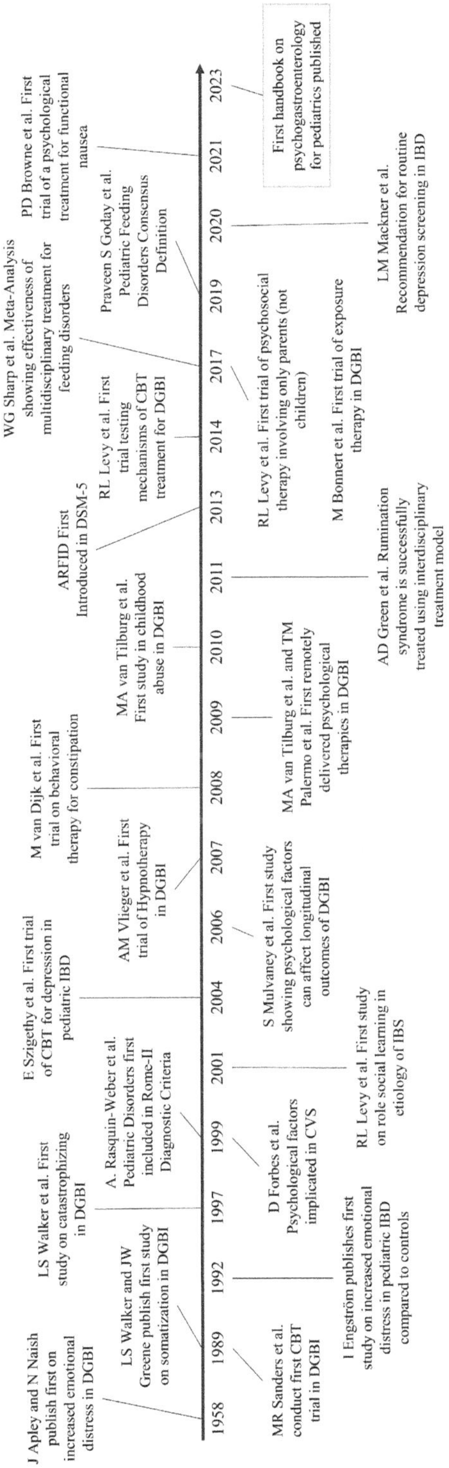

Figure 0.1 Historic timeline on the rise of pediatric psychogastroenterology.

The rationale for the book

As identified above, research relating to pediatric Psychogastroenterology has increased at a rapid rate. The knowledge gained from this research includes the growing understanding of the brain-gut axis, and its associated bi-directional pathways (brain-gut, gut-brain) in relation to gastrointestinal conditions and mental health.

Understandably, the evidence-based psychological approaches that are derived from pediatric Psychogastroenterology research are therefore increasingly relevant. While there is a growing number of publications demonstrating the relevant of psychological interventions in relation to better outcomes for those youth living with GI symptoms, due to their breadth and number, for many mental health professionals this area of work can be daunting. Further, despite the depth of knowledge in relation to the relevance and application of psychological interventions for youth living with a GI condition, few outside hospital-based university GI clinics have access to this information. This edited book represents the first attempt to provide mental health professionals with an evidence-based, practical handbook for working with youth living with a GI condition.

Due to the nature of the work, mental health professionals need more than the usual set of skills required when working with youth who present with GI symptoms and associated mental and behavioral difficulties. Basic additional knowledge relating to GI anatomy and functions, and the methods of diagnosis and ongoing management of GI conditions are needed. Further, knowledge regarding evidence-based psychological interventions, and how to apply them for youth with GI conditions is essential. To date, there is not a single source for mental health professionals that provides both a comprehensive introduction to the science of pediatric Psychogastroenterology and practical "how to" psychological protocols for working with GI cohorts. We hope that this handbook, written by experts across psychology, psychiatry, and gastroenterology, helps fill this gap and encourages others to follow.

The structure of the book

It is well established that the experience of psychotherapy leads to successful outcomes when mental health professionals are unconditionally positive towards patients, utilize microskills and apply evidence-based interventions. Aligned with successful therapy is the ability and need for mental health professionals to adapt interventions based on patient presentation, needs, and resources. To do this in pediatric psychogastroenterology settings, mental health professionals also need to be able to adapt their assessment and interventional skillset around a youth's condition/s and symptom/s.

Although, the current book aims to produce a handbook that is both comprehensive and practical, several compromises needed to be undertaken. Given the diversity and number of pediatric GI conditions, it was not possible to cover each of them. Nor was it feasible to provide case studies, as this would likely never appropriately reflect the diversity of GI conditions and associated psychological and behavioral presentation seen in pediatric gastroenterology practice. This current book is organized around the most common GI symptoms seen in pediatric GI youth presentations, namely feeding difficulties, nausea and vomiting, pain, and constipation and soiling.

Part I of the book is entitled "*Introduction to pediatric gastrointestinal physiology and conditions, the brain-gut axis, and working within health care teams*" The chapters in the first part of the handbook provides essential core aspects to the practice of pediatric psychogastroenterology, including GI physiology and common GI symptoms and conditions (Chapters 1 and 2). This part of the handbook also provides an overview of medical procedures and testing used in pediatric gastroenterology (Chapter 4) and recommendations to help youth manage them (Chapter 5). In addition, this part covers important practical aspects of pediatric psychogastroenterology, including case conceptualization (Chapter 6), how to work and promote multi-disciplinary approaches (Chapter 7), and working with parents of youth living with a GI condition (Chapter 8). The final chapter in this part, covers working with complex patients and psychological concerns (Chapter 9).

Entitled *Psychological approaches in pediatric Psychogastroenterology,* Part II provides readers with detailed recommendations and strategies in relation to the assessment and treatment of psychological issues often reported by youth with GI conditions. This part is has four main sections, broken down by the predominant presentations seen in pediatric GI youth, specifically feeding difficulties (Chapters 10–13), nausea and vomiting (Chapter 14), pain disorders (Chapters 15–17), and constipation and soiling (Chapters 18 and 19).

The last part of the book, Part III entitled *Transition and future challenges in pediatric Psychogastroenterology*, includes two chapters (Chapters 20 and 21) that explores the process of adaption to living with a chronic GI condition and recommendations associated with transitioning from pediatric to adult-based care. The final chapter provides recommendations relating to supervision of psychological trainees and an overview of the future challenges in pediatric psychogastroenterology.

We hope that this handbook, written by experts, will be an indispensable resource of information, guidance, and materials which enhance your knowledge of, and practice in, pediatric psychogastroenterology.

MvT, BR, and SK
Chapel Hill, Atlanta, and Melbourne
April 2023

References

1. Korterink JJ, Diederen K, Benninga MA, Tabbers MM. Epidemiology of pediatric functional abdominal pain disorders: A meta-analysis. *PloS One*. 2015;10(5):e0126982.
2. Ye Y, Manne S, Treem WR, Bennett D. Prevalence of inflammatory bowel disease in pediatric and adult populations: Recent estimates from large national databases in the United States, 2007–2016. *Inflamm Bowel Dis*. 2020;26(4):619–25.
3. Varni J, Bendo C, Nurko S, Shulman R, Self M, Franciosi J, et al. Pediatric Quality of Life Inventory (PedsQL) Gastrointestinal symptoms module testing study consortium. Health-related quality of life in pediatric patients with functional and organic gastrointestinal diseases. *J Pediatr.* 2015;166(1):85–90.
4. Mackner LM, Bickmeier RM, Crandall WV. Academic achievement, attendance, and school-related quality of life in pediatric Inflammatory Bowel Disease. 2012; 33(2):106–11.
5. Donovan E, Martin SR, Lung K, Evans S, Seidman LC, Cousineau TM, et al. Pediatric irritable bowel syndrome: Perspectives on pain and adolescent social functioning. *Pain Med (United States)*. 2019;20(2):213–22.
6. Hoekman DR, Rutten JM, Vlieger AM, Benninga MA, Dijkgraaf MG. Annual costs of care for pediatric irritable bowel syndrome, functional abdominal pain, and functional abdominal pain syndrome. *J. Pediatr.* 2015;167(5):1103–8. e2.
7. Newton E, Schosheim A, Patel S, Chitkara DK, van Tilburg MAL. The role of psychological factors in pediatric functional abdominal pain disorders. *Neurogastroenterol. Motil.* 2019; 31(6):e13538.

8. Reed B, Buzenski J, van Tilburg MA. Implementing psychological therapies for gastrointestinal disorders in pediatrics. *Expert Rev Gastroenterol Hepatol.* 2020;14(11):1061–7.
9. Knowles SR, Keefer L, Mikocka-Walus AA. *Psychogastroenterology for Adults: A Handbook for Mental Health Professionals.* Routledge; 2019.
10. Sterba E. Analysis of psychogenic constipation in a two-year-old child. *Psychoanal Study Child.* 1947;3(1):227–52.
11. Glenn J. Psychoanalysis of a constipated girl: Clinical observations during the fourth and fifth years. *J Am Psychoanal Assoc.* 1977;25(1):141–61.
12. Salvati EP. Psychogenic constipation. *Dis Colon Rectum.* 1966;9(4):293–4.
13. Schlesinger B, Platt J. Ulcerative colitis in childhood and a follow-up study. *Proc R Soc Med.* 1958;51(9):733–5.
14. Kirsner JB. Historical origins of current IBD concepts. *World J. Gastroenterol.* 2001;7(2):175–84.
15. Apley J, Naish N. Recurrent abdominal pain: A field study of 1000 school children with recurrent abdominal pain. *Arch. Dis. Child.* 1958;46:337–40.
16. Recurrent abdominal pain in children. *Br Med J.* 1970;4(5727):66–7.
17. Engstrom I. Inflammatory bowel disease in children and adolescents: Mental health and family functioning. *J. Pediatr. Gastroenterol. Nutr.* 1999;28(4):S28–33.
18. Walker LS, Greene JW. Children with recurrent abdominal pain and their parents: More somatic complaints, anxiety, and depression than other patient families? *J Pediatr Psychol.* 1989;14(2):231–43.
19. Levy RL, Langer SL, Van Tilburg MA, Romano JM, Murphy TB, Walker LS, et al. Brief telephone-delivered cognitive-behavioral therapy targeted to parents of children with functional abdominal pain: A randomized controlled trial. *Pain.* 2017;158(4):618.

Part 1

Introduction to pediatric gastrointestinal physiology and conditions, the brain-gut axis, and working within health care teams

Chapter 1

Gastrointestinal anatomy and physiology

Jordan M. Shapiro

Chapter aims

The aim of this chapter is to provide an introduction to the gastrointestinal (GI) tract, specifically in relation to its key structures and functions, including the mechanical and biochemical processes associated with normal digestion. The chapter also provides an overview of the microbiome and immunologic components and their role in the GI tract.

Learning points

- Introduction to key GI anatomy and physiology, including biological, chemical, and physical processes to break down, move, and absorb nutrients and eliminate waste.
- Introduction to the GI microbiome and immune system as they relate to normal function and disease states.
- Practical recommendations relating to psychoeducation about the GI tract.

Background

The GI tract is a complex group of organs with functions that range from digestion and absorption, maintaining fluid and electrolyte balance, immune function, as well as housing and mediating the interactions between the gut microbiome and human health.

Basic structure and function of the GI system

The GI tract is comprised of a tubular tract running from the mouth to the anus and accessory organs connected to the tubular structure (pancreas and liver). Each segment is highly specialized to carry out specific functions, see Figure 1.1 depicting key structures of the GI tract.

The esophagus facilitates the passage of food from the mouth to the stomach, where it is mechanically and biochemically broken down into smaller, more digestible components. The small intestine is made up of three segments – duodenum, jejunum, and ileum – and is the site of absorption of nutrients. The liver has many functions, such as detoxification, protein synthesis, energy storage, and cholesterol synthesis, but from the standpoint of digestion, it is primarily involved in the production of bile, which helps break down fat to help make it more easily digestible. Bile is also stored in the gallbladder to aid in the digestion of meals with higher fat content. The pancreas has endocrine (i.e., insulin production) and exocrine (i.e., digestive enzymes) functions. Enzymes are proteins that accelerate biochemical reactions such as digestion. Both

DOI: 10.4324/9781003308683-2

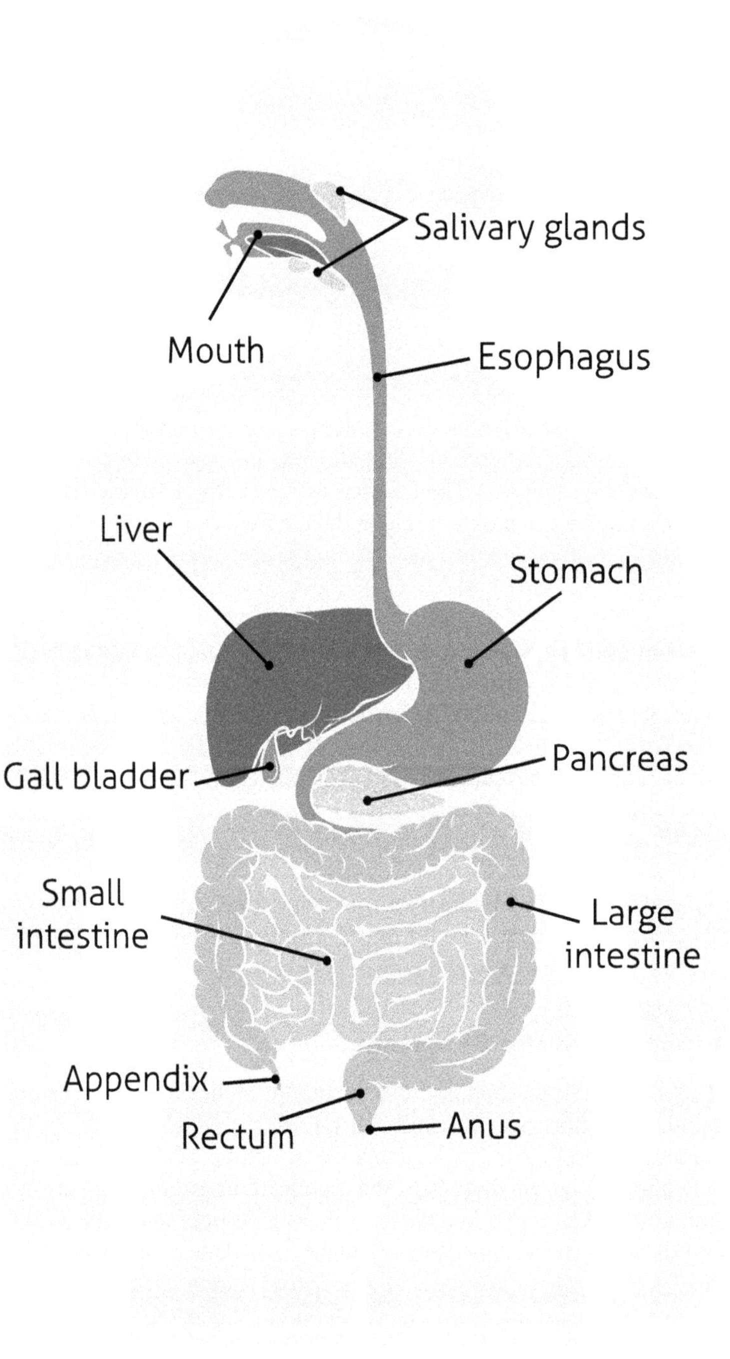

Figure 1.1 The anatomy of the GI tract (Source: Christos Georghiou/Shutterstock.com).

bile and pancreatic digestive enzymes travel in their respective bile and pancreatic ducts and are released into the duodenum via a common opening – the ampulla of Vater – to mix with and further digest food. The large intestine, or colon, absorbs water to create formed stools, and the pelvic floor and anorectal muscles help to hold stool until it is possible to defecate (otherwise known as "having a bowel movement" or "pooping").

Layers of the GI tract

The tubular portion of the GI tract consists of four layers (see Figure 1.2):

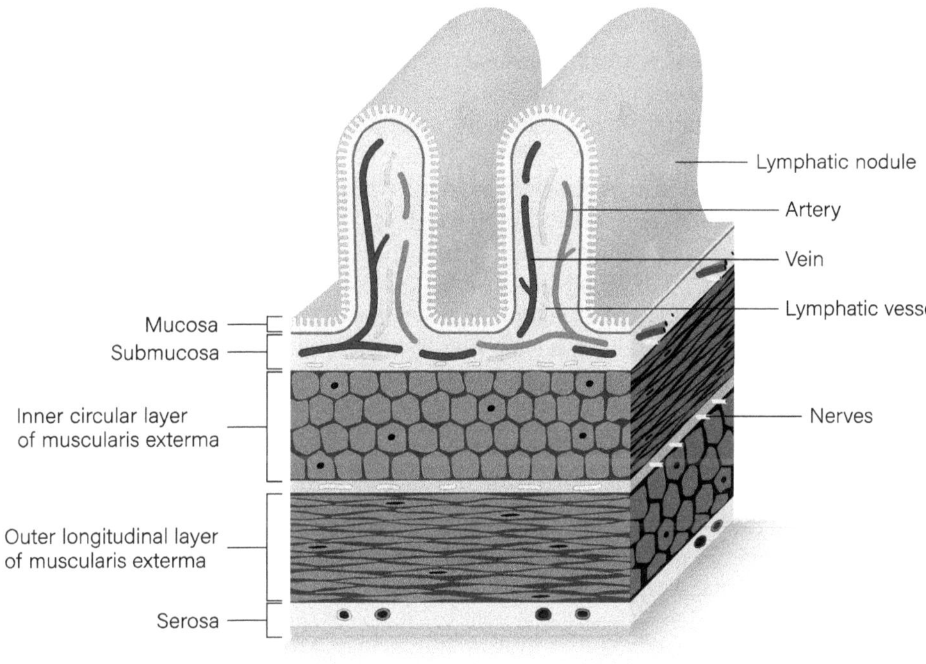

Figure 1.2 Layers of the GI tract (Source: Dee-sign/Shutterstock.com).

- The mucosa is the innermost layer of the GI tract (i.e., the layer in direct contact with food contents in the lumen) and consists of several different types of specialized epithelial (or surface lining) cells with different functions, such as secretion, absorption, or production of hormones.
- The submucosa is a connective tissue layer beneath the mucosa and contains blood vessels, lymphatics, and nerves (including the submucosal nerve plexus of Meissner) which provide both afferent (i.e., receiving signals from the lining of the GI tract and carrying them back to the central nervous system (CNS)) and efferent (i.e., sending signals to muscles to move or cells to secrete) innervation to the mucosa and its epithelial cells.
- The muscular layer consists of inner circular muscle and outer longitudinal muscle which allow the GI tract to contract and move contents from mouth to anus. The myenteric nerve plexus of Auerbach lies between the circular and longitudinal layers of muscle and regulates

these movements, often collectively referred to as "motility". In addition, the stomach has a third innermost layer called the oblique muscle layer. A common pattern of movement of the GI tract is peristalsis, which involves coordinated involuntary smooth muscle contractions above and relaxations below the food bolus in a sequential fashion to propel the contents of the GI tract forwards.

- The serosa is the outermost connective tissue covering of the GI tract, consisting of a thin layer of connective tissue reinforcement of the GI tract and covered by epithelium which protects the GI tract and reduces the friction of the organs as they move in the abdomen.

Blood supply of the GI tract

Oxygen-rich blood from the lungs returns to and is pumped from the left side of the heart to the body through the aorta, the largest artery in the body. The aorta rises from atop the heart to form an arch and then descends through the diaphragm (the large, dome-shaped muscle that flattens with inspiration to pull air into the lungs and which separates the chest and the abdomen) and into the abdomen, where three branches supply the GI tract: (1) the celiac artery, (2) the superior mesenteric artery, and (3) the inferior mesenteric artery. Most blood from the GI tract returns to the liver through the portal vein, then flows through the liver to the hepatic veins, which drain into the inferior vena cava, and ultimately back to the right side of the heart before being pumped to the lungs to pick up oxygen and repeat the cycle. The cycle occurs each heartbeat, which ranges from 100 to 160 beats per minute in newborns to 60 to 100 beats per minute in older children and young adults. Blood traveling from the intestines to the liver carries nutrients for further processing and is used in and by the liver.

The nervous system of the GI tract

The GI tract also includes the enteric nervous system (ENS). The ENS is often referred to as "the second brain" due to its highly complex organization and function, which includes over 500 million nerves, more than 20 different neurotransmitters, and bidirectional communication with the central nervous system (i.e., brain and spinal cord) [1]. There are two main nerve plexuses (i.e., bundles of condensed nerves where many nerves intersect and/or run together) in the GI tract: the submucosal plexus of Meissner and the myenteric plexus of Auerbach. The former lies in the submucosa layer, regulates local blood flow and secretion, and contains sensory nerve fibers to relay information from the gut to the brain. The latter lies between the circular and longitudinal layers of muscle and is the major player in the motility, or movement, of the GI tract. Throughout the GI tract, pacemaker cells (interstitial cells of Cajal) generate intrinsic nerve impulses and cause the GI tract to move. The interstitial cells of Cajal are akin to the pacemaker cells found in the sinoatrial node of the heart, which initiates each heartbeat.

The ENS can operate largely independently to propel food from the mouth to the anus. A classic physiology experiment by Bayliss and Starling in 1899 demonstrated that the tubular GI tract will squeeze a pellet of food from the end of the mouth to the anus with the bowel completely disconnected from the rest of the body, known as "the law of the intestine". Despite its independence, the GI tract is also innervated by the autonomic nervous system, composed of the sympathetic ("fight, flight, or freeze") and parasympathetic ("rest or digest") divisions. Sympathetic nervous system (SNS) activation diverts blood away from and slows the movement of food contents through the GI tract, while parasympathetic nervous system (PNS) activation increases blood flow to and movement of food contents through the GI tract. The vagus nerve (cranial nerve X) is the major nerve involved in carrying efferent (from central towards the periphery) signals from the PNS to the GI tract to cause actions such as muscular contractions of the intestines. However, 85% of the nerve fibers in the vagus nerve are afferent and carry information from the GI tract back to the brain and brain stem in the central nervous system. The communication between the brain and the gut constitutes what is referred to as the brain–gut axis (BGA) and underlies many disorders of gut–brain interaction (DGBI) such as functional dyspepsia and irritable bowel syndrome (IBS). For more information about the gut–brain interaction, see Chapter 2.

An integrated review of GI physiology: A journey through the GI tract

Swallowing (mouth and esophagus)

Swallowing, also known as *deglutition*, is comprised of three phases: (1) oral, (2) pharyngeal, and (3) esophageal. These phases prepare and carry portions of food from the mouth down the esophagus to the stomach. Of note, prior to food entering the GI tract, a "pre-oral" phase triggered by the mere thought, smell, and/or sight of food causes salivation to begin in anticipation of food entering the oral cavity. This so-called "cephalic" (head) phase of salivation was highlighted in the infamous psychological research by Nobel Prize winner Isaac Pavlov that led to the discovery of the behavioral procedure called classical conditioning [1]. In the experiments, Pavlov paired the salivation that occurred with the sight and smell of food with the ringing of a bell and then demonstrated the ability to induce salivation without the sight and smell of food just by ringing the bell.

Oral phase: In the oral phase of swallowing, food and drink enter the oral cavity, where the tongue and teeth begin to mechanically break food into smaller pieces. Different types of teeth serve different roles in the chewing process, with incisors cutting, canines tearing, and premolars and molars grinding food. The muscles of mastication (chewing) include the strongest muscle per weight in the body, the masseter, which forcefully closes the jaw to facilitate chewing. Chewing includes both voluntary and involuntary (reflexive) mechanisms, with stretching of the muscles of mastication leading to their rhythmic contraction followed by relaxation to grind up food. In addition, the salivary glands produce saliva, which contains water, mucin (a protein that contributes to the lubricating, softening, and wetting properties of saliva), and the digestive enzymes salivary amylase and lingual lipase. The latter contribute to the chemical digestion of carbohydrates and fats, respectively. Total unstimulated (continuous) saliva production ranges from 145 ml per day in children to 600 ml per day in adults, with decreases during sleep and increases with eating and non-nutritive chewing (e.g., gum). The tongue sections off a small portion of the chewed, moistened food into a bolus, forms a ramp with a depression in the midline by sealing it against the hard palate, and then propels the bolus into the back of the oropharynx.

Pharyngeal phase: When food contacts the highly innervated posterior palatopharyngeal arch – the more posterior of the two arches visible when looking in the back of the throat – the bolus enters the pharyngeal phase of swallowing. This marks the last volitional portion of the entire trip of food through the GI tract until defecation occurs. The food bolus is kept from entering the nasopharynx by the lifting and closure of the soft palate located on the posterior portion of the roof of the mouth, which occurs reflexively in response to food touching the posterior oropharynx. Simultaneously, the epiglottis folds backwards and closes the airway to prevent swallowed food from entering the lungs, also referred to as "aspiration". The upper esophageal sphincter prevents the entry of excessive air into the stomach and the reflux of stomach contents into the airway. The upper esophageal sphincter is contracted at rest and opens to allow passage of the food bolus into the esophagus, marking the end of the pharyngeal phase of swallowing. The pharyngeal phase of swallowing is the quickest and lasts roughly one second.

Esophageal phase: As the food bolus enters the esophagus, coordinated muscular contractions move food down the esophagus by peristalsis, see Figure 1.3.

The speed of transit through the esophagus depends in part on what is swallowed, as liquids often reach the stomach before the peristaltic wave. Primary peristalsis occurs when a normal swallow is initiated and the food bolus is moved into and through the esophagus (i.e., from oral to pharyngeal to esophageal). Secondary peristalsis is an intrinsic capability of the esophagus to start additional waves of peristalsis in the upper esophagus without the oral or pharyngeal phases to clear something that should not be there after the initial swallow such as a large food bolus, sticky foods such as peanut butter, a pill, or acid that has refluxed from the stomach into the esophagus. The esophageal phase is also contributed to, in part, by gravity. However, peristalsis of a food bolus through the esophagus and to the stomach can occur even when an individual is upside down.

The length of the esophagus at birth is 7 in. (18 cm) and in adults is 10–13 in. (25–33 cm), with widths of 6 mm and 20 mm in newborns and adults, respectively. As food nears the end of the esophagus, the lower esophageal sphincter (LES) – which is tonically contracted at baseline – relaxes to allow food to enter the stomach. The LES is contributed to by muscle fibers from the phrenoesophageal ligament, the diaphragmatic crura, and circular muscle layer of the distal esophagus. In addition to relaxing in response to a swallow, the LES periodically relaxes in what is called a transient lower esophageal sphincter relaxation (TLESR). TLESRs also help to vent gas from the stomach.

TLESRs – not overproduction of acid – are the primary mechanism that leads to gastroesophageal reflux disease (GERD), which manifests as the cardinal symptoms of heartburn and reflux (see Figure 1.4). Gastroesophageal reflux is common in infants as the LES does not mature until approximately two years of age. In addition, most infantile reflux is nonacid. Therefore, most cases of infantile GERD can be managed without the use of acid-suppressing medications [2].

Belching (burping) is the audible escape of air from the esophagus or stomach. Belching is a normal physiologic event that can occur dozens of times per day. Belching can be classified as supragastric (above the stomach) or gastric (from within the stomach). Supragastric belching involves increased swallowing of air (termed aerophagia) and evacuation of the air prior to it reaching the stomach. Gastric belching occurs when gaseous distention of the stomach causes stretch receptors to send signals to the LES to relax and the stomach to contract to force air out of the esophagus and mouth.

Stomach

As food travels down the esophagus and approaches the stomach, a nerve-mediated reflex results in receptive relaxation of the upper portion of the stomach (the fundus) to make room for incoming food (see Figure 1.5). The newborn stomach is approximately the size of a marble and can hold roughly 30 ml of food. The adult stomach is approximately the size of a cantaloupe (also known as rockmelon) and holds an average volume of 1 L after meals. However, it can expand to hold up to 4 L. Once all food has entered the stomach, the lower esophageal sphincter (inflow to the stomach) and pylorus (ring of muscle that serves as the outflow of the stomach) contract to close and the stomach begins to rhythmically grind the food against the antrum (the portion of the stomach closest to the outflow) and pylorus resulting in mechanical

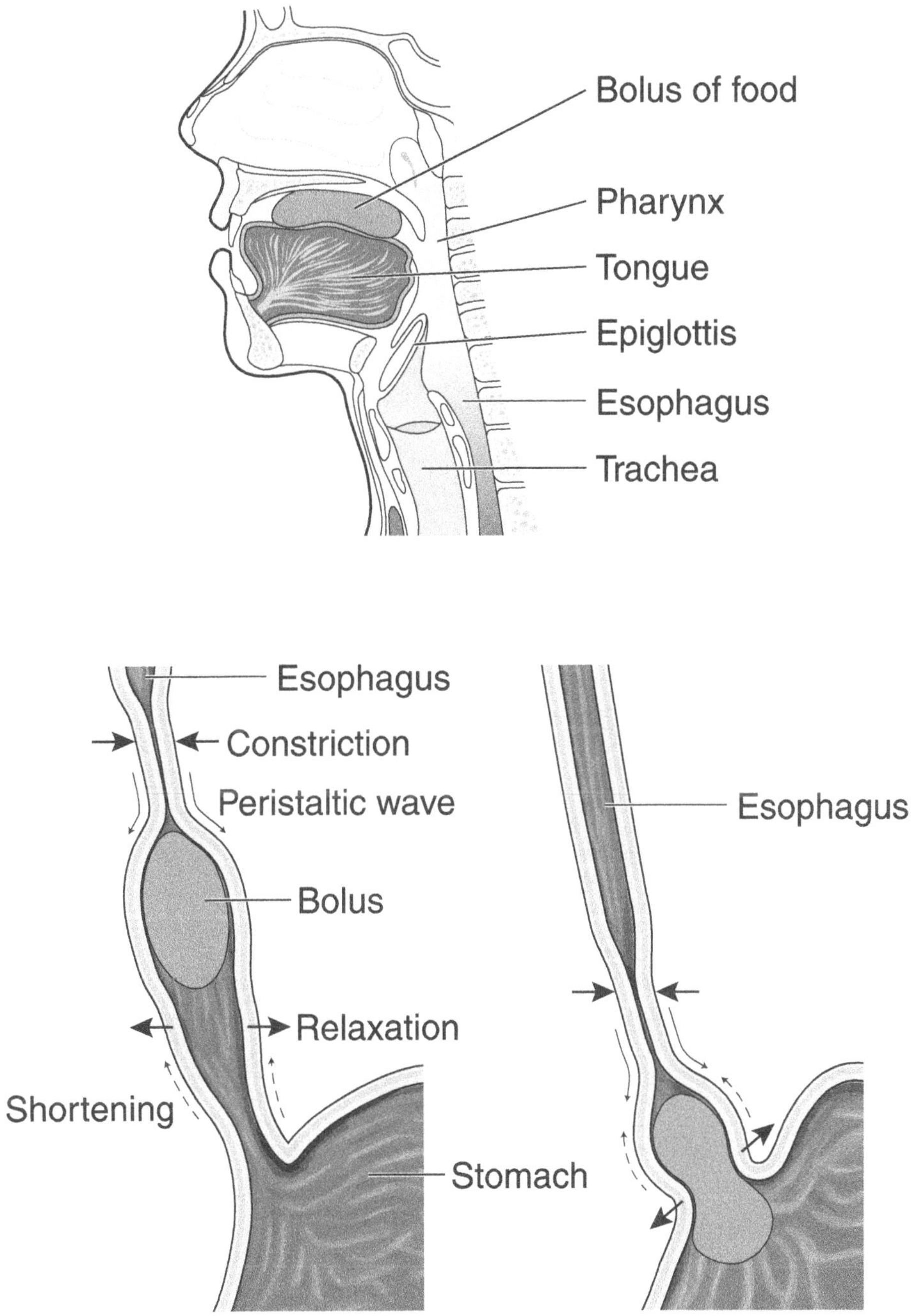

Figure 1.3 Esophageal phase of swallowing (Source: Blamb/Shutterstock.com).

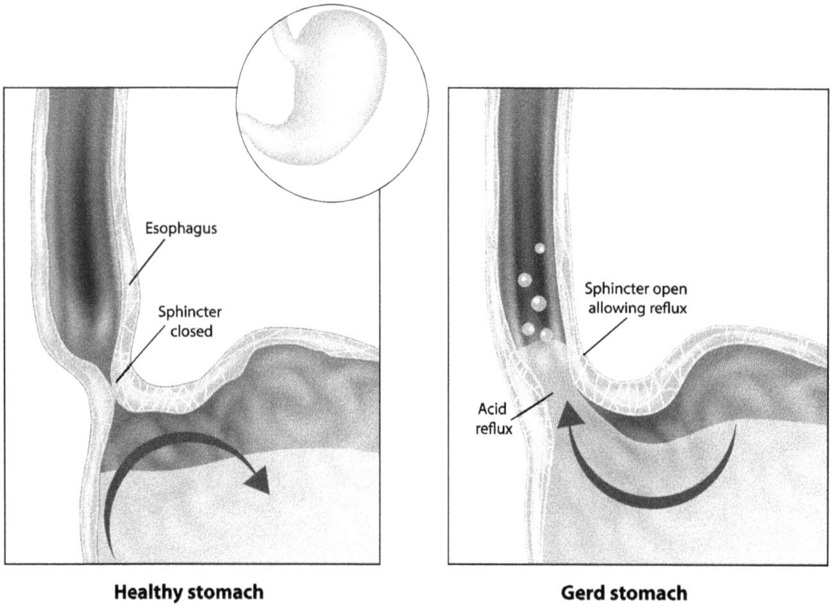

Figure 1.4 The role of the lower esophageal sphincter in gastroesophageal reflux disease (Source: Sakurra/Shutterstock.com).

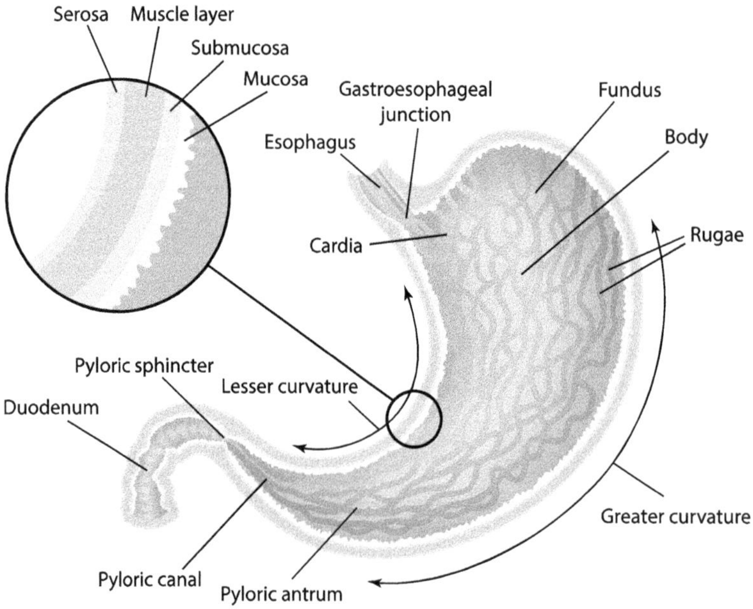

Figure 1.5 Anatomy of the stomach (Source: Olga Bolbot/Shutterstock.com).

digestion of food content. Chemical digestion occurs simultaneously as food is exposed to gastric juices containing acid and pepsin (a digestive enzyme) made in the stomach, which begin breaking down proteins. The pH of the human body is 7.4 (slightly alkaline); however, the pH of the stomach is 1–2 (highly acidic).

The mucosa of the stomach contains many specialized cells which secrete different substances involved in the digestive process and collectively make up "gastric juices":

- Parietal cells are in the body and fundus of the stomach and produce hydrochloric acid and intrinsic factors.
- Acid helps in the digestion of protein, kills bacteria that are ingested, and inactivates salivary amylase. Acid secretion occurs continuously in a basal fashion at about 10–15% of the maximum capacity. Parietal cells have multiple different receptors for stimuli that can trigger increased acid secretion: (1) muscarinic acetylcholine receptors are stimulated by acetylcholine from the parasympathetic nervous system, (2) histamine type 2 receptors are stimulated by histamine released by enterochromaffin-like cells, and (3) gastrin receptors are stimulated by gastrin released by G-cells in the antrum of the stomach. Gastrin and acetylcholine directly cause parietal cells to secrete acid. Gastrin indirectly causes acid secretion by stimulating enterochromaffin-like cells to make histamine, which then stimulates histamine receptors to cause acid secretion. Histamine potentiates the effects of gastrin and acetylcholine on parietal cells so that smaller amounts are necessary to increase acid secretion.
- Intrinsic factor is required for the absorption of vitamin B_{12} and is the only product of secretion made by the stomach which humans cannot live without (i.e., supplementation with vitamin B_{12} injections is required when the body is unable to produce intrinsic factor as in autoimmune gastritis, or when the segment of the small intestine required for absorption of vitamin B_{12}, the ileum, is inflamed, as in Crohn's disease, or surgically resected).
- Chief cells produce pepsinogen, the inactive form of the enzyme pepsin. Acid converts pepsinogen to pepsin, which is involved in the breakdown of protein.
- Mucus cells produce mucus, which along with bicarbonate, forms a layer that protects the stomach from acid.
- G-cells are located in the antrum and secrete the hormone gastrin in response to stretch of the stomach, protein, or increased pH (i.e., less acidity) in the stomach. Gastrin is a major stimulus of the parietal cells to make acid.
- Enterochromaffin-like cells make histamine which potentiates the effects of the neurotransmitter acetylcholine and gastric hormone gastrin to stimulate parietal cells to make acid.
- D-cells are located in the antrum (as well as the duodenum and pancreas) and release somatostatin, which inhibits gastric secretion, gastric emptying, and intestinal motility in addition to several other non-GI hormones (e.g., thyroid-stimulating hormone, prolactin, and growth hormone).

Gastric secretion occurs in three phases:

(1) The cephalic phase, which occurs before food is ingested, accounts for 30–50% of gastric secretions and is stimulated by special senses such as sight, smell, and thought. Most of these special senses lead to vagal nerve outputs with acetylcholine-stimulating parietal

cells to secrete acid, chief cells to make pepsinogen (which in an acidic environment is cleaved into the active form pepsin), and enterochromaffin-like cells to make histamine. Vagal efferents (nerves sending signals away from the central nervous system and towards the peripheral body) stimulate G-cells using gastrin-releasing peptide (not acetylcholine) to cause gastrin release. Inhibitors of the cephalic phase include anything that stimulates the sympathetic nervous system, such as physical or psychological distress.

(2) The gastric phase, which occurs when food enters the stomach, accounts for roughly 40–60% of gastric secretions. Stimuli for the gastric phase of secretion include stretch/distention and breakdown products from proteins (i.e., amino acids and peptides). Food entering the stomach stretches the stomach and buffers the acidity (i.e., makes it less acidic or the pH increase), which both trigger acid secretion. Stretch primarily triggers nerve reflexes that directly stimulate acid secretion via the vagal nerve. Increased pH triggers G-cells to secrete gastrin which stimulates acid secretion. D-cells shut down acid production by producing somatostatin in response to decreased pH (i.e., increased acidity), which directly inhibits acid production by parietal cells, histamine production by enterochromaffin-like cells, and gastrin production by G-cells.

(3) The intestinal phase, which accounts for 5–10% of gastric secretions, is triggered by increased concentrations of partially digested proteins reaching the duodenum where duodenal G-cells secrete gastrin and other hormones that simulate gastric acid secretion.

The process of gastric emptying is highly regulated. For example, fatty acids longer than 12 carbon molecules long stimulate the production of a peptide called cholecystokinin (CCK) in the duodenum which slows gastric emptying by increasing the tone of the pylorus and decreasing contractions of the antrum and fundus. When the food is sufficiently broken down into a sludge called “chyme”, the pylorus begins to act as a sieve allowing the only particles of food that are 2–3 mm or smaller to exit the stomach into the small intestine. The stomach usually empties within 2–4 hours, with liquids emptying more rapidly than solids. Delayed emptying of the stomach is known as gastroparesis, with youth experiencing symptoms such as nausea, vomiting, pain, and early satiety.

Small intestine

The small intestine receives partially broken down and digested food from the stomach in the form of chyme. There are three parts of the small intestine (top to bottom): (1) duodenum, (2) jejunum, and (3) ileum. The small intestine is the primary site of absorption of both macronutrients (proteins, fats, and carbohydrates) and micronutrients (e.g., vitamins and minerals). The majority of nutrients are absorbed in the duodenum and jejunum. However, the terminal (final part of) ileum is the site of absorption of vitamin B_{12}, as well as the four fat-soluble vitamins: vitamins A, D, E, and K (see Figure 1.6). In addition, 95% of bile acids released into the small intestine are reabsorbed in the terminal ileum and recycled. Normal transit time through the small intestine is 2–6 hours.

The small intestine is approximately 9–10 ft (270–300 cm) in length in newborns and 15–22 ft (450–670 cm) in adults. The surface area of the adult small intestine is nearly the size of a tennis court due to not only its length but also small finger-like projections called microvilli that cover the surface of the small intestine. Each villus contains a capillary and lacteal – small blood vessel and lymphatic vessel – with glucose and amino acids absorbed into the former and fatty acids in the latter. Capillaries ultimately drain into the portal vein and then to the liver, while lacteals drain into the thoracic duct which then empties into subclavian and/or jugular

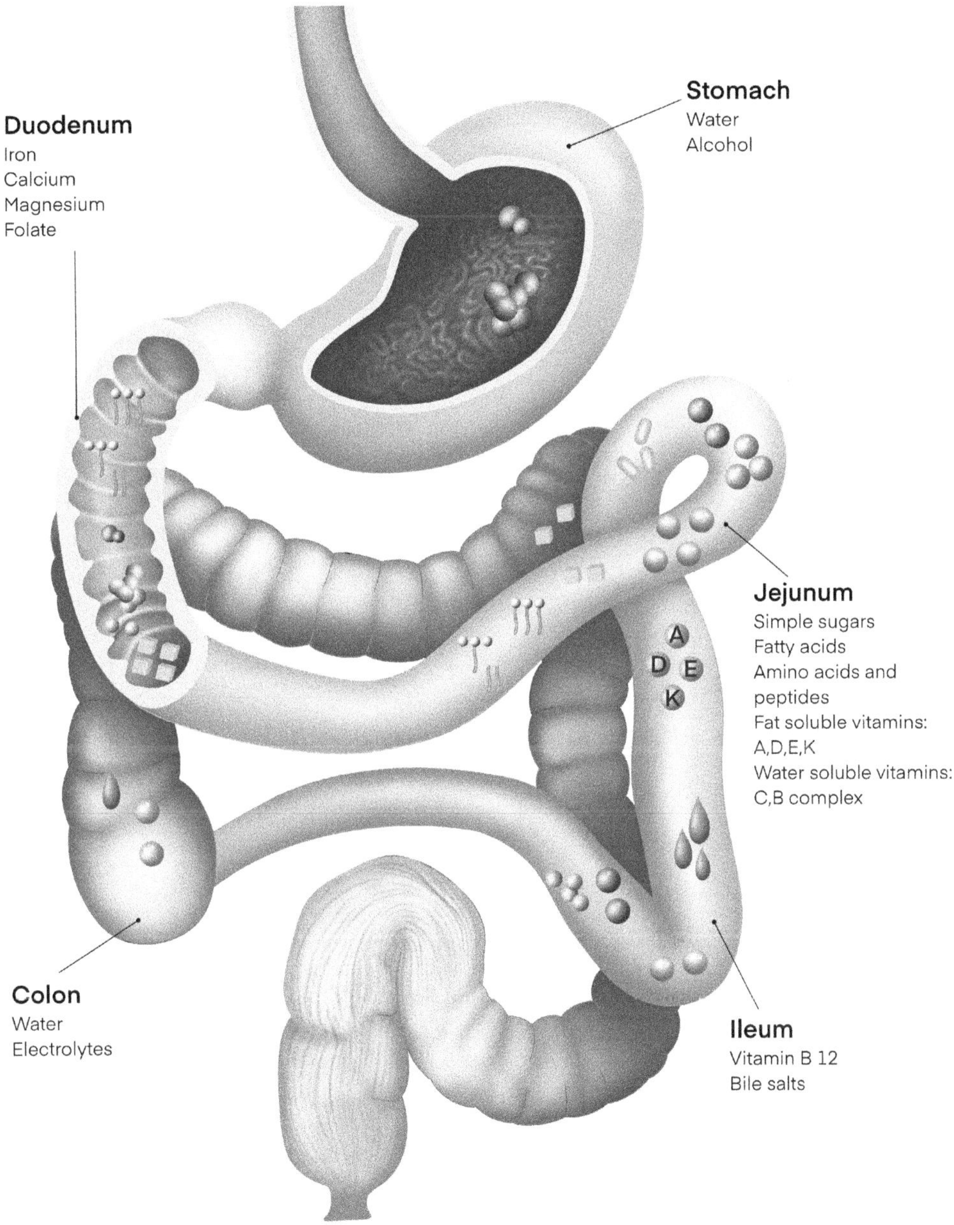

Figure 1.6 Sites of absorption of macronutrients and micronutrients along the GI tract (Source: Jordan Shapiro).

veins on the left side of the chest and neck. Several different contraction patterns occur in the small and large intestine. Peristalsis is the propulsion of bowel contents forward, segmentation breaks the contents into smaller portions for easier digestion, and mixing movements cause a to-and-fro movement of contents to mix chyme with digestive enzymes and maximize contact with the microvilli.

Pancreas

The pancreas releases the enzymes lipase, trypsin (secreted as the inactive trypsinogen and activated to trypsin which then breaks down protein and activates other pancreatic enzymes), and amylase to digest fat, protein, and carbohydrates, respectively. Pancreatic enzymes are secreted into the pancreatic duct which empties into the duodenum via an opening called the ampulla of Vater (see Figure 1.7).

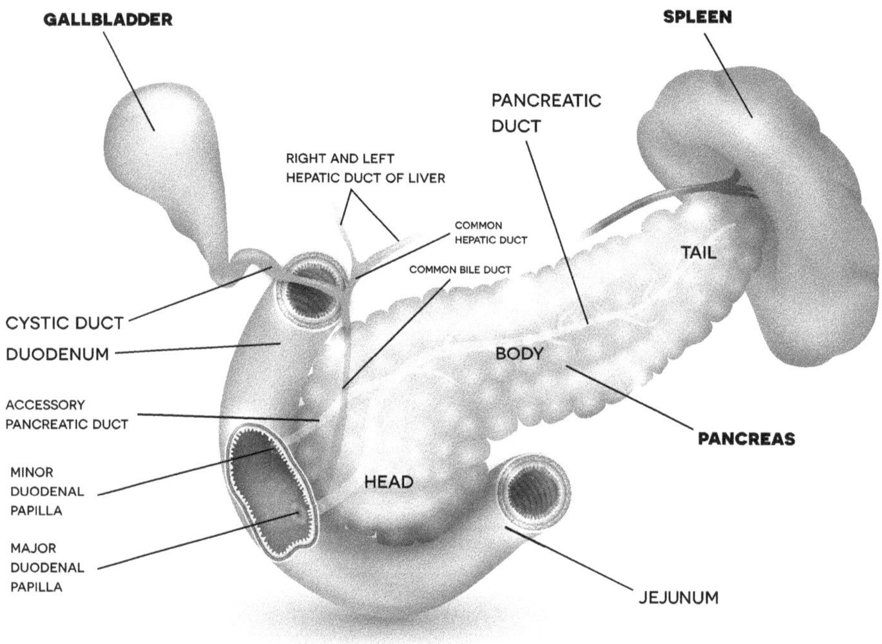

Figure 1.7 Pancreatobiliary system (Source: TimeLineArtist/Shutterstock.com).

In addition to the production of digestive enzymes (exocrine function), the pancreas also produces two hormones – insulin and glucagon – which are released into the bloodstream to act on other organs (endocrine function). These hormones tightly regulate blood sugar levels and are involved in energy storage and metabolism. Insulin is secreted after meals in response to elevated blood sugar and facilitates the storage of glucose as glycogen in cells around the body, reducing blood sugar levels. Glucagon is released in response to a low blood sugar level and primarily acts in the liver to break down glycogen to release glucose into the bloodstream for energy.

Liver and gallbladder

The liver has many roles including the production of bile, which acts as a detergent to break fats into smaller constituents. These smaller constituents are then broken down further by pancreatic lipase into glycerol and fatty acids, see Figure 1.8. Bile flows down the series of bile ducts within the liver, to those from the right and left sides of the liver (the left and right hepatic ducts), and ultimately to the common bile duct, which empties into the duodenum via the ampulla of Vater, alongside the pancreatic duct. Bile acts like a detergent, emulsifying fats so that lipase can better act to break them down into fatty acids and glycerol. Some bile is stored in the gallbladder in preparation for ingestion of higher fat-containing meals that may require extra bile. Fat in the duodenum causes the release of the hormone cholecystokinin (CCK), which causes the gallbladder to contract and squeeze extra bile into the small intestine.

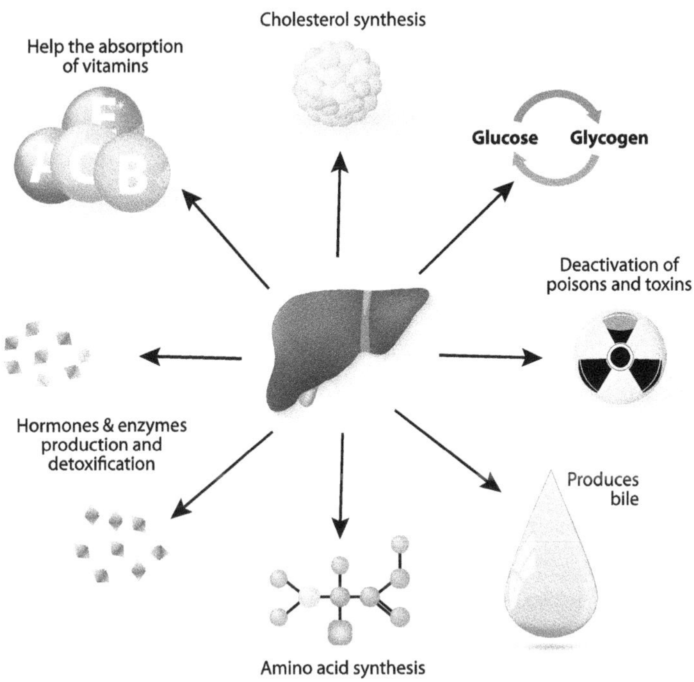

Figure 1.8 Functions of the liver (Source: Designua/Shutterstock.com).

In addition to the production of bile for fat digestion, the liver has many other vital functions:

- Protein synthesis (putting amino acid building blocks together into proteins) and degradation occur in the liver. The liver produces factors that help the blood clot and those that break down clots, carrier proteins for various other substances, and makes thrombopoietin, the protein that stimulates the bone marrow to make platelets (a component of blood that helps with initial clot formation).
- Cholesterol production primarily occurs in the liver (only about 20% of cholesterol comes from the diet). Cholesterol is a critical component of cell membranes, signaling between cells, and serves as the chemical precursor for vitamin D and all steroid hormones including cortisol, aldosterone, progesterone, estrogen, and testosterone.

- Detoxification from environmental toxins and drugs by modifying these substances to be excreted in the urine (water soluble) or stool (fat soluble).
- Storage of nutrients such as glycogen (the storage form of glucose), vitamin A, vitamin D, vitamin E, vitamin K, and vitamin B_{12}, as well as iron and copper.
- Immune functions of the liver are carried out by its rich supply of immunologically active cells that help remove bacteria and other pathogens from the blood that flows from the intestines back to the liver.
- Red blood cell production (erythropoiesis) occurs in the liver, spleen, and yolk sac of the fetus and shifts the bone marrow prior to birth.

Large intestine (colon)

The large intestine is divided into the cecum (portion where the appendix is attached and which is connected to the end of the small intestine, the ileum), ascending colon, transverse colon, descending colon, and sigmoid colon. connected to the end of the small intestine (the ileum) by a valve referred to as the ileocecal valve. The primary job of the colon is to absorb water and propel feces to the rectum for defecation. However, the bacteria of the colon also produce several B vitamins, vitamin K, and short-chain fatty acids. The length of the colon is 1.5 ft at birth (50 cm) and 5 ft (150 cm) in adults. Normal transit time through the colon averages 30–40 hours but ranges from 10 to 59 hours.

Bloating (feeling of abdominal swelling or pressure) and distention (visible increase in abdominal size) are common symptoms. Excess of these symptoms may occur due to dietary intake, excessive air swallowing, medications, abnormal sensation (feeling the stretch of the intestines at normal volumes of gas), overgrowth of bacteria in the small or large intestine, abnormal motility, or pelvic floor dysfunction preventing normal evacuation of stool. The passing of gas (flatus) is normal, with an average of 5–15 episodes per day.

Anorectal/pelvic floor muscles

Multiple mechanisms prevent stool from falling out of our bottoms uncontrollably. The ability of the anus and rectum to feel the subtle differences between solid, liquid, and gas allows for the passing of gas without accidents. The degree of sensation and coordination required to handle feces parallels or exceeds that of our hands and fingers. There are two circular sphincter muscles at the anorectal junction that are contracted (i.e., closed) at baseline (see Figure 1.9) depicting the anorectal canal. The external anal sphincter is under our voluntary control and can be contracted by squeezing as if to hold in a bowel movement. The internal anal sphincter is controlled involuntarily. In addition to the sphincters, a sling-like muscle called the puborectalis extends from the pubic bone posteriorly and around the anorectal junction to form an angle that further prevents leakage of stool when it is contracted. When the rectum fills with stool, the stretch causes two things to occur: (1) the urge to defecate, and (2) the relaxation of the puborectalis and internal anal sphincter muscles so that stool can travel towards the anus. The external anal sphincter can be contracted until an individual is in an appropriate place to defecate. With all of the sphincters relaxed and anorectal canal straightened by the relaxation of the puborectalis muscle, a gentle increase in intraabdominal pressure by contraction of the abdominal wall muscles pushes stool down and out the anus.

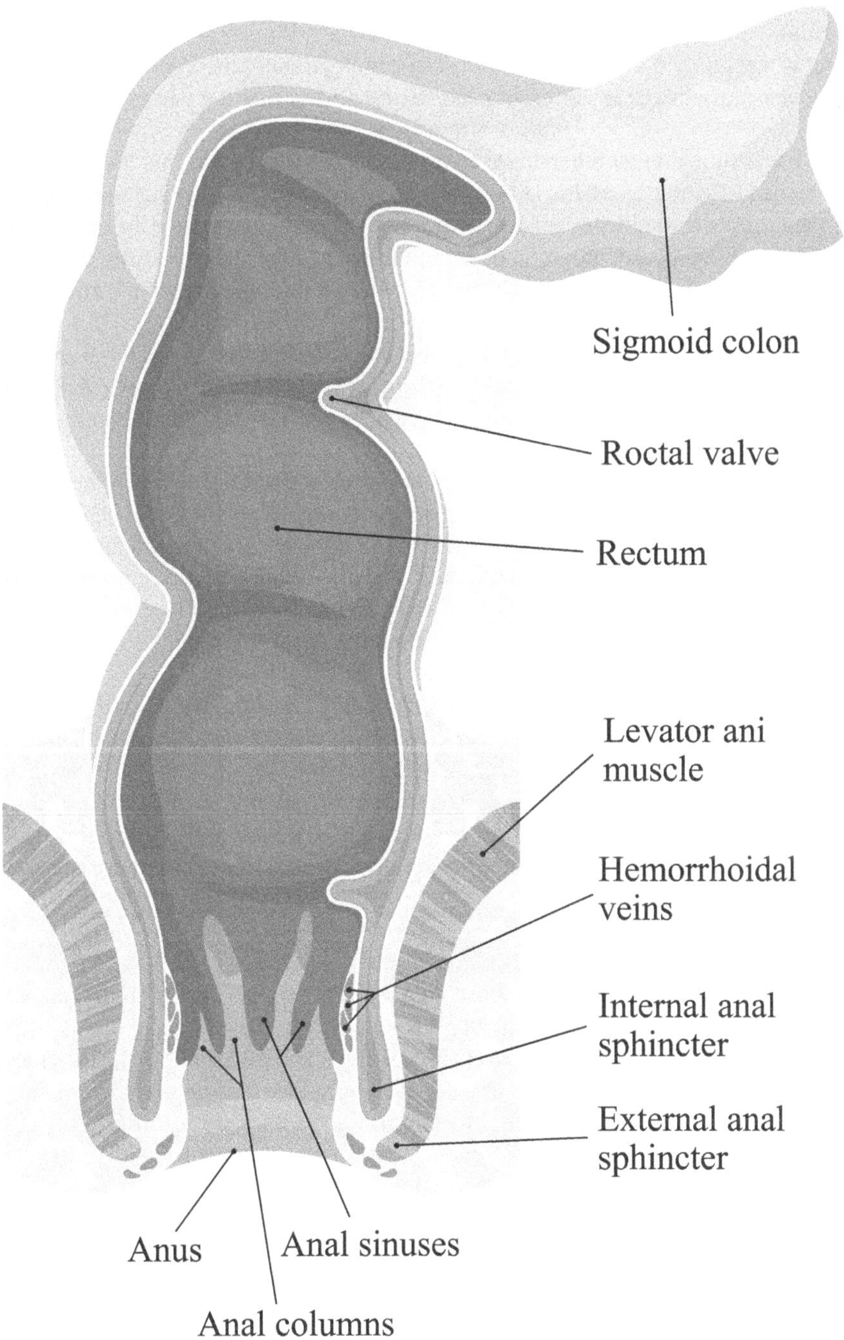

Figure 1.9 The anatomy of the anorectal canal (Source: logika600/Shutterstock.com).

Gut microbiota

The gut microbiome consists of over 30–40 trillion bacteria – the same as the number of human cells – but weighs only 0.2 kg (0.4 pounds). The composition of the microbiome varies significantly between individuals, in different parts of the GI tract, and changes throughout the lifespan [3].

Until recently, it was thought that the in utero environment was sterile and that the intestinal microbiome developed after birth. There is now emerging evidence suggesting the in utero colonization of the GI tract through studies demonstrating bacterial colonization of meconium (newborn stool), the umbilical cord, amniotic fluid, and the placenta [4]. After birth, the newborn microbiome changes significantly towards that of the adult microbiome from birth to the first two years of age.

The acidity of the stomach is inhabitable for most bacteria and limits bacterial counts to 10^2–10^3, with *Lactobacillus*, *Streptococcus*, *Staphylococcus*, and *Enterobacteriaceae* being the predominant species. Colonic bacterial counts reach 10^9–10^{12}, and *Bacteroides*, *Peptostreptococcus*, *Streptococcus*, *Bifidobacterium*, *Fusobacterium*, *Lactobacillus*, *Clostridium*, and *Enterobacteriaceae* are the predominant species. Bacterial counts of the small intestine increase in a gradient from 10^2 to 10^3 in the duodenum to 10^4 to 10^7 in the ileum, with predominant species of the duodenum similar to those in the stomach and predominant species in the ileum similar to many of those found in the colon. The microbiome plays significant roles in health and disease, including nutrient metabolism, drug and toxin metabolism, maintenance of the structural integrity of the gut mucosal barrier, modulation of the immune system, and protection against pathogens.

Diet is thought to be the biggest modifiable factor influencing the composition of the microbiome. Changes in the microbiome have been noted in multiple disease states, though there are more often general changes in composition such as reduced diversity of bacteria rather than disease-specific microbiome patterns. For this reason, the brain–gut axis is often expanded to the brain–gut–microbiome axis (see Chapter 2 for a more detailed description). In addition, it is unclear in many disease states if the microbiome changes drive disease states or if these changes occur as a result of these conditions.

Despite the interest in changes in the microbiome in various disease states, the microbiome is incredibly resilient. In most cases of antibiotic exposure, GI infections, and use of colon-cleansing medications used to prepare for colonoscopies, the gut microbiome is briefly altered (referred to as "dysbiosis") but bounces back to its prior state within 10–14 days.

Finally, fecal microbiota transplantation (FMT) is a well-established and very efficacious treatment for antibiotic refractory *Clostridium difficile* infections [5]. This involves instillation of donor stool into the youth with *C. difficile* infection using frozen capsules or liquid stool dispensed into the colon during colonoscopy. Potential stool donors are screened with extensive questionnaires about disorders associated with disruption of normal gut microbiota (e.g., personal history of chronic GI diseases, cancer, autoimmune conditions, neurologic or psychiatric conditions, and obesity or body mass index > 30), drugs that can alter gut microbiota (e.g., antibiotics, proton pump inhibitors, immunosuppressant agents, and chemotherapy) and laboratory testing for infectious diseases and antibiotic-resistant bacteria. Ongoing studies are assessing the potential benefits of age-matched stool donors for FMT.

GI immune system

The GI tract is open and exposed to the external environment at both ends – mouth and anus – and several mechanisms of defense against pathogens exist. Physical barriers include the epithelial cell layer lining the GI tract, mucin, and stomach acid. The GI tract is also rich in immune cells – up to 70% of the body's immune system cells are found in the GI tract – that serve a variety of roles. Immune cells protect the ability of the surface epithelium to digest and absorb nutrients by defending it from infection, ingesting and neutralizing harmful pathogens (e.g., bacteria and viruses), and maintaining tolerance (i.e., preventing the GI immune system cells from reacting to food and healthy GI bacteria as foreign pathogens). The immune system cells of the GI tract influence and are influenced by the enteric nervous system and the microbiome through a complex series of chemical signals that maintain homeostasis. The common causes of disruption of this equilibrium between systems (i.e., the GI enteric nervous system, immune system cells, and microbiome) are disruptions that occur after GI infections leading to post-infectious IBS. Individuals with post-infectious IBS suffer from pain, changes in stool frequency and consistency (most commonly diarrhea), bloating, and gas that may last weeks to years after the infection itself has resolved.

Implications of GI anatomy/physiology in GI disorders

It is important to note the distinction between symptoms (subjective complaints reported by youth/caregivers) and signs (physical, objective findings reported by youth/caregivers and/or discovered on examination by providers). Youth and parents largely present to providers with symptoms.

Many common GI conditions ultimately have concrete, identifiable abnormalities in anatomy/physiology that can be elucidated through history taking, physical exams, laboratory tests (e.g., blood, stool, breath testing), radiology tests (e.g., X-rays, computed tomography (CT) scans, magnetic resonance imaging (MRI)), and endoscopy (e.g., upper endoscopy or colonoscopy to look directly into the GI tract). Examples of these conditions include inflammatory bowel diseases (Crohn's disease and ulcerative colitis), peptic ulcer disease (ulcers in the stomach or duodenum), and symptomatic gallstones (see Chapter 3). Such conditions are conceptually easier to discuss with youth and families and allow a more direct application of anatomy/physiology for treatment, monitoring, and making sense of symptoms.

However, many of the most common GI conditions presenting in children, adolescents/young adults, and adults are DGBI. These include functional nausea/vomiting, functional abdominal pain, IBS (with subtypes including constipation-predominant, diarrhea-predominant, and mixed stool types), functional dyspepsia (with subtypes including epigastric pain syndrome and postprandial distress syndrome), and functional constipation (see Chapter 3). These conditions typically manifest with significant symptom burdens that are often as or more severe than disorders with more clearly identifiable structural or inflammatory drivers of symptoms, such as Crohn's disease or a stomach ulcer. Youth and families often go through significant amounts of testing before DGBI are diagnosed.

To add to the complexity, many youth with conditions such as Crohn's disease may also have DGBI such as IBS (in this case highlighted by ongoing symptoms after youth have achieved remission from inflammation in their intestines). In addition, there is a clear bidirectional impact of physical health on mental health and mental health on physical health symptoms, which is perhaps clearer in the GI tract than in most other organ systems.

Given the complexity of the GI tract, the challenges that often arise in linking even severe symptoms to abnormalities on exam or diagnostic tests, and the crossroads of the GI tract and psychological health, many youth and caregivers may reach the care of a GI mental health professional with frustrations, lack of satisfying answers, and seeking validation, as much as alleviation of their suffering.

Pearls of wisdom

- Understanding the structures and functions of the GI tract can help providers to understand GI conditions that ail youth and to educate youth about their conditions.
- Many GI symptoms occur in the absence of structural abnormalities, inflammation, or infections and may instead be problems of motility, gut–brain interaction, or the microbiome.

Summary

The GI tract serves to efficiently physically and chemically digest food to facilitate the absorption of nutrients from food. Digestion begins before food enters the mouth. Most macronutrients, water, electrolytes, and vitamins and minerals are absorbed in the small intestine. The large intestine further absorbs electrolytes and water and produces waste products for expulsion via defecation. The enteric nervous system (ENS), or "second brain", can function independently in many respects but is also influenced by the central nervous system (CNS).

Recommended readings

For youth and caregivers:

- Enders, G. (2015). *Gut: the inside story of our body's most under-rated organ.* Brunswick, VIC: Scribe Publications.
- Mayer, E.A. (2016). *The mind-gut connection: how the hidden conversation within our bodies impacts our mood, our choices, and our overall health* (1st ed.). Harper Wave, an imprint of HarperCollins Publishers.

For mental health professionals:

- Barrett, K.E. (2014). *Gastrointestinal Physiology* (2nd ed.). New York, USA: Lange/McGraw-Hill Education.
- Keshav, S., & Bailey, A. (2013). *The gastrointestinal system at a glance (2nd ed.).* Chichester, UK: Wiley-Blackwell.

References

1. Fleming MA, Ehsan L, Moore SR, Levin DE. The enteric nervous system and its emerging role as a therapeutic target. *Gastroenterol Res Pract.* 2020; Sep 8;2020:8024171.

2. Rosen R, Vandenplas Y, Singendonk M, Cabana M, DiLorenzo C, Gottrand F, et al. Pediatric gastroesophageal reflux clinical practice guidelines: Joint recommendations of the North American Society for Pediatric Gastroenterology, Hepatology, and Nutrition and the European Society for Pediatric Gastroenterology, Hepatology, and Nutrition. *J Pediatr Gastroenterol Nutr.* 2018;66(3):516–54.
3. Wilmanski T, Diener C, Rappaport N, Patwardhan S, Wiedrick J, Lapidus J, et al. Gut microbiome pattern reflects healthy ageing and predicts survival in humans. *Nat Metab.* 2021;3(2):274–86.
4. Ihekweazu FD, Versalovic J. Development of the pediatric gut microbiome: Impact on health and disease. *Am J Med Sci.* 2018;356(5):413–23.
5. Baunwall SMD, Lee MM, Eriksen MK, Mullish BH, Marchesi JR, Dahlerup JF, et al. Faecal microbiota transplantation for recurrent. *EClinicalMedicine*. 2020;29–30:100642.

Chapter 2

Stress, psychological factors, and the brain–gut axis

Julie Snyder Christiana and Samuel Nurko

Chapter aims

This chapter introduces the brain–gut axis (BGA), including its physiology and biochemical processes, within the context of the biopsychosocial model. Evidence for the role of the BGA on the bidirectional interactions between gastrointestinal (GI) and psychological conditions and symptomatology is also reviewed.

Learning points

- The BGA refers to a bidirectional communication system involving multiple systems of the body.
- The biopsychosocial model suggests that psychological and environmental factors, such as stress, anxiety, depression, and family modeling, in conjunction with biological factors, may contribute to miscommunication within the BGA and the onset, maintenance, and exacerbation of chronic GI symptoms.
- A basic understanding of the BGA by both parents and youth is crucial for the successful treatment of chronic GI conditions.

The biopsychosocial model and the brain–gut axis

Over the course of childhood and adolescence, it is inevitable that youth will experience a wide array of GI symptoms. Symptoms may emerge due to an acute infection or a chronic disease. The strong connection between the brain and the gut may also result in the development of GI symptoms in anticipation of an exciting or stressful event. For example, it is common to hear reports of "knots" or "butterflies" in the stomach right before giving a class presentation or when preparing to step out on a sports field.

The remittance of symptoms within a reasonably short period of time following a known trigger, such as a stomach "bug", a bout of constipation, or the start of a new school year typically results in a return to baseline functioning without the need or thought to pursue medical evaluation. Symptoms that persist and that result in physiological (i.e., weight loss, fatigue, decreased appetite), psychological (i.e., anxiety related to not being able to find a bathroom in time), and/or social (i.e., missed school, absence from extracurricular activities) consequences may prompt visits to the pediatrician and, ultimately, a pediatric gastroenterology subspecialty practice. For many families, the assumption is that a visit to the doctor will include a physical exam and testing in order to determine the reason why symptoms are occurring and to arrive at

DOI: 10.4324/9781003308683-3

a medical diagnosis that has a clearly defined medical treatment. But what happens when this linear plan fails to take place?

Medical evaluation and testing that is reassuringly normal in youth who present with GI symptoms or that fails to demonstrate active inflammation in youth diagnosed with a chronic GI illness may result in families feeling confused and upset. One of the reasons for this is because Western medicine practices tend to follow what is known as the biomedical model of disease, which posits that symptoms are linked to a biological or organic cause [1]. That is the case for inflammatory bowel disease (IBD), eosinophilic esophagitis, and other inflammatory conditions of the GI tract (see Chapter 3 for a review of common GI conditions). The "absence" of an organic etiology, according to this model, infers that symptoms are the result of a psychological process. Gastroenterologists who ascribe to this model, who suggest that the absence of a clinical finding means that a youth's symptoms are "all in their head", and who therefore recommend termination of medical care in order to solely pursue psychological treatment have neglected to consider the impact of illness on one's social and emotional functioning [2]. Failure to consider these factors and to discuss the interrelationship between the mind and the body may have negative consequences, including reduced satisfaction with the medical provider, increased parental anxiety, the pursuit of costly and invasive testing, and worsening of symptoms [3–5].

In contrast to the biomedical model, the biopsychosocial model [1] explains how biological, psychological, and environmental processes interact and impact health and disease. Conceptualizing diagnoses in accordance with this model affords medical providers the opportunity to discuss with families how a youth's symptom presentation is influenced by multiple factors, which in turn requires a treatment approach that is multidisciplinary in nature and that may include both medical and psychologically focused therapies.

In recent years, the biopsychosocial model has been well received within the field of gastroenterology. It is viewed as the primary way of understanding the pathophysiology of disorders of gut–brain interaction (DGBI), including irritable bowel syndrome (IBS) and functional abdominal pain, and plays an integral role in comprehending disease onset, maintenance, and exacerbation in nearly all other GI illnesses [6]. This is because the bidirectional relationship and communication between the brain and the gut, referred to as the BGA, is influenced by all facets of the biopsychosocial model. More specifically, human emotions and experiences impact gut functioning, but what is happening in the gut can also impact one's state of mind and being [2, 7, 8].

Understanding the brain–gut axis (BGA)

Within the BGA, the central nervous system (CNS), consisting of the brain and the spinal cord, communicates with the enteric nervous system (ENS), which is oftentimes referred to as the gut's own nervous system (see Figure 2.1 and Chapter 1) [9].

The ENS is sometimes referred to as the "second brain of the body" and is comprised of millions of neurons that exist within the entire GI tract [10]. The BGA allows for *gut*-to-brain (ascending) communication, whereby gut stimuli trigger a response within the emotional and cognitive centers of the brain [7]. Inversely, in a *brain*-to-gut (descending) fashion, the BGA allows for central regulation of bowel function and facilitates intestinal responses to emotions and cognitions. These central processes are carried out via dynamic, interactive brain networks [11, 12]. Studies using functional magnetic resonance imaging in both children and adults with pain-associated GI conditions consistently demonstrate both regional and connectivity-related differences compared with healthy controls in several important networks related to pain control,

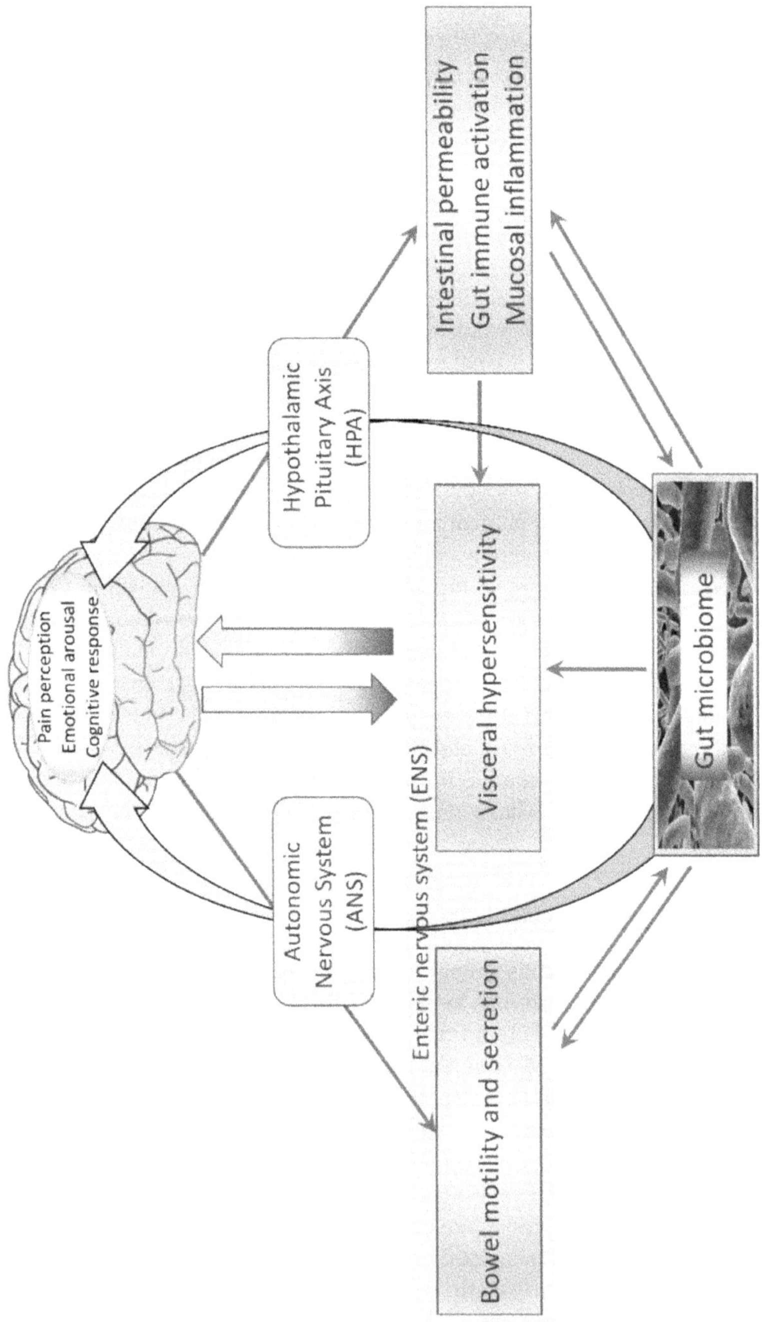

Figure 2.1 The brain–gut axis. (Source: Adapted from Tait et al. [9]).

including the amygdala and the limbic system [11, 12]. It can therefore be inferred that youth with pain-predominant GI disease have visceral hypersensitivity, with increased pain perception and a diminished ability to process and control pain. This is usually associated with certain psychological responses such as catastrophizing, which will be described in more detail later in this chapter [7]. The recognition of the altered functions of these brain networks therefore provides a biologic basis for the efficacy of psychological interventions.

The influence of stress on the BGA

The BGA also communicates with the autonomic nervous system (ANS) (consisting of the sympathetic and parasympathetic nervous systems) and both the neuroimmune and neuroendocrine systems. The ANS plays a significant role in brain–gut functioning [9]. This system, consisting of both the sympathetic ("fight or flight") and parasympathetic ("rest and digest") branches, is responsible for regulating the involuntary processes taking place within the body, one of which includes digestion [13]. When the ANS is working properly, these two branches work side by side to provide balance within the body; should a danger or stress present, the sympathetic nervous system becomes activated. When this activation occurs, changes in the GI tract and in other areas of the body are initiated in an effort to assist the body in adequately managing the stressor. These changes may include slowed emptying of food from the stomach to the intestine or overstimulation of the bowel and result in symptoms of nausea and increased urgency to have a bowel movement [14]. Once the stressor is no longer present, the "rest and digest" component of the ANS takes action and assists the body once again with achieving homeostasis.

The hypothalamic–pituitary–adrenal axis (HPA) and the sympathetic–adrenal–medullary (SAM) axis are also important components involved in stress response [15–17] (see Figure 2.1). The SAM provides the first response to stress mediated by catecholamine release, resulting in short-lasting responses, such as alertness, vigilance, and appraisal of the situation, enabling a strategic decision to face the challenge in the initial phase of a stressful event [17]. The HPA system is mediated by cortisol release and provides a secondary delayed response and falls within the limbic system, an area of the brain responsible for behavioral and emotional responses and a key influencer in ANS activation [17]. When a stimulus is perceived by the brain to be stressful, and regardless of whether the stress is perceived as good (for example, getting ready to attend a birthday party) or bad (for example, being bullied at school), both the SAM and the HPA axes are activated. This activation of the ANS aids in the effective initiation of the fight or flight system mentioned above, including temporarily altering digestive functioning in the GI tract.

In certain situations, such as in the case of significant, solitary life stress or repeated exposure to the same stressor, the sympathetic nervous system and HPA axis may remain activated [18, 19]. Constant activation of the fight or flight response and the continued release of cortisol can result in the maintenance of GI symptoms and the development of visceral hypersensitivity, a term used to describe a lowered pain/sensation threshold in the internal organs of the body [20]. When this occurs, messages are constantly transported to the brain via the spinal cord and chronic GI symptoms, as well as heightened anxiety about experiencing symptoms may ultimately ensue. This is why a child with a hypersensitive gut may find a "normal meal" painful.

Research has shown that significant life stressors at a young age, often referred to as Adverse Childhood Experiences (ACEs), are risk factors for the development of chronic pain and chronic GI symptoms in adults [21, 22] and in children [23]. A retrospective study by Nelson and colleagues demonstrated the presence of at least one ACE in over 80% of youth presenting for a multidisciplinary, chronic pain evaluation [23]. Early life medical events that stress bodily systems may also contribute to visceral hypersensitivity and disrupt the development and functioning of the BGA [21, 22]. Not only do these findings provide evidence to suggest that stressful experiences and chronic activation of the stress response in childhood may impact the brain–gut axis, but they also point to the consideration of providing trauma-focused psychological treatments in conjunction with pain-focused interventions to this subset of youth diagnosed with chronic pain [18]. See Chapter 9 for a more detailed review of this topic.

Psychological factors and the BGA

A multitude of psychological processes have been identified as playing a role in the onset, maintenance, and exacerbation of GI symptoms. These include psychiatric diagnoses, such as anxiety, depression, and post-traumatic stress disorder (PTSD), in addition to pain/symptom catastrophizing and coping, and somatization [24]. Given that the BGA is bidirectional, psychological factors may contribute to a worsening of GI symptoms via activation of the ANS or misinterpretation of symptoms as threatening; alternatively, psychological symptoms may present due to the persistent nature of GI symptoms and the impact that symptoms have on daily functioning.

Anxiety

There is a high prevalence of anxiety in children and adolescents diagnosed with GI conditions [25–29]. Children and adolescents who are anxious demonstrate a tendency to look for the dangerous components of a situation; as such, it is common for them to interpret neutral stimuli, such as the sight of a school building, as a threat. This in turn contributes to both the development of unhelpful thought patterns and feelings in addition to activation of the fight or flight response as well as avoidance of activities to reduce the perceived threat. Symptoms of anxiety may be more generalized or illness-specific, and it is especially important to assess for symptoms of illness-specific anxiety.

According to the gate control theory of pain [16], repeated or frequent activation of the sympathetic nervous system in an anxious child or adolescent can result in the onset and exacerbation of chronic GI discomfort. The gate control theory of pain posits that pain (in the case of GI disorders, the term "pain" also refers to other symptoms such as nausea and urgency) messages are more easily transported from the stomach to the brain via an open "pain gate", which refers to a mechanism by which chronic activation of the sympathetic nervous system due to anxiety and the false alarm signaling that occurs in chronic pain results in a wide open "gate" allowing messages to be easily carried from the spinal cord to the brain.

When GI messages are continuously received by the brain due to this open gate, it becomes much more difficult to tune them out. Though youth with premorbid anxiety may certainly struggle with this constant messaging, it is also possible for youth with no past history of worry to become anxious about uncomfortable sensations experienced in the gut or the possibility of re-experiencing symptoms in the future. In fact, research has shown that GI-specific anxiety and avoidance are far better predictors of child outcomes than general anxiety.

Catastrophizing

The term "catastrophizing" is commonly used throughout the chronic pain literature to describe a tendency to expect the worst to happen, while feeling unable to control this negative outcome

[30]. For example, even when pain is minor, a child may expect the pain to become debilitating in hours and that he/she will have no tools to reduce pain. Youth who present with high levels of catastrophizing demonstrate increased levels of disability in addition to prolonged duration of pain [31, 32]. Research examining this construct has demonstrated that pain catastrophizing mediates the relationship between anxiety and pain severity in youth diagnosed with IBS [24]. Pain catastrophizing has also been studied in youth diagnosed with IBD; there is some evidence to suggest that this style of coping is a predictor of increased disability in this population [33, 34].

Depression

Depressive symptoms are also highly prevalent in youth diagnosed with GI conditions [35] and contribute to more severe disruptions in functioning [36, 37] and treatment non-adherence [38]. The onset of depression, either prior to or following the development of chronic GI symptoms, may negatively influence one's ability to cope. Faulty and unhelpful thought patterns commonly associated with depression, including rumination (perseverating on symptoms or negative experiences), may contribute to the persistent over-communication between the gut and the brain [7]. There is also evidence to suggest that the effect of catastrophizing on functional disability is mediated by the presence of depressive symptoms [39].

Somatization

Somatization, or increased focus on unpleasant sensations in the body, is highly prevalent in youth diagnosed with various GI diseases [40–43]. This type of hypervigilance to bodily sensations may result in heightened anxiety and distress and serve to further exacerbate GI symptoms. Although somatization is sometimes explained as "unexpressed psychological stress", there is no evidence of this, and currently this is an outdated concept.

Somatization is likely explained by an interplay between biological factors and psychosocial factors. Biological factors include changes in the ANS and HPA axis in response to physical or emotional stress (as mentioned above), as well as central sensitization, a term used to describe changes in the way that the brain processes pain [44]. Psychosocial factors, contributing to the onset of somatization include anticipatory worry about physiological sensations and implementation of more passive coping (i.e., withdrawing from activities when symptoms are present) [36] in combination with social–environmental factors (see below).

Trauma/PTSD

Youth diagnosed with GI conditions who are also exposed to adverse childhood experiences may meet the diagnostic criteria for PTSD [45]. Invasive testing and surgical procedures may also contribute to the onset of traumatic stress symptoms in youth diagnosed with GI illnesses. In a cohort of youth diagnosed with IBD, pancreatitis, and cystic fibrosis, over one-third were identified as experiencing symptoms consistent with pediatric medical traumatic stress (PMTS) [46], a term used to describe a set of intense psychological distress symptoms that occur in response to stressful medical treatments [47]. See Chapter 5 for further detail and suggestions for managing distress during procedures in order to reduce the potential onset of PMTS.

Environmental factors and the BGA

Environmental factors, most notably parental modeling of disease management and functioning and parental response to a child or adolescent's diagnosis, can also influence the brain–gut axis and contribute to the onset and maintenance of chronic GI symptoms in the pediatric population. See Chapter 8 for more information on this topic.

Other factors that influence the BGA

Evidence also suggests that changes in inflammatory pathways can have an influence on symptom development and symptom perception. The gut microbiota (the bacterial flora colonizing the bowel) also have an important role in the facilitation of gut–brain messaging. Most consistent findings have included alterations in the ratio of Firmicutes to Bacteroidetes, and a diminished presence of *Lactobacillus* and *Bifidobacterium* [48].

In summary, multiple factors can contribute to a disruption in homeostasis and altered communication between the brain and the gut. In addition to biological factors (e.g., genetic predisposition, exposure to sensitizing medical events, microbiome changes), psychological and environmental factors can contribute to the dysfunctional relationship between the brain and the gut and the onset, maintenance, and exacerbation of chronic GI symptoms [6, 7]. Examples of these include the ability to manage acute or chronic stress [49], exposure to traumatic events [50], anxiety or depression that predates or is exacerbated by GI symptoms [51], stress within a family system as a result of a youth's GI illness [52], and difficulty coping with the chronicity of an illness and associated absences from academic and social events [53].

Discussing the BGA and influencing psychological factors during therapy

Educating youth and families regarding the BGA and the role of psychological processes is a critical component of brain–gut behavior therapy for the treatment of GI disease. It is, however, imperative for a GI mental health professional to understand that providing this information is inherently different from the psychoeducation that is provided at the start of therapy when the reason for referral is primarily psychological in nature.

Youth referred to a mental health practice for the management of GI symptoms may struggle to fully comprehend the reason why they are seeing a mental health professional when their symptoms are primarily physical (i.e., nausea, abdominal pain, vomiting) in nature. It is up to the mental health professional to focus the initial sessions on understanding these symptoms, the impact that symptoms have on functioning, and potential triggers for symptom maintenance and exacerbation. Following this information gathering, GI mental health professionals can begin to provide psychoeducation on the biopsychosocial model, the BGA, and the impact of stress, psychological, and environmental processes on GI symptoms. Providing this information and ensuring that youth and their families comprehend this material pave the way to discuss the use of psychological interventions for the management of symptoms.

The following outline illustrates steps for providing the psychoeducation component during therapy. Handout 2.1 (Sample dialogue) expands on this, providing specific language for a mental health professional to use during the initial sessions. It is also recommended that mental health professionals use Handouts 2.2 (BGA diagram) and 2.3 (therapist–patient worksheet) alongside Handout 2.1 to ensure understanding. Finally, Table 2.1 outlines specific metaphors to further explain the BGA that are helpful to use to ensure understanding. Metaphors can be an effective educational tool when discussing chronic GI discomfort, such as abdominal pain, nausea, and urgency. It has been suggested that the use of metaphors may also reduce defensiveness, as the notion of chronic discomfort and the biopsychosocial conceptualization of this disease can be difficult for families to comprehend and believe [54]. The use of this type of

Table 2.1 Developmentally appropriate metaphors to explain the brain–gut connection, nervous system hypersensitivity, and the concept of chronic GI symptoms

Children (ages 4–9)	*Adolescents (ages 10–18)*
Sunburn: When you have a sunburn on your skin it hurts if someone touches it; however, once it is healed you can touch that area without experiencing pain. GI symptoms that last longer than they should result in your body becoming very sensitive to the experience of pain and other feelings in your stomach, similar to what a sunburn feels like when it first happens. It's like you have a constant sunburn in your belly; we need to figure out ways to heal this.	**Software vs. hardware**: Your GI symptoms have stuck around for far longer than you have wanted them to be there! This is because the "software" or nerves in your stomach are not working as they should. To help explain this, think about the computer that you have at home and what happens when it freezes. You typically turn it off, and then restart it. If you would look inside the computer at the "hardware" when it just froze, you would find that it looks okay; this is because the problem was with the "software" or one of the programs you had running. The same is the case for you. We know that your "hardware", meaning your stomach, intestines, etc., looks okay, but the problem lies in the nerves or your "software" having become overly sensitive.
Chit-chat: Your brain and your belly have started to talk to one another WAY too much! This is similar to your teacher assigning your seat right next to a classmate who always talks to you while you are trying to get your work done! We need to help your brain and your belly learn that they don't *always* have to talk to one another, much in the same way that you might politely ask that classmate to not bother you while you are doing your work!	**Too much texting**: Your stomach and your brain are doing a bit too much talking. It's similar to a friend of yours who won't stop texting you as you are trying to fall asleep at night or get your homework done. The goal is to help your brain and your stomach resume their normal communication habits, much in the same way that you might have to set limits with your friend regarding when/how often they can text you!
Rock concert: You have had these yucky feelings in your belly for way longer than you need to! It's like you have a rock concert going on in there, when what we really want is for your belly to be "listening" to soft, calming music.	**Speakerphone:** The sensitivity in your stomach is like the speakerphone setting on your phone has been turned on in your stomach, resulting in you experiencing feelings there in a much "louder" way. The goal is to find ways to help turn that "speaker" setting off so that the brain and the gut can communicate normally.
False alarm: These feelings in your belly have been there for a really long time, even though we know that what might have made them happen in the first place is no longer there. It's like a false alarm is going off in your body, where your brain is sending messages down to your belly to keep having pain! You can think of this like a smoke alarm that goes off in your house every time someone burns toast even though there's no fire, or a car alarm that goes off in the grocery store parking lot because the alarm system is really sensitive when someone just lightly brushes past the car.	

Note. All the examples used in the younger children may also be used in the older group.

language can be particularly helpful for a mental health professional to use in order to dismiss the preconceived notion that symptoms are due solely to psychological processes [16].

Step 1: Explain the biopsychosocial model

- Provide education regarding the difference between biomedical conceptualization of illness and biopsychosocial model.
  - For children under the age of 5, discuss only with caregivers.

Step 2: Explain the BGA

- Psychoeducation about the connection between the brain and the gut provided in developmentally appropriate terms.
  - For children under the age of 5, discuss only with caregivers.
  - Refer to Table 2.1 for metaphors to incorporate when explaining the BGA to school-aged children and adolescents.

Step 3: Explain how stress, psychological, and environmental factors can impact the BGA

- Assist youth and families in understanding different triggers that can contribute to the onset, maintenance, and exacerbation of GI symptoms.
  - For children under the age of 5, discuss only with caregivers.
  - For school-aged children and adolescents along with their caregivers, consider the incorporation of the following key points:
    - Impact of stress on the GI tract, with reference to the fight or flight response and consequence of repeated activation of this response.
    - Impact of psychological factors (e.g., anxiety, changes in mood) on activation of fight or flight response and the response of the GI tract.
    - Impact of caregiver factors on maintenance of GI symptoms in youth, including caregiver history of pain, caregiver anxiety about a youth's symptoms, and caregiver response to a youth's GI symptoms (e.g., granting special privileges, permitting youth to stay home).

Pearls of wisdom

- Education regarding the BGA is a key component of treatment for youth diagnosed with GI conditions. It is important for a GI mental health professional to spend time providing this education in order to ensure that youth and their families understand the diagnosis and the rationale behind using psychological strategies for the management of symptoms and to enhance functioning.
- Information pertaining to the BGA must be tailored to the developmental level of the child or adolescent. It is often helpful to ask youth living with a GI condition to provide their own understanding of the information provided, in their words, once the mental health professional has provided education on this topic.
- Youth living with a GI condition may be more open to the use of psychological strategies for the management of chronic GI symptoms and less likely to feel that a provider is suggesting that symptoms are "all in their head" following BGA education.

Summary

The brain and the gut engage in bidirectional communication with the assistance of the central and enteric nervous systems. Multiple factors can influence this communication, including visceral hypersensitivity, response to stressors, psychological symptoms, and environmental influences. A GI-focused mental health professional should aim to further a youth and family's understanding of the BGA at the start of psychotherapy. Doing so can increase the willingness to accept a biopsychosocial treatment model for the management of GI disease, thereby opening the door for engagement in psychological interventions.

Recommended readings

For youth and caregivers:

- Weston, G. Zeltzer, L.K., & Zeltzer, P.M. (2021). *The smart brain pain syndrome: The primer for teens & young adults*. Shylisca Press.
- Coakley, R. (2016). *When your child hurts*. New Haven, CT: Yale University Press.
- Zeltzer, L.K., Blackett Schlank, C. (2005). *Conquering your child's chronic pain: A pediatrician's guide for reclaiming a normal childhood.* New York, NY: HarperCollins Publishers.

For mental health professionals:

- Van Oudenhove, L., Levy, R.L., Crowell, M.D., Drossman, D.A., Halpert, A.D., Keefer, L., Lackner, J.M., Murphy, T.B., & Naliboff, B.D. (2016). Biopsychosocial aspects of functional gastrointestinal disorders: How central and environmental processes contribute to the development and expression of functional gastrointestinal disorders. *Gastroenterology*, 150, 1355–1367.
- Reed-Knight, B., Maddux, M.H., Deacy, A.D., Lampyrk, K., & Stone, A. (2017). Brain-gut interactions and maintenance factors in pediatric gastrointestinal disorders: Recommendations for clinical care. *Clinical Practice in Pediatric Psychology*, 5(1), 93–105.

References

1. Engel GL. The clinical application of the biopsychosocial model. *Am J Psychiatry*. 1980;137(5):535–44.
2. Ballou S, Feingold JH. Stress, resilience, and the brain-gut axis: Why is psychogastroenterology important for all digestive disorders? *Gastroenterol Clin North Am.* 2022;51(4):697–709.
3. Williams SE, Smith CA, Bruehl SP, Gigante J, Walker LS. Medical evaluation of children with chronic abdominal pain: Impact of diagnosis, physician practice orientation, and maternal trait anxiety on mothers' responses to the evaluation. *Pain*. 2009;146(3):283–92.
4. Schechter NL, Coakley R, Nurko S. The golden half hour in chronic pediatric pain-feedback as the first intervention. *JAMA Pediatr.* 2021;175(1):7–8.
5. Dhroove G, Chogle A, Saps M. A million-dollar work-up for abdominal pain: Is it worth it? *J Pediatr Gastroenterol Nutr.* 2010;51(5):579–83.
6. Van Oudenhove L, Crowell MD, Drossman DA, Halpert AD, Keefer L, Lackner JM, et al. Biopsychosocial aspects of functional gastrointestinal disorders. *Gastroenterology*. 2016.
7. Thapar N, Benninga MA, Crowell MD, Di Lorenzo C, Mack I, Nurko S, et al. Paediatric functional abdominal pain disorders. *Nat Rev Dis Primers*. 2020;6(1):89.
8. Carabotti M, Scirocco A, Maselli MA, Severi C. The gut-brain axis: Interactions between enteric microbiota, central and enteric nervous systems. *Ann Gastroenterol.* 2015;28(2):203–9.

9. Tait C, Sayuk GS. The brain-gut-microbiotal axis: A framework for understanding functional GI illness and their therapeutic interventions. *Eur J Intern Med.* 2021;84:1–9.
10. Fleming MA, 2nd, Ehsan L, Moore SR, Levin DE. The enteric nervous system and its emerging role as a therapeutic target. *Gastroenterol Res Pract.* 2020;2020:8024171.
11. Mayer EA, Labus J, Aziz Q, Tracey I, Kilpatrick L, Elsenbruch S, et al. Role of brain imaging in disorders of brain-gut interaction: A Rome working team report. *Gut.* 2019;68(9):1701–15.
12. Hubbard CS, Becerra L, Heinz N, Ludwick A, Rasooly T, Wu R, et al. Abdominal pain, the adolescent and altered brain structure and function. *PLoS One.* 2016;11(5):e0156545.
13. Tougas G. The autonomic nervous system in functional bowel disorders. *Gut.* 2000;47 Suppl 4:iv78–80; discussion iv7.
14. Drossman DA. Functional gastrointestinal disorders: History, pathophysiology, clinical features and Rome IV. *Gastroenterology.* 2016;150(6):1262–79.
15. Khlevner J, Park Y, Margolis KG. Brain-Gut Axis: Clinical implications. *Gastroenterol Clin North Am.* 2018;47(4):727–39.
16. Coakley R, Schechter, N. Chronic pain is like...The clinical use of analogy and metaphor in the treatment of chronic pain in children. *Pediatric Pain Letter.* 2013;15:1–8.
17. Godoy LD, Rossignoli MT, Delfino-Pereira P, Garcia-Cairasco N, de Lima Umeoka EH. A comprehensive overview on stress neurobiology: Basic concepts and clinical implications. *Front Behav Neurosci.* 2018;12:127.
18. Nelson S, Borsook D, Bosquet Enlow M. Targeting the stress response in pediatric pain: Current evidence for psychosocial intervention and avenues for future investigation. *Pain Rep.* 2021;6(3):e953.
19. Chang L. The role of stress on physiologic responses and clinical symptoms in irritable bowel syndrome. *Gastroenterology.* 2011;140(3):761–5.
20. Devanarayana NM, Rajindrajith S. Irritable bowel syndrome in children: Current knowledge, challenges and opportunities. *World J Gastroenterol.* 2018;24(21):2211–35.
21. Rosenblat JD, Mansur RB, Brietzke E, Kennedy SH, Carvalho AF, Lee Y, et al. Association of history of adverse childhood experiences with irritable bowel syndrome (IBS) in individuals with mood disorders. *Psychiatry Res.* 2020;288:112967.
22. Zia JK, Lenhart A, Yang PL, Heitkemper MM, Baker J, Keefer L, et al. risk factors for abdominal pain-related disorders of gut-brain interaction in adults and children: A systematic review. *Gastroenterology.* 2022;163(4):995–1023 e3.
23. Nelson S, Simons LE, Logan D. The incidence of Adverse Childhood Experiences (ACEs) and Their association with pain-related and psychosocial impairment in youth with chronic pain. *Clin J Pain.* 2018;34(5):402–8.
24. Hollier JM, van Tilburg MAL, Liu Y, Czyzewski DI, Self MM, Weidler EM, et al. Multiple psychological factors predict abdominal pain severity in children with irritable bowel syndrome. *Neurogastroenterol Motil.* 2019;31(2):e13509.
25. Dufton LM, Dunn MJ, Compas BE. Anxiety and somatic complaints in children with recurrent abdominal pain and anxiety disorders. *J Pediatr Psychol.* 2009;34(2):176–86.
26. Newton E, Schosheim A, Patel S, Chitkara DK, van Tilburg MAL. The role of psychological factors in pediatric functional abdominal pain disorders. *Neurogastroenterol Motil.* 2019;31(6):e13538.
27. Thavamani A, Umapathi KK, Khatana J, Gulati R. Burden of psychiatric disorders among pediatric and young adults with inflammatory bowel disease: A population-based analysis. *Pediatr Gastroenterol Hepatol Nutr.* 2019;22(6):527–35.
28. Harris RF, Menard-Katcher C, Atkins D, Furuta GT, Klinnert MD. Psychosocial dysfunction in children and adolescents with eosinophilic esophagitis. *J Pediatr Gastroenterol Nutr.* 2013;57(4):500–5.
29. Germone M, Phu T, Slosky C, Pan Z, Jones A, Stahl M, et al. Anxiety and depression in pediatric patients with celiac disease: A large cross-sectional study. *J Pediatr Gastroenterol Nutr.* 2022;75(2):181–5.

30. Lalouni M, Ljotsson B, Bonnert M, Hedman-Lagerlof E, Hogstrom J, Serlachius E, et al. Internet-delivered cognitive behavioral therapy for children with pain-related functional gastrointestinal disorders: Feasibility study. *JMIR Ment Health.* 2017;4(3):e32.
31. Walker LS, Sherman AL, Bruehl S, Garber J, Smith CA. Functional abdominal pain patient subtypes in childhood predict functional gastrointestinal disorders with chronic pain and psychiatric comorbidities in adolescence and adulthood. *Pain.* 2012;153(9):1798–806.
32. Miller MM, Meints SM, Hirsh AT. Catastrophizing, pain, and functional outcomes for children with chronic pain: A meta-analytic review. *Pain.* 2018;159(12):2442–60.
33. Wojtowicz AA, Greenley RN, Gumidyala AP, Rosen A, Williams SE. Pain severity and pain catastrophizing predict functional disability in youth with inflammatory bowel disease. *J Crohns Colitis.* 2014;8(9):1118–24.
34. van Tilburg MA, Claar RL, Romano JM, Langer SL, Walker LS, Whitehead WE, et al. Role of coping with symptoms in depression and disability: Comparison between inflammatory bowel disease and abdominal pain. *J Pediatr Gastroenterol Nutr.* 2015;61(4):431–6.
35. Szigethy EM, Youk AO, Benhayon D, Fairclough DL, Newara MC, Kirshner MA, et al. Depression subtypes in pediatric inflammatory bowel disease. *J Pediatr Gastroenterol Nutr.* 2014;58(5):574–81.
36. Campo JV. Annual research review: Functional somatic symptoms and associated anxiety and depression – Developmental psychopathology in pediatric practice. *J Child Psychol Psychiatry.* 2012;53(5):575–92.
37. Sinclair CM, Meredith P, Strong J, Feeney R. Personal and contextual factors affecting the functional ability of children and adolescents with chronic pain: A systematic review. *J Dev Behav Pediatr.* 2016;37(4):327–42.
38. Hommel KA, Franciosi JP, Gray WN, Hente EA, Ahrens A, Rothenberg ME. Behavioral functioning and treatment adherence in pediatric eosinophilic gastrointestinal disorders. *Pediatr Allergy Immunol.* 2012;23(5):494–9.
39. Brosbe MS, Thompson CC, Flanders XC, Day A, Ward C, Slifer KJ. Pain catastrophizing and functional disability in youth with chronic pain: An examination of indirect effects. *J Clin Psychol Med Settings.* 2022;29(3):546–56.
40. Boerner KE, Green K, Chapman A, Stanford E, Newlove T, Edwards K, et al. Making sense of "somatization": A systematic review of its relationship to pediatric pain. *J Pediatr Psychol.* 2020;45(2):156–69.
41. Spatuzzo M, Chiaretti A, Capossela L, Covino M, Gatto A, Ferrara P. Abdominal pain in children: The role of possible psychosocial disorders. *Eur Rev Med Pharmacol Sci.* 2021;25(4):1967–73.
42. Mackner LM, Greenley RN, Szigethy E, Herzer M, Deer K, Hommel KA. Psychosocial issues in pediatric inflammatory bowel disease: Report of the North American Society for Pediatric Gastroenterology, Hepatology, and Nutrition. *J Pediatr Gastroenterol Nutr.* 2013;56(4):449–58.
43. Mazzone L, Reale L, Spina M, Guarnera M, Lionetti E, Martorana S, et al. Compliant gluten-free children with celiac disease: An evaluation of psychological distress. *BMC Pediatr.* 2011;11:46.
44. Adams L, Turk, DC. Central sensitization and the biopsychosocial approach to understanding pain. *Journal of Applied Behavioral Research.* 2018;23:e12125.
45. Nelson S, Cunningham N. The impact of posttraumatic stress disorder on clinical presentation and psychosocial treatment response in youth with functional abdominal pain disorders: An exploratory study. *Children (Basel).* 2020;7(6):56.
46. Cuneo AA, Abu-El-Haija M, Marsac ML, Verstraete S, Heyman MB, Ly N, et al. Pediatric medical traumatic stress in inflammatory bowel disease, pancreatitis, and cystic fibrosis. *J Pediatr Gastroenterol Nutr.* 2022;75(4):455–61.
47. Price J, Kassam-Adams N, Alderfer MA, Christofferson J, Kazak AE. Systematic review: A reevaluation and update of the integrative (trajectory) model of pediatric medical traumatic stress. *J Pediatr Psychol.* 2016;41(1):86–97.
48. Singh P, Lembo A. Emerging role of the gut microbiome in irritable bowel syndrome. *Gastroenterol Clin North Am.* 2021;50(3):523–45.

49. Labanski A, Langhorst J, Engler H, Elsenbruch S. Stress and the brain-gut axis in functional and chronic-inflammatory gastrointestinal diseases: A transdisciplinary challenge. *Psychoneuroendocrinology*. 2020;111:104501.
50. Glynn H, Moller SP, Wilding H, Apputhurai P, Moore G, Knowles SR. Prevalence and impact of post-traumatic stress disorder in gastrointestinal conditions: A systematic review. *Dig Dis Sci*. 2021;66(12):4109–19.
51. Yacob D, Di Lorenzo C, Bridge JA, Rosenstein PF, Onorato M, Bravender T, et al. Prevalence of pain-predominant functional gastrointestinal disorders and somatic symptoms in patients with anxiety or depressive disorders. *J Pediatr*. 2013;163(3):767–70.
52. Lewandowski AS, Palermo TM, Stinson J, Handley S, Chambers CT. Systematic review of family functioning in families of children and adolescents with chronic pain. *J Pain*. 2010;11(11):1027–38.
53. Varni JW, Bendo CB, Nurko S, Shulman RJ, Self MM, Franciosi JP, et al. Health-related quality of life in pediatric patients with functional and organic gastrointestinal diseases. *J Pediatr*. 2015;166(1):85–90.
54. Gallagher L, McAuley J, Moseley GL. A randomized-controlled trial of using a book of metaphors to reconceptualize pain and decrease catastrophizing in people with chronic pain. *Clin J Pain*. 2013;29(1):20–5.

Chapter 3

Common gastrointestinal conditions in pediatrics

Ashish Chogle

Chapter aims

This chapter aims to provide an introduction to the common pediatric gastrointestinal (GI) conditions and symptoms associated with the GI tract (i.e., structural, inflammatory, and disorders of gut–brain interaction). The chapter will also provide a summary of common treatment methods and associated side effects.

Learning points

- Pediatric GI conditions can be classified into structural, inflammatory, or disorders of gut–brain interaction (DGBI), with conditions and symptoms often overlapping.
- Red flags indicating organic conditions need to be watched out for, and appropriate investigations must be initiated if they are present.
- An integrative, multidisciplinary holistic approach with medications, diet, integrative therapies, and psychology works well for DGBI.

The common presenting symptoms of GI conditions that affect youth include abdominal pain, constipation, diarrhea, nausea, vomiting, and feeding problems. Various GI conditions can present with similar symptoms, and more than one condition can coexist in a single patient. The diagnosis depends upon a thoughtful investigative process including a detailed history and physical examination; see Chapter 1 for an overview of GI physiology and Chapter 4 for common medical procedures/testing in youth.

GI conditions can have an impact on the psychosocial functioning of the child and their quality of life [1]. Conversely, psychological distress that is either pre-existing or results from illness can adversely affect the child's disease activity and severity. A chronic GI condition can also affect the entire family and not only the patient. It is helpful for mental health professionals to have a basic understanding of the common GI conditions so that they can help the families have a better understanding and acceptance of their medical diagnosis, and incorporate the necessary psychological interventions in the treatment plan.

A summary of the common GI disorders in youth and related symptoms associated with the GI tract is outlined in Table 3.1 (see also Handout 3.1). For simplicity, GI conditions have been categorized into either structural, inflammatory, or DGBI:

DOI: 10.4324/9781003308683-4

Table 3.1 Common GI conditions in youth

Structural	*Inflammatory*	*Disorders of gut–brain interaction (DGBI)*
• Esophageal atresia and tracheoesophageal fistula • Hirschsprung disease • Anorectal malformations	• Gastroesophageal reflux disease (GERD) • Eosinophilic esophagitis (EoE) • Peptic ulcer disease • Inflammatory bowel disease (IBD): Crohn's disease and ulcerative colitis • Celiac disease	• Functional dyspepsia • Rumination syndrome • Aerophagia • Abdominal migraines • Irritable bowel syndrome • Functional abdominal pain • Functional nausea • Cyclic vomiting syndrome • Functional constipation • Nonretentive fecal incontinence

- Structural GI conditions are either congenital or acquired and cause obstructive symptoms.
- Inflammatory GI conditions are acquired and result from infections, chemical irritation, and/or immune reactions in the GI tract.
- DGBI occur secondary to dysfunction of the brain–gut axis (BGA) that causes visceral hypersensitivity and changes in GI motility.

Symptoms are not specific to particular conditions. For example, dysphagia can be present in inflammatory conditions such as eosinophilic esophagitis (EoE) and in structural conditions such as esophageal atresia. Diarrhea can be present in DGBI such as irritable bowel syndrome but can also be the main symptom in inflammatory conditions such as celiac disease. Commonly used medications to treat these common pediatric GI conditions have been summarized in Table 3.2 (see also Handout 3.1).

Structural GI conditions

Esophageal atresia (EA) and tracheoesophageal fistula (TEF)

EA with TEF is among the most common birth defects requiring surgery in infancy [2]. In EA, the upper esophagus does not connect (atresia) to the lower esophagus and stomach. Almost 90% of babies born with esophageal atresia also have a TEF, in which the esophagus and the trachea are abnormally connected [3]. Approximately 1 in 3,000 infants is born with an EA–TEF defect [4]. See Figure 3.1 for an overview of the five types of EA. Of these variants, Type C TEF is common, comprising more than 80% of cases. About 50% of infants with EA–TEF will have another birth defect, cardiac being the most common one [2]. Classically, infants with EA–TEF present with coughing and choking after their initial feeding. After surgery, patients can have complications including leakage of esophageal contents, narrowing, vocal cord injury, or breakdown of the surgery site [5]. Most youth with esophageal narrowing respond to repeated stretching, but some need steroid injections at the narrowed sites. Tracheomalacia or weakness of the trachea is a common problem in youth with EA–TEF [6]. Tracheomalacia can present with a barking cough or trouble breathing. Gastroesophageal reflux disease (GERD) is very common in youth with EA–TEF (mainly due to impaired esophageal movement [7]), with symptoms tending to worsen with increasing age [8]. The mainstay treatment of GERD is antacids [9]. Youth

Table 3.2 Commonly used medications for GI conditions in youth

Type of medication	*Medications*	*Indications*	*Comments relating to medication*
Antacids	Famotidine, omeprazole, esomeprazole, pantoprazole	GERD	Stopping antacids suddenly can lead to rebound hyperacidity.
Pro-motility	Erythromycin, reglan	GERD	Can cause diarrhea as a side effect. Reglan can cause neurological side effects especially if continued for a prolonged duration.
Topical steroids	Fluticasone, budesonide	EoE	These medications have minimal absorption in the body, so do not cause side effects of the same magnitude as prednisone.
Anti-inflammatory	5-ASA drugs, prednisone	IBD	Use of prednisone needs to be minimized to the shortest duration to reduce chances of serious side effects including impact on growth.
Immunomodulator	Azathioprine, mercaptopurine, methotrexate	IBD	Possible side effects on the bone marrow and liver need to be monitored.
Gastric relaxer	Cyproheptadine	DGBI	Increases appetite, rarely causes mood swings.
Antispasmodic	Hyoscyamine, dicyclomine	Abdominal pain	Excessive use can cause constipation.
Antinausea	Ondansetron, granisetron, scopolamine, aprepitant	Nausea, vomiting	Scopolamine can occasionally cause drowsiness, blurring of vision.
Osmotic laxative	Miralax, milk of magnesia, lactulose	Constipation	Can cause increased leakage of stools if there is an uncleared hard stool mass in the rectum.
Stimulant laxative	Senna, dulcolax	Constipation	Contrary to popular belief, these medications are not habit forming.
Antidiarrheal	Loperamide	Diarrhea	Can be abused to achieve a high similar to opioids if taken in large doses.

with severe reflux undergo fundoplication, which involves wrapping the top of the stomach around the lower end of the esophagus [9]. Given the disease process associated EA–TEF, youth have an increased risk of Barrett's esophagus, and subsequently require lifelong endoscopic surveillance [7]. More than half of those living with EA–TEF report swallowing difficulty, which can occur secondary to post-surgical esophageal narrowing, associated heart defects, or esophageal movement issues [10]. Chronic respiratory issues are common and include issues with aspiration, pneumonia, choking, wheezing, cough, asthma, and reactive airway disease [6].

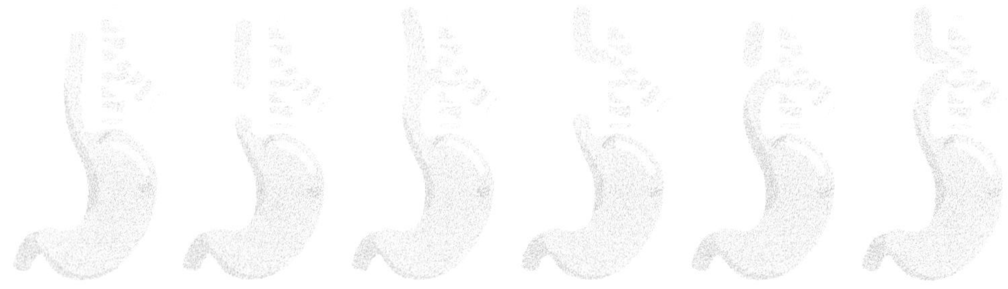

Figure 3.1 Classification of esophageal atresia (Type A isolated EA, Type B EA with proximal TEF, Type C EA with distal TEF, Type D EA with proximal and distal TEF, and Type E isolated TEF [H-type]) (Source: Inspiring/Shutterstock.com).

Hirschsprung disease

Hirschsprung disease is a birth defect that is characterized by the absence of ganglion cells (type of nerves) in parts of the bowel, leading to impaired gut movement. The incidence is approximately one in every 5,000 live births per year [11]. The most common type, affecting 80–85% of children, is short-segment Hirschsprung disease, in which the distal-most part of the colon (the last 10% of the bowel) lacks the ganglion cells [12]. Most children with Hirschsprung disease are diagnosed within the first month of life [13]. Babies can present with delayed passage of stools (>24 hours but especially >48 hours) with feeding issues, abdominal distension, vomiting, and constipation. If the diagnosis is made later in childhood, the presenting symptoms include constipation that does not improve with medications, abdominal distension, vomiting, failure to thrive, and enterocolitis (inflammation of the intestines and colon) [13]. Hirschsprung disease is a lifelong condition. Even after surgery, patients can experience complications narrowing at the surgical site, stool leakage, constipation, and enterocolitis [14]. Several studies have shown impaired bowel function in a majority of youth, even when they reach adolescence or early adult life [14, 15]. Hirschsprung disease negatively affects the quality of life of these youth, including their physical and psychosocial well-being [14]. Youth have reported issues such as impaired bowel function, food intolerances, embarrassment of surgical scars, emotional effects from impaired bowel function, feelings of being different/loneliness, lack of knowledge about Hirschsprung disease, concerns about sexuality and fertility, and limited access to adult services. Therefore, long-term care with a multidisciplinary team that includes a mental health professional, and a good transition plan, is important.

Anorectal malformations

Anorectal malformations are birth defects that occur due to the improper formation of the anus and rectum. Anorectal malformations could be of various types. There could be a membrane covering the anal opening; the rectum may not connect to the anus (rectal atresia); the anal passage may be narrow or located in the wrong place (recto-perineal fistula); there can be an abnormal passage from the rectum, located behind the vagina (recto-vestibular fistula); the rectum may connect to a part of the urinary tract or the reproductive system through an abnormal opening, and an anal opening is not present; there could be no anus and no connection to the urinary tract or reproductive system (imperforate anus without a fistula); the urethra, vagina, and rectum are joined together as a common channel instead of three separate ones (cloaca) [16]. Approximately one in 5,000 children are born with an anorectal malformation [17]. It can present with the inability to pass stools at birth, severe constipation in infancy, and passage of stools via the abnormal openings in the urinary or reproductive tracts, or with recurrent urinary tract infections [17].

Around half of those born with anorectal malformations have other congenital defects in their spine or kidneys, heart, airways, esophagus, or limbs [16]. Anorectal malformations are usually diagnosed at birth and surgically treated. These youth can have continued medical problems even after their surgery. Common short-term and long-term issues that have been reported include stool leakage, chronic constipation, urinary leakage, issues with ejaculation, and erectile dysfunction [18]. The presence of these issues significantly affects the quality of life and social development in the teenage and young adult period [19].

Inflammatory GI conditions

Gastroesophageal reflux disease (GERD)

Gastroesophageal reflux (GER) is a physiological process by which contents from the stomach go into the esophagus. There is episodic relaxation of the lower esophagus sphincter and it is the most common reason for GER to occur. When GER becomes excessive and causes troublesome symptoms and/or esophageal damage, then it is called GERD [20]. GERD is present in more than 25% of infants and the incidence decreases with increasing age. GERD is observed in more than 10% of toddlers, children, and adolescents. The symptoms of GERD can vary by age of presentation from fussiness, pain, back arching, refusal to eat, weight loss, and pneumonia in infants to heartburn, chest pain, vomiting, and pain on eating in older children and adolescents.

GER does not need treatment and will typically resolve on its own with time. However, GERD should be treated, and the treatment varies with age. In infants, non-medication approaches such as a change in position after feeding, thickening of formula, and change in the type of formula are initially utilized. If these do not help, then medications that reduce the acid production in the stomach and/or make the stomach move faster are used. In adolescents, lifestyle and dietary changes can be helpful as an initial approach, followed by medications if symptoms persist. For severe cases of GERD, a surgery in which the upper part of the stomach is wrapped around the lower end of the esophagus to increase pressure (Fundoplication) is occasionally performed [21].

Eosinophilic esophagitis (EoE)

EoE is a chronic inflammatory disease of the esophagus. The inflammation is caused by eosinophils, which accumulate in the esophagus in response to certain food and possibly airborne allergens. EoE is now increasingly diagnosed, with an estimated 19 per 100,000 children and adolescents affected [22]. Youth with EoE commonly have a history of other allergic diseases such as asthma, eczema, and rhinitis [23]. Esophageal inflammation can lead to symptoms that may vary depending on age. Infants and toddlers often refuse to eat and can have trouble growing optimally. School-age youth may present with vomiting, abdominal pain, and trouble swallowing [24]. They also may have a history of chewing their food for a long time and eating slowly. Adolescents and adults commonly present with painful swallowing and food getting stuck in their esophagus. The food can get stuck due to esophageal swelling from the inflammation, poor movement, and/or narrowing of the esophagus (stricture). The two main treatments recommended for EoE are dietary change (food elimination diets) and medications [25]. Youth with EoE need upper GI endoscopies with biopsies to monitor the effectiveness of the treatment plan. If the esophagus becomes narrowed due to prolonged inflammation, then the youth undergoes esophageal stretching using a balloon or a tube that is inserted into the narrowed section of the esophagus [26].

Peptic ulcer disease (PUD)

A peptic ulcer forms when stomach acid and digestive enzymes damage the walls of the stomach or duodenum. There are many causes of peptic ulcers, but the most common include *Helicobacter pylori* (*H. pylori*) infection and excessive acid production [27]. Other factors such as being on non-steroidal anti-inflammatory drugs make the stomach and duodenum susceptible to the corrosive effects of stomach acid and digestive enzymes [28]. PUD is seen in about 8% of youth, equally in males and females, with the incidence increasing after 10 years of age [29]. PUD can be asymptomatic but typically presents with a burning pain in the stomach, bloating, nausea and/or vomiting, decreased appetite, weight loss, and occasionally GI bleeding causing anemia. Sometimes, peptic ulcers can bleed profusely or perforate, requiring emergency medical care including endoscopy or surgery [29].

PUD caused by *H. pylori* infection is treated with antibiotics to kill the bacteria and antacids to minimize the production of stomach acid [30]. Youth living with PUD benefit from lifestyle changes such as avoidance of trigger foods such as fried foods, spicy foods, chocolate, coffee, and carbonated drinks. Losing excessive weight, avoiding tight clothes, and sleeping with the head elevated can help reduce PUD symptoms [29].

Inflammatory bowel disease (IBD): Crohn's disease and ulcerative colitis

IBD is an inflammatory condition of the GI tract that has a rising incidence in North America, estimated to be 77 per 100,000 in the pediatric population [31, 32]. Twenty-five percent of individuals with IBD are diagnosed before 18 years of age, most commonly between 10 and 12 years [31]. IBD is also increasingly being diagnosed in younger children (very early onset IBD, or VEO-IBD) and these children usually have the more severe, treatment-resistant form of the disease, with higher chances of surgery and frequent hospital readmissions [33]. The exact cause of IBD is not well understood, but it is thought to be a dysfunctional response of the immune system to intestinal microbes in a genetically predisposed individual, whereby the body produces inflammation and does not know how to switch it off. There seems to be a role for environmental factors such as infections, exposure to antibiotics, and stress in triggering the inflammatory response [34, 35].

There are two forms of IBD – Crohn's disease (CD) and ulcerative colitis (UC). CD manifests in the entire GI tract and anus and is characterized by inflammation across the intestinal mucosa (GI tract lining), patchy disease activity, segments with inflammation alternating with normal areas, and the presence of strictures and/or fistulas. Crohn's disease most commonly affects the small and large intestine, although it can also affect the upper GI tract [36]. UC is typically confined to the colon and is characterized by continuous inflammation and sores (ulcers) in the rectum that extends toward the anus [36]. CD can present with symptoms such as abdominal pain, diarrhea, rectal bleeding, anemia, fatigue, fevers, weight loss, growth failure, delayed sexual development, pus collection, or tears around the anus. Similarly, UC can present with abdominal pain, especially during defecation, bloody diarrhea, fatigue, anemia, and weight loss. IBD can also affect parts of the body other than the GI tract such as eyes, bones, skin, liver, pancreas, and kidneys [37]. For some youth, IBD inflammation is fairly minor, and they may spend months to years in remission before the inflammation rises again. For others, the inflammation can be severe, with life-threatening complications requiring the removal of parts of the bowel after which some youth will have to wear a stoma.

Treatment of IBD focuses on minimizing inflammation and preventing disease-related complications while optimizing nutrition to improve growth and improve quality of life [38]. Medications such as steroids and other immunosuppressants slow down the disease progression by reducing and controlling inflammation in the body, leading to the healing of the GI tract [39]. Nutritional rehabilitation is important in these youth to help resolve nutritional deficiencies that have resulted from malabsorption and poor food intake. There are diets such as specific carbohydrate diet, Crohn's disease exclusion diet, and exclusive enteral nutrition, which have been found to help reduce GI inflammation in certain patient populations. All changes in diet should be medically monitored if chosen as a treatment strategy in youth with IBD. For those with severe IBD, surgery may be necessary to remove the diseased portion of the GI tract [40].

Celiac disease

Celiac disease is a common digestive disorder that is caused by eating foods that contain gluten (the protein found in grains such as wheat, rye, and barley). It is present in 1 in 100–200 people in North America. Celiac disease can occur at any age, from infancy to old age. It is more common in people of northern European descent [41]. There is a higher risk of developing celiac disease if there is a first-degree relative with celiac disease. When youth living with celiac disease consume foods containing gluten, it leads to an autoimmune reaction that causes inflammation in the small intestines and other parts of the body. The GI inflammation causes flattening of the absorptive surface of the small intestines (villi) resulting in malabsorption of nutrients [42]. The symptoms of celiac disease vary widely and may include abdominal pain, nausea, vomiting, constipation, diarrhea, rashes, sores in the mouth, headaches, fatigue, loss of appetite, weight loss, growth failure, joint pain, and infertility. Treatment of celiac disease includes strict elimination of gluten from the youth's diet. It is very important for youths to be seen by a dietician who can guide the family on gluten elimination and help recommend alternate foods to ensure optimal nutritional intake [43].

Disorders of gut–brain interaction (DGBI)

This section provides a summary of DGBI, formally known as functional gastrointestinal disorders (FGID) seen in youth. These conditions are common in 12–29% of youth worldwide [44]. DGBI have a major impact on quality of life and cause significant functional disability, higher rates of anxiety and depression, and school absenteeism [45]. The pathophysiology of DGBI in youth can be explained using the biopsychosocial model of chronic diseases involving a complex interplay of genetic, physiological, psychological, and environmental factors (see Chapter 6 for case conceptualization and assessment). These factors cause a disruption in the functioning of the gut–brain axis (BGA; see Chapter 2). Contrary to popular belief, DGBI are not diagnoses of exclusion and can be established positively using a set of clinical criteria (Rome IV criteria), without any testing [46]. These conditions require a detailed history and physical exam, ruling out red flags (alarm signs) for organic conditions (see Box 3.1) for diagnosis. Diagnostic testing is optional and is indicated only if red flags are present in the history or physical examination. Symptom development is sometimes associated with a preceding event, for example, an infection [47]. Youth with DGBI are vulnerable to the development of mental health issues such as anxiety that begins in childhood and persists into late adolescence and early adulthood, even if abdominal pain resolves [48, 49]. There is evidence that stress is increased in children with a DGBI such as functional abdominal pain disorder [50–53], and in turn stress can exacerbate DGBI symptoms. For example, traumatic stress in childhood may not only affect the child now but may also have long-lasting effects on gut functioning and symptoms into adulthood [54].

BOX 3.1 RED FLAGS SUGGESTIVE OF ORGANIC CONDITIONS

- Family history of IBD, celiac disease, or peptic ulcer disease
- Persistent right upper quadrant pain
- Dysphagia
- Persistent vomiting
- GI bleeding
- Nocturnal diarrhea
- Arthritis
- Perirectal disease
- Involuntary weight loss
- Slow height gain
- Delayed puberty
- Unexplained fevers
- Oral sores

The presence of red flags could point towards organic conditions (with inflammation or tissue injury). Normal or negative test results in youth with DGBI are common since there is no actual inflammation or injury occurring presently in the GI tract. Parents often get frustrated with the normal testing and think that the health professional does not know the exact cause of their child's symptoms and hence their child is given a diagnosis of a DGBI. The family's expectations need to be set for the high likelihood of normal testing and they need to be educated about the positive diagnosis of DGBI based on clinical criteria. Also, spending time explaining the two-way interaction between the GI tract and the brain (i.e., BGA) to the family is of paramount importance and the most vital step in starting a good therapeutic relationship; see Chapter 2 for example dialogue and methods explaining the BGA. It is critical that the child starts receiving treatment for the likely DGBI even while the investigations are ongoing to avoid delaying treatment.

The treatment of DGBI is multifaceted and includes lifestyle interventions, nonpharmacologic treatments (e.g., herbal medications, psychotherapy modalities, acupuncture, diets), pharmacologic medications, and neuromodulation with peripheral electrical nerve field stimulation (PENFS) [55]. Psychosocial stressors and triggers need to be identified with a plan to reintegrate the youth back into their routine. These youth benefit from coping and symptom-reducing tools such as cognitive behavioral therapies, clinical hypnotherapy, and other psychological techniques; for a detailed review of these conditions, see the Rome IV publications [56–58] and Chapters 16 and 17. Although an extensive review is not possible, the following text provides a brief overview of several DGBI, including functional dyspepsia, rumination syndrome, aerophagia, functional abdominal pain, abdominal migraines, functional nausea, cyclic vomiting syndrome, functional constipation, and nonretentive fecal incontinence.

Functional dyspepsia (FD)

Youth with FD present with abdominal pain or discomfort in the upper middle region of the abdomen (above the belly button). The discomfort can be a sensation of excessive fullness after meals, an early feeling of having had enough to eat, bloating, belching, retching, nausea, vomiting, regurgitation, or loss of appetite [56, 57]. The prevalence of FD in youth has been reported to range from 0.2% to 26%. Little is known about the cause of FD; however, there is some evidence that stomach motility issues and GI nerve hypersensitivity may be involved [55]. Psychological factors such as psychosocial stressors (e.g., difficulties at school) can exacerbate symptoms. Treatment of FD includes dietary changes such as reduction or avoidance of acidic, spicy, fatty, or caffeine-containing, food or drinks. Acid-blocking medications and those that change the motility of the stomach have been used with some success. Medications such as antidepressants (e.g., Amitriptyline, Citalopram) can be used to reduce visceral hypersensitivity. Relaxation techniques, psychotherapies such as biofeedback and hypnotherapy, can also be helpful in these youth [55, 58].

Rumination syndrome

Rumination syndrome is a condition where children bring up food from their stomach soon after eating, without retching, and either vomit or re-swallow the food [56, 57]. The symptoms do not occur while the youth is asleep. There is often a history of some "triggering" event such as a viral infection, some other GI disease, or psychological stress. Even after the triggering event has subsided, the rumination persists. Rumination syndrome is thought to be like a tic or a habit. The abdominal muscles contract and push the food or liquid from the stomach up into the esophagus and the mouth [59]. Youth living with rumination syndrome may report abdominal pain, nausea, or a feeling of discomfort before the rumination begins. Due to the nature of rumination syndrome, youth living with this condition are at risk for malnutrition, dehydration, and weight loss. Treatment of rumination syndrome includes counseling families regarding the condition's pathophysiology since it is often confused with GERD or vomiting [60].

Treating symptoms such as abdominal pain, nausea, or bloating that occur after eating can reduce rumination. Eating small meals initially and then gradually increasing the meal volumes can help the stomach's ability to tolerate larger amounts of foods and fluids. Learning to keep the abdominal muscles relaxed and preventing them from contracting using techniques such as diaphragmatic breathing, biofeedback, and gut-directed therapy can be effective [61, 62]. Medications such as Baclofen that increases the tone of the lower esophageal sphincter, and low-dose antidepressants that reduce visceral hypersensitivity, are used occasionally for the treatment of rumination syndrome [63]. Youth with rumination syndrome and malnutrition are started on the nasojejunal tube (commonly referred to as NJ tube) feeds to improve nutrition prior to starting definitive treatment of this condition [64]. The NJ tube feeds deliver food directly into the small intestines and prevent the food from being regurgitated out into the mouth.

Aerophagia

Aerophagia involves excessive air swallowing by a child resulting in progressive abdominal distension. The average prevalence of aerophagia has been estimated to be around 3% worldwide

[65, 66]. A typical child with aerophagia will start the day with a soft, non-distended abdomen and then has progressive abdominal distension that worsens by evening [56, 57]. Observation will often identify audible air swallowing, frequent belching, and excessive flatus. There is a higher incidence of aerophagia in developmentally delayed children [67]. GI symptoms can be associated with a reduction in oral intake due to decreased appetite and feeling full all the time. There are no treatment trials that have been performed in youth with aerophagia. Possible treatment approaches include relaxation techniques and diaphragmatic breathing [68]. The education of parents about the gulping movements and sounds suggestive of air swallowing is considered an important part of the therapy and helps assuage their concerns about a more serious organic disease being missed by the health professional. Youth with aerophagia are asked to avoid carbonated beverages, hard candy, and chewing gum to reduce the volume of gas in the GI tract. Drugs such as simethicone can decrease abdominal discomfort/pain by preventing gas bubble formation [69].

Abdominal migraine

Youth with abdominal migraines have episodes of acute onset and intense abdominal pain that lasts for an hour or more and prevents them from participating in normal activities. These episodes occur every few weeks or months [57]. The child is typically symptom-free between these episodes. The pain can be associated with decreased appetite, nausea, vomiting, headaches, pale skin, and sensitivity to light. Abdominal migraines are seen most in youth under 10 years of age, in more girls than boys, and affect 1–4% of school-aged youth [70]. More than half the youth with this condition no longer have abdominal migraines by their late teenage years. About 70% of the youth with a previous history of abdominal migraines eventually develop headache migraines [71].

Foods such as chocolate, monosodium glutamate, and nitrites (meat preservatives) can trigger abdominal migraines. Psychological stress and lack of adequate/restful sleep can worsen abdominal migraines. Specific foods that can initiate an attack are removed from the diet. Stress management is taught to youth via relaxation techniques and psychotherapy. Improvement of sleep can help reduce abdominal migraines. Medications that are used for the treatment of headache migraines such as cyproheptadine and triptans (e.g., sumatriptan, rizatriptan) are also used for abdominal migraines [55].

Irritable bowel syndrome (IBS)

IBS is a condition that includes chronic abdominal pain along with changes in form and frequency of stool. It occurs in about 5% of youth [53, 72], with presenting symptoms including abdominal discomfort or pain with diarrhea and/or constipation, and bloating. There may be other symptoms such as early feeling of fullness on eating, nausea, heartburn, and less commonly vomiting [57]. Based on the symptoms, three main IBS classifications are (1) IBS with constipation (IBS-C), (2) IBS with diarrhea (IBS-D), and (3) mixed IBS with alternating constipation and diarrhea (IBS-M). A characteristic of IBS-C is that the abdominal pain does not resolve with the treatment of constipation. Like other DGBI, psychosocial stressors can exacerbate IBS symptoms. The goal of treatment of IBS is to reduce symptoms so the child can resume daily activities. The treatment may include lifestyle interventions, nonpharmacologic treatments, psychotherapy, diets, acupuncture, neuromodulation, and pharmacological medications [55].

Functional abdominal pain (FAP)

FAP, also known as chronic abdominal pain, is an episodic or persistent stomachache that occurs for at least 2 months and does not meet clinical criteria for functional dyspepsia, IBS, or abdominal migraines [56, 57]. The prevalence of functional abdominal pain in youth has been noted to be between 0.3% and 5.3% worldwide [73]. Youth living with abdominal pain can have coexisting conditions such as nausea, headaches, joint pain, fatigue, sleep disorders, anxiety, and depression [74–76]. Treatment approaches include reduction of visceral hypersensitivity with antidepressant medications (e.g., amitriptyline, citalopram) and non-pharmacological medications such as peppermint oil, identification and treatment of specific pain triggers, dietary changes, and psychotherapies such as cognitive behavioral therapy, hypnotherapy, and neuromodulation with PENFS [55].

Functional nausea

Youth are said to have functional nausea when they have the predominant symptom of nausea not explained by any other medical condition. It is an accompanying symptom in about half of FAP disorders, occurring more commonly in Caucasian females and is associated with worse GI symptoms, anxiety, depression, low self-esteem, family stress, and impaired functioning [75]. Functional nausea occurs in about 16% of all school-aged youth [77]. Nausea is commonly seen in other DGBI such as abdominal migraines and cyclic vomiting syndrome and in conditions with autonomic dysfunction such as postural orthostatic tachycardia syndrome. Its pathophysiology is multifactorial and likely involves disturbances in the BGA, including dysfunction of the autonomic nervous system and disturbances of stomach motility coupled with psychological comorbidity. Treatment of functional nausea can be challenging. Traditional antiemetic medications such as ondansetron have little benefit. Herbal medications such as ginger, peppermint oil, and STW5 (iberogast) can have some beneficial effects on meal-related nausea [78–80]. In addition to medications, the treatment of nausea needs a multimodal approach with the education of families about the role of brain–gut connections and stress in the generation of nausea. Acupressure has also been shown to help reduce nausea [79]. Early involvement of a GI mental health professional for relaxation strategies, hypnotherapy, cognitive behavioral therapy, and biofeedback may be of great benefit. A diet that is low in fat, with small portion sizes multiple times a day, can help those experiencing nausea after meals [81].

Cyclic vomiting syndrome (CVS)

CVS is a condition that presents as stereotypical, recurrent episodes of vomiting which last hours to days with symptom-free intervals lasting weeks to months when the youth resumes completely normal or baseline health [56, 57]. CVS affects 1–2% of youth with an increased prevalence between 2 and 7 years [82]. CVS has a distinctive on–off pattern of vomiting that is an essential criterion for diagnosis. For many youth with CVS, the onset of episodes occurs during the early morning hours. Over two-thirds of youth living with CVS identify prodromal symptoms, such as increased sweating, pallor, abdominal pain, and headaches. For those experiencing severe or prolonged CVS episodes (i.e., lasting beyond 1 week), hospitalization may be required for fluid and nutritional support.

CVS likely occurs because of DGBI and has a strong resemblance to migraine disorders. In fact, most of the youth with CVS will transition to having migraine headaches as they grow older, typically around 10 years of age. Mitochondrial dysfunction, hyperactive hypothalamic–pituitary–adrenal (HPA) axis, genetic predisposition, and imbalance of the autonomic nervous system may play a role in the pathophysiology of CVS [83]. Evidence indicates that for youth, psychological, infectious, and physical stressors can precipitate CVS episodes [84]. Even positive stressors such as holidays, birthdays, and vacations are known to trigger CVS in some youth.

CVS treatment consists of four approaches: (1) lifestyle modifications, such as improvement of sleep routine, stress reduction with improvement of coping skills with the help of psychotherapy, avoidance of exhausting schedules, regular eating times, identification, and elimination of likely food triggers, (2) treatments that stop the episode right when it is starting, such as antimigraine medications, antiemetic medications, and sedatives (such as diphenhydramine), (3) supportive or rescue therapy (during episodes), such as fluids, electrolytes, antiemetic medications, and sedatives, and (4) preventative treatment (prevent or decrease future episodes), such as cyproheptadine, tricyclic antidepressants (e.g., amitriptyline), beta blockers (e.g., propranolol), antiseizure medications (e.g., topiramate), and mitochondrial supplements (e.g., coenzyme Q10, riboflavin, L-carnitine) [83].

Functional constipation

Functional constipation in youth is described as having difficult or infrequent bowel movements, the passage of painful or hard stools, sometimes large in diameter, often with leakage of stools in the underwear, and demonstration of withholding behaviors [56, 57]. There are no anatomical issues or systemic diseases causing constipation. The prevalence of functional constipation in youth is around 13–31% [85]. Ninety-five percent of youth with a history of constipation have functional constipation [86]. Refusing to pass stools due to current or past experiences of pain during defecation leads to stool accumulation. The colon absorbs water from stool making it harder and difficult to pass. As stool accumulates, the rectum and colon stretch, and become less effective in pushing the stools forward. As the rectum stretches, it begins to lose sensations and the child is not able to tell when they need to go to the toilet to defecate. The stretching, poor motility, and loss of sensations lead to the formation of a hard stool mass in the rectum and the soft stool often starts leaking around the plug into the diaper or underwear resulting in soiling of underwear, also called encopresis. This means that a child who is constipated can have dirty underwear multiple times a day.

Treatment of functional constipation consists of medications to address the child's constipation and behavior modification strategies to promote and maintain appropriate defecation. Treatment of constipation should always include the removal of the fecal mass (if present) from the rectum using enemas or oral laxatives. This is followed by maintenance treatment with osmotic laxatives with or without stimulant laxatives. Stimulant laxatives are useful in youth who withhold to give them the intense urge to stool and help overcome the habit of withholding. They are also useful when the colon and rectum have decreased motility from excessive stool accumulation and stretching. Youth are asked to maintain a normal intake of fiber and fluids. Physical activity also helps in the improvement of constipation. Youth should be encouraged to sit on the toilet after meals with their feet resting on a step stool, to take advantage of the natural gastrocolic reflex (an increase in colon activity in response to ingested food). Reward systems for effort and successful toileting can be helpful for positive reinforcement [87]. For a detailed overview of constipation and soiling, see Chapters 18 and 19.

Nonretentive fecal incontinence

Nonretentive fecal incontinence is a condition in which youth of at least 4 years of age have bowel movements in places and at times that are inappropriate, without signs of fecal retention [57]. There is no clinical history of constipation. They will have small or entire bowel movements in their underwear during waking hours. Nonretentive fecal incontinence can be associated with emotional disturbances in a school-aged child or behavioral issues such as oppositional defiant disorder. Some youth can use the threat of having incontinence for secondary gain. Parents need to be counseled about the nonmedical nature of this condition. They need guidance to understand that this type of stool incontinence is a symptom of underlying psychological issues and that their child needs help from a mental health professional to address the emotional disturbances and behavioral disorders [88].

Pearls of wisdom

- GI conditions can present with overlapping symptoms; it is important to know the red flags to rule out organic conditions.
- Mental health professionals encountering these youth should have knowledge of the Rome IV criteria for diagnosis of DGBI and help the youth accept these diagnoses which are given in the absence of any positive test results.
- Many parents of youth with DGBI consider normal test results (child is healthy) less reassuring than abnormal test results (child is sick). When the test results are negative, parents tend to worry about having missed an important diagnosis causing the child's symptoms. The family's expectations need to be set when ordering these investigations.
- Spending time explaining the conditions, along with the two-way interaction between the GI tract and the brain to the youth and family, is of paramount importance and the most vital step in starting a good therapeutic relationship with the youth.
- It is important to treat the whole individual rather than focus on just one bodily system.
- Psychosocial aspects and brain–gut treatments are often considered for youth with DGBI, but should equally be considered for youth with other GI disorders.

Summary

Pediatric GI conditions can be classified into structural, inflammatory, or DGBI, with conditions and symptoms often overlapping. Mental health professionals should be aware of the general symptom presentations of each condition and the red flags that warrant further investigation. For youth with DGBI, parents should be reassured that testing has limited value and is usually not needed (unless there are red flags). There is a significant role that mental health professionals can play in the treatment of most pediatric GI conditions. An integrative, multidisciplinary holistic approach with medications, diet, integrative therapies, and psychotherapy works well for DGBI.

Recommended readings

For youth and caregivers:

- GI Kids: https://gikids.org/
- International Foundation for Gastrointestinal Disorders: https://iffgd.org/
- The Rome Foundation: https://theromefoundation.org/

For mental health professionals:

- The Rome Foundation: https://theromefoundation.org/
- NASPGHAN: https://naspghan.org/professional-resources/medical-professional-resources/

References

1. Varni JW, Bendo CB, Nurko S, Shulman RJ, Self MM, Franciosi JP, et al. Health-related quality of life in pediatric patients with functional and organic gastrointestinal diseases. *J Pediatr*. 2015;166(1):85–90.e2.
2. Walk RM. Esophageal atresia and tracheoesophageal fistula: Overview and considerations for the general surgeon. *The Surgical clinics of North America*. 2022;102(5):759–78.
3. Achildi O, Grewal H. Congenital anomalies of the esophagus. *Otolaryngol Clin North Am.* 2007;40(1):219–44, viii.
4. Shaw-Smith C. Oesophageal atresia, tracheo-oesophageal fistula, and the VACTERL association: Review of genetics and epidemiology. *J Med Genet.* 2006;43(7):545–54.
5. Lal DR, Gadepalli SK, Downard CD, Ostlie DJ, Minneci PC, Swedler RM, et al. Challenging surgical dogma in the management of proximal esophageal atresia with distal tracheoesophageal fistula: Outcomes from the midwest pediatric surgery consortium. *J Pediatr Surg.* 2018;53(7):1267–72.
6. Porcaro F, Valfre L, Aufiero LR, Dall'Oglio L, De Angelis P, Villani A, et al. Respiratory problems in children with esophageal atresia and tracheoesophageal fistula. *Ital J Pediatr.* 2017;43(1):77.
7. Connor MJ, Springford LR, Kapetanakis VV, Giuliani S. Esophageal atresia and transitional care – Step 1: A systematic review and meta-analysis of the literature to define the prevalence of chronic long-term problems. *Am J Surg.* 2015;209(4):747–59.
8. Koivusalo A, Pakarinen MP, Rintala RJ. The cumulative incidence of significant gastrooesophageal reflux in patients with oesophageal atresia with a distal fistula – A systematic clinical, pH-metric, and endoscopic follow-up study. *J Pediatr Surg.* 2007;42(2):370–4.
9. Krishnan U, Mousa H, Dall'Oglio L, Homaira N, Rosen R, Faure C, et al. ESPGHAN-NASPGHAN Guidelines for the evaluation and treatment of gastrointestinal and nutritional complications in children with esophageal atresia-tracheoesophageal fistula. *J Pediatr Gastroenterol Nutr.* 2016;63(5):550–70.
10. Acher CW, Ostlie DJ, Leys CM, Struckmeyer S, Parker M, Nichol PF. Long-term outcomes of patients with tracheoesophageal fistula/esophageal atresia: Survey results from tracheoesophageal fistula/esophageal atresia online communities. *Eur J Pediatr Surg.* 2016;26(6):476–80.
11. Anderson JE, Vanover MA, Saadai P, Stark RA, Stephenson JT, Hirose S. Epidemiology of Hirschsprung disease in California from 1995 to 2013. *Pediatr Surg Int.* 2018;34(12):1299–303.
12. Heuckeroth RO. Hirschsprung disease – Integrating basic science and clinical medicine to improve outcomes. *Nat Rev Gastroenterol Hepatol.* 2018;15(3):152–67.
13. Bradnock TJ, Knight M, Kenny S, Nair M, Walker GM, British Association of Paediatric Surgeons Congenital Anomalies Surveillance S. Hirschsprung's disease in the UK and Ireland: Incidence and anomalies. *Arch Dis Child.* 2017;102(8):722–7.
14. Dai Y, Deng Y, Lin Y, Ouyang R, Li L. Long-term outcomes and quality of life of patients with Hirschsprung disease: A systematic review and meta-analysis. *BMC Gastroenterol.* 2020;20(1):67.
15. Fosby MV, Stensrud KJ, Bjørnland K. Bowel function after transanal endorectal pull-through for Hirschsprung disease – Does outcome improve over time? *Journal of Pediatric Surgery.* 2020;55(11):2375–8.
16. Wood RJ, Levitt MA. Anorectal malformations. *Clin Colon Rectal Surg.* 2018;31(2):61–70.
17. Levitt MA, Peña A. Anorectal malformations. *Orphanet J Rare Dis.* 2007;2:33.
18. Rigueros Springford L, Connor MJ, Jones K, Kapetanakis VV, Giuliani S. Prevalence of active long-term problems in patients with anorectal malformations: A systematic review. *Dis. Colon Rectum.* 2016;59(6):570–80.

19. Kyrklund K, Pakarinen MP, Rintala RJ. Long-term bowel function, quality of life and sexual function in patients with anorectal malformations treated during the PSARP era. *Semin Pediatr Surg.* 2017;26(5):336–42.
20. Fass R, Boeckxstaens GE, El-Serag H, Rosen R, Sifrim D, Vaezi MF. Gastro-oesophageal reflux disease. *Nat Rev Dis Primers.* 2021;7(1):55.
21. Lightdale JR, Gremse DA. Gastroesophageal reflux: Management guidance for the pediatrician. *Pediatrics.* 2013;131(5):e1684-95.
22. Arias Á, Pérez-Martínez I, Tenías JM, Lucendo AJ. Systematic review with meta-analysis: The incidence and prevalence of eosinophilic oesophagitis in children and adults in population-based studies. *Aliment Pharmacol Ther.* 2016;43(1):3–15.
23. Ruffner MA, Capucilli P, Hill DA, Spergel JM. Screening children for eosinophilic esophagitis: Allergic and other risk factors. *Expert Rev Clin Immunol.* 2019;15(4):315–8.
24. Ruffner MA, Capucilli P, Hill DA, Spergel JM. Screening children for eosinophilic esophagitis: Allergic and other risk factors. *Expert Rev Clin Immunol.* 2019;15(4):315–8.
25. Munoz-Persy M, Lucendo AJ. Treatment of eosinophilic esophagitis in the pediatric patient: An evidence-based approach. *Eur J Pediatr.* 2018;177(5):649–63.
26. Barni S, Arasi S, Mastrorilli C, Pecoraro L, Giovannini M, Mori F, et al. Pediatric eosinophilic esophagitis: A review for the clinician. *Ital J Pediatr.* 2021;47(1):230.
27. Mladenova I. Clinical Relevance of *Helicobacter pylori* Infection. *J Clin Med.* 2021;10(16):3473.
28. Harirforoosh S, Asghar W, Jamali F. Adverse effects of nonsteroidal antiinflammatory drugs: An update of gastrointestinal, cardiovascular and renal complications. *J Pharm Pharm Sci.* 2013;16(5):821–47.
29. Sierra D, Wood M, Kolli S, Felipez LM. Pediatric gastritis, gastropathy, and peptic ulcer disease. *Pediatr Rev.* 2018;39(11):542–9.
30. Lai HH, Lai MW. Treatment of pediatric *Helicobacter pylori* infection. *Antibiotics (Basel, Switzerland).* 2022;11(6):757.
31. Borowitz SM. The epidemiology of inflammatory bowel disease: Clues to pathogenesis? *Front Pediatr.* 2022;10:1103713.
32. Ye Y, Manne S, Treem WR, Bennett D. Prevalence of inflammatory bowel disease in pediatric and adult populations: Recent estimates from large national databases in the United States, 2007–2016. *Inflamm Bowel Dis.* 2020;26(4):619–25.
33. Arai K. Very early-onset inflammatory bowel disease: A challenging field for pediatric gastroenterologists. *Pediatr Gastroenterol Hepatol Nutr.* 2020;23(5):411–22.
34. de Souza HSP. Etiopathogenesis of inflammatory bowel disease: Today and tomorrow. *Curr Opin Gastroenterol.* 2017;33(4):222–9.
35. Kellermayer R, Zilbauer M. The gut microbiome and the triple environmental hit concept of inflammatory bowel disease pathogenesis. *J Pediatr Gastroenterol Nutr.* 2020;71(5):589–95.
36. North American Society for Pediatric Gastroenterology H, Nutrition, Colitis Foundation of A, Bousvaros A, Antonioli DA, Colletti RB, et al. Differentiating ulcerative colitis from Crohn disease in children and young adults: Report of a working group of the North American Society for Pediatric Gastroenterology, Hepatology, and Nutrition and the Crohn's and Colitis Foundation of America. *J Pediatr Gastroenterol Nutr.* 2007;44(5):653–74.
37. Jang HJ, Kang B, Choe BH. The difference in extraintestinal manifestations of inflammatory bowel disease for children and adults. *Transl Pediatr.* 2019;8(1):4–15.
38. Bouhuys M, Lexmond WS, van Rheenen PF. Pediatric inflammatory bowel disease. *Pediatrics.* 2023;151(1): e2022058037.
39. van Rheenen PF, Aloi M, Assa A, Bronsky J, Escher JC, Fagerberg UL, et al. The medical management of paediatric Crohn's disease: An ECCO-ESPGHAN guideline update. *J Crohns Colitis.* 2020; 15(2):171–94.
40. Rosen MJ, Dhawan A, Saeed SA. Inflammatory bowel disease in children and adolescents. *JAMA Pediatrics.* 2015;169(11):1053–60.

41. Barton SH, Murray JA. Celiac disease and autoimmunity in the gut and elsewhere. *Gastroenterol Clin North Am.* 2008;37(2):411–28, vii.
42. Hill ID, Dirks MH, Liptak GS, Colletti RB, Fasano A, Guandalini S, et al. Guideline for the diagnosis and treatment of celiac disease in children: Recommendations of the North American Society for Pediatric Gastroenterology, Hepatology and Nutrition. *J Pediatr Gastroenterol Nutr.* 2005;40(1):1–19.
43. Jimenez J, Loveridge-Lenza B, Horvath K. Celiac disease in children. *Pediatr Clin North Am.* 2021;68(6):1205–19.
44. Lewis ML, Palsson OS, Whitehead WE, van Tilburg MAL. Prevalence of functional gastrointestinal disorders in children and adolescents. *J Pediatr.* 2016;177:39–43.e3.
45. Varni JW, Bendo CB, Nurko S, Shulman RJ, Self MM, Franciosi JP, et al. Health-related quality of life in pediatric patients with functional and organic gastrointestinal diseases. *J Pediatr.* 2015;166(1):85–90.
46. Drossman DA. Functional gastrointestinal disorders: History, pathophysiology, clinical features and Rome IV. *Gastroenterology.* 2016;150(6):1262–79.
47. Saps M, Pensabene L, Di Martino L, Staiano A, Wechsler J, Zheng X, et al. Post-infectious functional gastrointestinal disorders in children. *J Pediatr.* 2008;152(6):812–6, 6.e1.
48. Shelby GD, Shirkey KC, Sherman AL, Beck JE, Haman K, Shears AR, et al. Functional abdominal pain in childhood and long-term vulnerability to anxiety disorders. *Pediatrics.* 2013;132(3):475–82.
49. Waters AM, Schilpzand E, Bell C, Walker LS, Baber K. Functional gastrointestinal symptoms in children with anxiety disorders. *J Abnorm Child Psychol.* 2013;41(1):151–63.
50. Phavichitr N, Koosiriwichian K, Tantibhaedhyangkul R. Prevalence and risk factors of dyspepsia in Thai schoolchildren. *J Med Assoc Thai.* 2012;95 Suppl 5:S42–7.
51. Devanarayana NM, Mettananda S, Liyanarachchi C, Nanayakkara N, Mendis N, Perera N, et al. Abdominal pain-predominant functional gastrointestinal diseases in children and adolescents: Prevalence, symptomatology, and association with emotional stress. *J Pediatr Gastroenterol Nutr.* 2011;53(6):659–65.
52. Miranda A. Early life stress and pain: An important link to functional bowel disorders. *Pediatr Ann.* 2009;38(5):279–82.
53. Zia JK, Lenhart A, Yang PL, Heitkemper MM, Baker J, Keefer L, et al. Risk factors for abdominal pain-related disorders of gut-brain interaction in adults and children: A systematic review. *Gastroenterology.* 2022;163(4):995–1023.e3.
54. Ju T, Naliboff BD, Shih W, Presson AP, Liu C, Gupta A, et al. Risk and protective factors related to early adverse life events in irritable bowel syndrome. *J Clin Gastroenterol.* 2020;54(1):63–9.
55. Thapar N, Benninga MA, Crowell MD, Di Lorenzo C, Mack I, Nurko S, et al. Paediatric functional abdominal pain disorders. *Nat Rev Dis Primers.* 2020;6(1):89.
56. Benninga MA, Faure C, Hyman PE, St James Roberts I, Schechter NL, Nurko S. Childhood functional gastrointestinal disorders: neonate/toddler. *Gastroenterology.* 2016.
57. Hyams JS, Di Lorenzo C, Saps M, Shulman RJ, Staiano A, van Tilburg M. Functional disorders: Children and adolescents. *Gastroenterology.* 2016:150(6):1456–68.
58. Waseem S, Rubin L. A comprehensive review of functional dyspepsia in pediatrics. *Clin J Gastroenterol.* 2022;15(1):30–40.
59. Chial HJ, Camilleri M, Williams DE, Litzinger K, Perrault J. Rumination syndrome in children and adolescents: Diagnosis, treatment, and prognosis. *Pediatrics.* 2003;111(1):158–62.
60. Levine DF, Wingate DL, Pfeffer JM, Butcher P. Habitual rumination: A benign disorder. *Br Med J (Clin Res Ed).* 1983;287(6387):255–6.
61. Chitkara DK, Van Tilburg M, Whitehead WE, Talley NJ. Teaching diaphragmatic breathing for rumination syndrome. *Am J Gastroenterol.* 2006;101(11):2449–52.
62. Murray HB, Zhang F, Call CC, Keshishian A, Hunt RA, Juarascio AS, et al. Comprehensive cognitive-behavioral interventions augment diaphragmatic breathing for rumination syndrome: A proof-of-concept trial. *Dig Dis Sci.* 2021;66(10):3461–9.

63. Pauwels A, Broers C, Van Houtte B, Rommel N, Vanuytsel T, Tack J. A randomized double-blind, placebo-controlled, cross-over study using baclofen in the treatment of rumination syndrome. *Am J Gastroenterol.* 2018;113(1):97–104.
64. Martinez M, Rathod S, Friesen HJ, Rosen JM, Friesen CA, Schurman JV. Rumination syndrome in children and adolescents: A mini review. *Front Pediatr.* 2021;9:709326.
65. Boronat AC, Ferreira-Maia AP, Matijasevich A, Wang YP. Epidemiology of functional gastrointestinal disorders in children and adolescents: A systematic review. *World J Gastroenterol.* 2017;23(21):3915–27.
66. Rajindrajith S, Gunawardane D, Kuruppu C, Dharmaratne SD, Gunawardena NK, Devanarayana NM. Epidemiology of aerophagia in children and adolescents: A systematic review and meta-analysis. *PloS One.* 2022;17(7):e0271494.
67. Ramirez JM, Karlen-Amarante M, Wang JJ, Bush NE, Carroll MS, Weese-Mayer DE, et al. The pathophysiology of Rett syndrome with a focus on breathing dysfunctions. *Physiology (Bethesda, Md).* 2020;35(6):375–90.
68. Cigrang JA, Hunter CM, Peterson AL. Behavioral treatment of chronic belching due to aerophagia in a normal adult. *Behav Modif.* 2006;30(3):341–51.
69. Morabito G, Romeo C, Romano C. Functional aerophagia in children: A frequent, atypical disorder. *Case Rep. Gastroenterol.* 2014;8(1):123–8.
70. Winner P. Abdominal migraine. *Semin Pediatr Neurol.* 2016;23(1):11–3.
71. Dignan F, Abu-Arafeh I, Russell G. The prognosis of childhood abdominal migraine. *Arch Dis Child.* 2001;84(5):415–8.
72. Saps M, Velasco-Benitez CA, Langshaw AH, Ramirez-Hernandez CR. Prevalence of functional gastrointestinal disorders in children and adolescents: Comparison between Rome III and Rome IV Criteria. *J Pediatr.* 2018;199:212–6.
73. Korterink JJ, Diederen K, Benninga MA, Tabbers MM. Epidemiology of pediatric functional abdominal pain disorders: A meta-analysis. *PloS One.* 2015;10(5):e0126982.
74. Murphy LK, Palermo TM, Tham SW, Stone AL, Han GT, Bruehl S, et al. Comorbid sleep disturbance in adolescents with functional abdominal pain. *Behav Sleep Med.* 2021;19(4):471–80.
75. Kovacic K, Kapavarapu PK, Sood MR, Li BUK, Nugent M, Simpson P, et al. Nausea exacerbates symptom burden, quality of life, and functioning in adolescents with functional abdominal pain disorders. *Neurogastroenterol Motil.* 2019;31(7):e13595.
76. Helgeland H, Van Roy B, Sandvik L, Markestad T, Kristensen H. Paediatric functional abdominal pain: Significance of child and maternal health. A prospective study. *Acta Paediatr.* (Oslo, Norway: 1992). 2011;100(11):1461–7.
77. Saps M, Velasco-Benítez C, Kovacic K, Chelimsky G, Kovacic K, Játiva Mariño E, et al. High prevalence of nausea among school children in Latin America. *J Pediatr.* 2016;169:98-104.e1.
78. Malfertheiner P. STW 5 (Iberogast) therapy in gastrointestinal functional disorders. *Dig Dis.* 2017;35 Suppl 1:25–9.
79. Lee A, Fan LT. Stimulation of the wrist acupuncture point P6 for preventing postoperative nausea and vomiting. *Cochrane Database Syst Rev.* 2009(2):CD003281.
80. Di Lorenzo C. Functional nausea is real and makes you sick. *Front Pediatr.* 2022;10:848659.
81. Kovacic K, Di Lorenzo C. Functional nausea in children. *J Pediatr Gastroenterol Nutr.* 2016;62(3):365–71.
82. Ertekin V, Selimoglu MA, Altnkaynak S. Prevalence of cyclic vomiting syndrome in a sample of Turkish school children in an urban area. *J. Clin. Gastroenterol.* 2006;40(10):896–8.
83. Kovacic K, Li BUK. Cyclic vomiting syndrome: A narrative review and guide to management. *Headache.* 2021;61(2):231–43.
84. Li BUK. Managing cyclic vomiting syndrome in children: beyond the guidelines. *Eur J Pediatr.* 2018;177(10):1435–42.
85. Baaleman DF, Velasco-Benítez CA, Méndez-Guzmán LM, Benninga MA, Saps M. Functional gastrointestinal disorders in children: Agreement between Rome III and Rome IV diagnoses. *Eur J Pediatr.* 2021;180(7):2297–303.

86. Khan L. Constipation management in pediatric primary care. *Pediatr Ann.* 2018;47(5):e180–e4.
87. Madani S, Tsang L, Kamat D. Constipation in children: A practical review. *Pediatr Ann.* 2016;45(5):e189–96.
88. Koppen IJ, von Gontard A, Chase J, Cooper CS, Rittig CS, Bauer SB, et al. Management of functional nonretentive fecal incontinence in children: Recommendations from the international children's continence society. *J. Pediatr. Urol.* 2016;12(1):56–64.

Chapter 4

Medical procedures/testing in pediatric gastroenterology

Shaunte McKay and Jose Garza

Chapter aims

This chapter describes laboratory tests, imaging modalities, and procedures that are used to diagnose common gastrointestinal (GI) disorders. It also elaborates on common concerns and expected adverse effects experienced during and sometimes after a test or procedure is completed.

Learning points

- Understand the breadth of routinely utilized diagnostic tests and procedures for GI symptoms.
- Describe the appropriate indications for diagnostic testing and procedures.
- Describe parental concerns and adverse effects associated with routine testing modalities.
- Describe the potential harms and contraindications for over-testing youth with GI symptoms.

There are a variety of GI disorders that are present in youth, and these include: (1) structural, (2) inflammatory, and (3) disorders of gut–brain interaction (DGBI) [1] (see Chapter 3). GI symptoms within youth can vary in presentation. Common concerns include poor weight gain, malnutrition, abdominal pain, nausea, vomiting, heartburn, diarrhea, constipation, difficulty swallowing, and food refusal. It can be difficult to discern whether the initial presentation of symptoms is due to a structural or inflammatory process or DGBI as the clinical history can overlap in these categories. DGBI differ from organic and structural GI disorders because there are typically no positive findings on routine blood tests, imaging, or procedural analysis. Instead, DGBI occur due to the signaling from the centers within the brain that communicate to the GI tract and vice versa (for more explanation, see Chapters 2 and 3). The gastroenterologist will often evaluate for a variety of GI disorders based on the youth's past medical history, clinical symptoms, clinical presentation, and physical exam findings. Diagnostic testing is often required to rule out or diagnose certain diseases and these tests may include blood or stool samples, imaging modalities, or motility testing. All studies are typically reviewed with the family and/or adolescent to relay whether testing is or is not suggestive of a particular disease process. A better understanding of the indications for testing can help GI mental health professionals partner with gastroenterologists to support youth being evaluated for chronic GI symptoms. A summary of common tests and procedures used in pediatric gastroenterology is outlined and

DOI: 10.4324/9781003308683-5

also provided in Handout 4.1. See also Chapter 5 (and associated handouts 5.1–5.4) for practical strategies to help youth manage these common medical procedures.

Blood tests

Blood tests are utilized by providers to evaluate for abnormalities that can contribute to common GI symptoms. Youth may be asked to fast 8–12 hours prior to a blood test if labs that are sensitive to fat, sugar, or hormone levels in the bloodstream are collected. For all pediatric age groups, blood drawn from the vein (venipuncture) is the preferred method to obtain a blood sample. Typically, a steel needle about 23 gauge in size with an extension tube (butterfly needle) is used to puncture the vein. The nurse or phlebotomist will first examine the child's arm or hand to determine which vessel will effectively produce the best sample of blood [2]. Parents may be asked to help immobilize infants and youth less than 7 years old to reduce sudden movements that could lead to a missed insertion of the needle into the vein or dislodgement of the needle while it is in place. Note that immobilization of fearful children is not recommended (see Chapter 5 for how to manage anxiety around venipunctures). Otherwise, the parent will be asked to hold the child close and extend the child's arm straight with the wrist and palm facing upward while firmly holding the child's shoulder in place to reduce movement [2]. A rubber band (tourniquet) is then tied tightly around the arm by the nurse/technician, which helps the vein fill with blood before the needle is stuck into the vein. The needle must stay inside the vein while the technician/nurse connects the syringe to the device to collect approximately 1–5 ml of blood for a single tube [3]. It is often not possible to use the same tube for all of the tests ordered by the provider. Therefore, multiple tubes of blood may need to be collected and the needle will need to stay in place until the last tube of blood is drawn. The collection of blood from multiple tubes may take 3–5 minutes or longer depending on the time needed to immobilize the child prior. Rarely, blood can be collected from a heel or finger stick which is called a capillary sample [2]. This method only collects a few drops of blood and is not adequate for the evaluation of common GI disorders. Infants of 0–6 months old or less than 10 kg can receive a heel stick and youth greater than 10 kg should receive a finger stick if indicated [2]. After either method of blood collection, a bandage will be placed over the area as a minimal amount of bleeding may occur afterwards. After the heel or finger stick, there may be a residual stinging sensation or soreness over the area where the needle was inserted. This sensation typically resolves after 24 hours.

Common blood tests to evaluate for markers of inflammation include a complete blood count (CBC; a test to look at blood cell counts), erythrocyte sedimentation rate (ESR; a measure of proteins that correlates with inflammation), and C-reactive protein (CRP; a measure of acute inflammation). For example, in an infectious process like an intra-abdominal abscess or in an inflammatory process like inflammatory bowel disease (IBD), the CBC would have a high white blood cell count, an elevated CRP, and an elevated ESR value. A basic metabolic panel (BMP; assesses basic metabolic function, e.g., glucose, calcium, sodium, potassium, chloride), magnesium, phosphorus, or lipase may be sent to evaluate for electrolyte abnormalities, kidney dysfunction, or pancreatitis that could contribute to vomiting or nausea. Celiac disease is a common chronic autoimmune condition that presents with a variety of GI symptoms caused by intestinal damage triggered by gluten [3, 4]. Providers may screen for this disease with celiac antibody testing (tissue transglutaminase (TTG) IgA/total IgA or celiac antibody panel) [3, 4]. For this test to be accurate, youth are required to eat at least one gluten-containing meal daily (e.g., a slice of bread) for at least 1 month prior to obtaining the test to reduce the risk of false negative results. Common clinical symptoms and associated testing are highlighted in Table 4.1.

Table 4.1 Common indications for laboratory testing

Clinical indications	*Blood tests*	*Stool tests*	*Breath tests*
Diarrhea, bloody stool, abdominal pain, weight loss	CBC, ESR, CRP, TTG IgA (celiac screen)	Fecal calprotectin, fecal alpha-1-antitrypsin, stool-reducing substances, fecal fat, stool bacterial cultures, stool ova, and parasite cultures	N/a
Bloating, nausea, vomiting, abdominal pain, flatulence, +/−diarrhea	BMP, magnesium, phosphorus, lipase	*H. pylori* stool antigen	*H. pylori* (urease) Hydrogen/methane lactose

Stool tests

Stool samples may be collected to evaluate for infection, malabsorption, or markers of intestinal inflammation. A spontaneous bowel movement during the clinic visit is usually unlikely due to time constraints and perceived pressure by the youth to stool outside of the home environment. Therefore, the provider will typically provide a stool kit including a stool hat, gloves, stick, and stool specimen container for collection to be done at home. A stool hat is placed into the toilet so that toilet-trained children can sit on the toilet and stool directly into the hat. The hat can then be removed and two to three spoonfuls of stool can be transported with a provided stick into a small stool specimen container. If the child is not yet toilet trained, the parent can collect the sample from the diaper or pull-up. The stool should ideally be brought into the laboratory within a 24-hour period, but if this does not align with the parent's schedule, then the sample can be stored in a plastic bag and refrigerated for up to 72 hours before being brought into the laboratory.

Common stool studies to evaluate for infection include a *Helicobacter pylori* (*H. pylori*) stool antigen test which detects a special bacteria that can cause stomach and duodenal intestinal damage due to inflammation [5]. An *H. pylori* stool antigen test is often used in settings where alternative modes of *H. pylori* testing such as the *H. pylori* breath test are not available. *H. pylori* stool antigen tests are the preferred screening test for *H. pylori* evaluation in youth with neurodevelopmental delay, autism, or toddlers as it does not require physical cooperation. In adults, *H. pylori* infection can cause stomach ulcerations and even stomach cancer [5]. However, youth rarely have these complications and can often have the bacteria present asymptomatically [5]. Recent studies have recommended against the treatment of *H. pylori* when present in youth with DGBI as it is typically unlikely the cause of the recurrent GI symptoms [5]. Viral, bacterial, or parasitic infections in the colon can cause abdominal pain and diarrhea. Parasitic infections are common in 50–60% of youth in the developing world. Therefore, depending on the provider's location and the youth's history, this may be investigated with a viral stool PCR test, stool culture, and stool ova and parasite test [6]. Generalized inflammation within the intestinal tract can be assessed with a fecal calprotectin test and may be sent if there is a high suspicion of IBD [7]. Common symptoms and associated testing are highlighted in Table 4.1.

If diarrheal illness is present with clinical symptoms of ongoing weight loss with no infectious or inflammatory findings, the provider may send stool tests to evaluate for poor intestinal absorption of fat, protein, or sugar utilizing stool samples. A quantitative fecal fat test is a stool test that is collected over a 72-hour period with an associated diary to track fat intake [8]. Parents will typically be asked to monitor the fat content by grams in each meal that the child is consuming for breakfast, lunch, dinner, and snacks within that 72-hour time period that the stool is being collected at home. A large amount of fat in the stool sample would inform providers that there is evidence of pancreas dysfunction as the pancreas helps to produce enzymes that break down fat. A fecal alpha-1 antitrypsin test is a stool test that can be collected to determine if there is protein loss in the stool rather than the normal reabsorption of protein that the body uses [8]. Losing protein in the stool may be a marker of intestinal damage as the intestines should not leak large amounts of protein into a stool sample. A stool-reducing substance test can determine if there are abnormalities in the enzymes that break down sugar for intestinal absorption [8].

Breath tests

A breath test can be utilized to evaluate for common causes of abdominal pain, bloating, flatulence, diarrhea, and early fullness, such as lactose intolerance, small intestinal bacterial overgrowth, and *H. pylori*. Prior to the breath test, youth may be asked to eliminate certain starches and carbohydrates from their diet. Instructions are given to fast 8–12 hours prior to testing. Non-adherence to fasting instructions will invalidate the breath test [9].

A breath test is a test in which the youth drinks a solution containing a common sugar such as lactose or sucrose [9]. After the youth drinks the solution, they are expected to blow air for a few seconds into a device that measures the quantity of gas produced (usually hydrogen) by digestion of the sugar (see Figure 4.1). A high quantity of gas suggests that the youth is not able

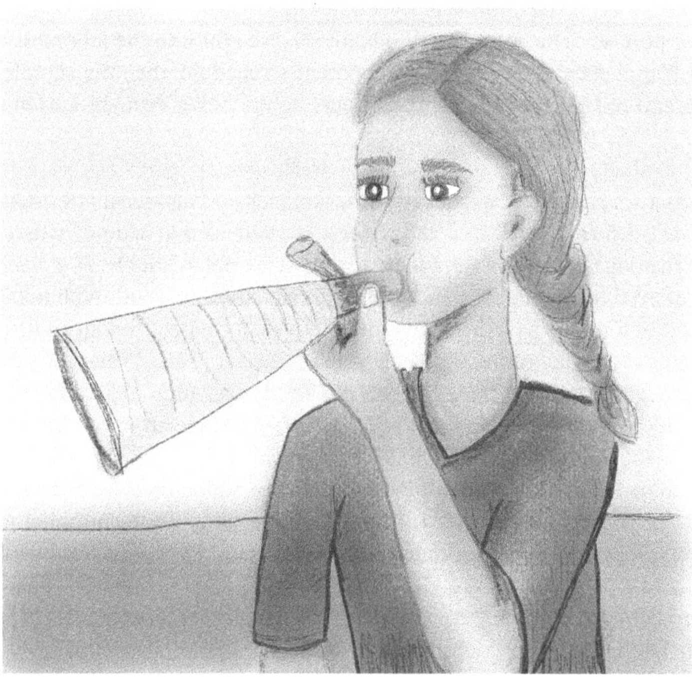

Figure 4.1 Child performing breath test (Source: Authors).

to digest that sugar appropriately. A breath test can also be used to assess for small intestine bacterial overgrowth. Our intestines have a normal concentration of bacterial flora; however, an overgrowth of certain bacteria in the small intestine can lead to clinical symptoms. After drinking the solution, the amount of hydrogen or methane exhaled in the breath can determine if there is bacterial overgrowth present in the small intestine [9]. A urease breath test is another noninvasive way to evaluate for *H. pylori* in youth 6–17 years old that are able to cooperate with the breath test method [9].

Imaging

Radiology studies are noninvasive tests used to look for structural, anatomical, or motility-associated GI disorders. These studies include abdominal X-ray, upper GI X-ray series, gastric emptying, and barium swallow studies. Abdominal X-ray is common in most countries, but more advanced imaging such as magnetic resonance abdominal imaging and computed tomography may be limited based on the availability of radiological equipment and radiology specialists at certain facilities. Families may often be concerned that exposure to ionizing radiation from X-ray studies can lead to increased risks of cancer. However, the risk of cancer from a single X-ray is low [10]. On average, an abdominal X-ray is about ~0.1 millisievert (mSv) and natural radiation exposure from day-to-day living is about 3 mSv per year. In females who are pregnant, there is a potential risk of teratogenic effects on the fetus and radiation should be minimized in this population [10]. A brief overview of the most common imaging modalities ordered by pediatric gastroenterologists for initial work-up of common GI symptoms is provided in Table 4.2.

Table 4.2 Summary of common imaging descriptions

Type of image	*Study time*	*Image description*	*Common indications*
Abdominal X-ray	15 minutes	Stationary image of the abdominal organs	Constipation, abdominal pain, abdominal distention, vomiting
Upper GI X-ray series	30 minutes if upper GI tract alone; 2–6 hours with upper GI tract with full small bowel analysis	Serial images showing the motion contrast moving through the GI tract	Reflux, vomiting, abdominal pain, prior surgical history, diarrhea
Gastric emptying study	4.5–5 hours	Imaging showing how fast radioactive isotope food empties from the stomach to the intestine	Early sensation of fullness, vomiting, nausea, abdominal pain

Abdominal X-ray

An abdominal X-ray is a common imaging study that a provider may use to evaluate the general anatomy of the bones, stomach, liver, and small and large intestines for possible causes of abdominal pain. An abdominal X-ray is a painless, non-invasive test that usually takes approximately 15 minutes to complete. There is no fasting needed prior to this exam. The study is performed while the youth is either standing or sitting. During the abdominal X-ray, youth are expected to stand still or lay flat on a board while the technician captures the X-ray image. Families should anticipate that the image may need to be taken more than once if the image is blurry or if there is movement while the X-ray film is being captured.

Upper GI X-ray

An upper GI X-ray series assesses the upper GI tract including the esophagus, stomach, and the first portion of the small intestine [11]. A barium swallow is a similar study to an upper GI X-ray used to evaluate active swallowing and the structure of the esophagus. These studies are completed within approximately 30 minutes to 1 hour and are often used for youth with recurrent vomiting, choking, poor feeding, abdominal pain, weight loss, or reflux. These studies utilize a special type of X-ray called fluoroscopy which allows the provider to assess the structure of the upper GI tract and/or esophagus in real time while it is in motion [11]. This differs from an abdominal X-ray which shows a stationary image of the GI structures including the lower GI tract. There is an expectation to fast the night before the procedure to ensure the procedure is completed on an empty stomach. If the child is developmentally able to follow commands, they will be instructed to drink approximately 1.5 cups of barium contrast, which will coat the inside of the GI tract for better visualization of its motion and structure ([11]; see Figure 4.2).

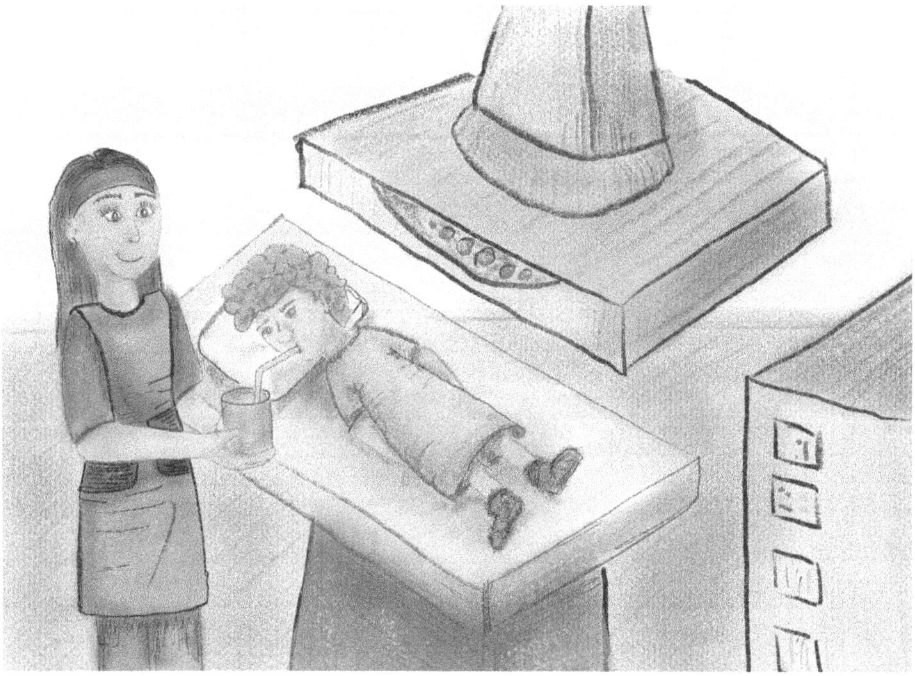

Figure 4.2 Child on tilt table drinking contrast for upper GI X-ray (Source: Authors).

To evaluate the structures of the entire small intestine, this test can be extended by 2–6 hours to monitor the contrast as it moves through the lower portions of the small intestines as well. If following commands are not possible, then a nasogastric tube (NG) will be temporarily placed through the nose down the throat into the stomach to administer the contrast. The NG will then quickly be removed after the barium is administered. The NG should not cause pain but may cause mild discomfort or a sensation that there is an object in the throat. There should not be difficulty breathing or choking with NG placement although this is a common concern of families. Youth may often find the barium to have a chalky thick texture despite the ability to add flavors to the contrast [11]. Youth may also feel pressure from the X-ray machine on the abdomen during the study. Youth are asked to lie down on a table that will be tilted during the study to capture images of the contrast coating the tract. It is possible that additional barium will need to be ingested throughout the study. After drinking barium contrast, youth may experience constipation followed by stools that have a gray or white color up to 72 hours after the study.

Gastric emptying studies

A gastric emptying study may be considered to evaluate youth who have persistent nausea, early sensation of fullness after meals, vomiting, and abdominal pain. Gastric emptying studies are X-ray studies that track whether the stomach is able to empty food within a normal time frame [12]. This study is used to determine if there are gastric motility anomalies. The gastric emptying study lasts for about 4.5–5 hours. Fasting is expected 8–12 hours prior to the study. A small 4 oz. meal of radioactive isotope scrambled eggs (or oatmeal if there is a known egg allergy) will be ingested to allow the food in the stomach to be seen on imaging [12]. The isotope should not change the taste of the eggs or oatmeal. X-rays will be taken on a strictly timed schedule immediately after, 1 hour after, 2 hours after, and finally 4 hours after eating. A study may be determined inconclusive if the youth is not able to complete the study. Delayed gastric emptying is diagnosed when greater than 60% of the meal is present at 2 hours, or greater than 10% of the meal present at 4 hours [12]. Although there have been consensus guidelines published in 2008 to standardize the protocol for gastric emptying studies, there are a variety of protocols between institutions [12].

Motility and pH testing

The GI tract utilizes a combination of relaxation and contractility throughout the esophagus, stomach, and small and large intestines to move food and subsequently stool through the tract effectively. Ineffective coordination of the muscles to relax or contract is called dysmotility. Manometry studies are minimally invasive studies utilized to evaluate the coordination of the muscles and sphincters within the GI tract. Accessibility to manometry testing is not readily available at every center or institution.

Esophageal manometry

Some diseases that occur in pediatrics due to esophageal dysmotility include reflux, achalasia, hypercontractile esophagus, and esophageal spasm. Esophageal manometry is used to evaluate esophageal motility by evaluating esophageal function and measuring the pressures of the esophageal sphincters and muscles [13]. The provider must have a high suspicion of disordered swallowing prior to ordering this test. Fasting is expected 8–12 hours prior to the test. To provide comfort for the youth, a numbing spray may be applied to the nose or back of the throat prior to starting the study. A catheter (tube) about 4 mm in diameter is then placed through the nose and esophagus with the end of the catheter ending in the stomach [13, 14]. Youth may be asked to swallow several times to mobilize the probe across the lower esophageal sphincter into the stomach. During the test, youth are expected to drink liquid (small sips at spaced intervals, multiple rapid swallows, or a rapid drink challenge) and may be expected to eat a solid snack to measure the function of the esophagus in the active swallowing state [13, 14]. Youth may have symptoms of sore throat, congestion, or mild nosebleed after the procedure is completed. This study is typically completed on youth who are able to follow commands.

Antroduodenal manometry

Common indications to pursue antroduodenal manometry in youth include suspicion for small intestinal pseudo-obstruction, unexplained abdominal pain, nausea/vomiting with feeding intolerance, or if a diffuse GI motility disorder is being evaluated. Common symptoms that prompt providers to consider testing include bloating, abdominal pain, nausea, vomiting, or diarrhea. Antroduodenal manometry is used to measure the movement of the stomach and the first portion of the small intestine. The test measures pressures with a catheter in both the fasting state and after eating a meal [15]. The catheter can be placed through the nose or G-tube using real-time X-ray guidance via fluoroscopy or it can be placed using an endoscope. Typically, catheter placement requires general anesthesia sedation; therefore, fasting is required prior to the procedure. The catheter will evaluate the pressures in the fasting state for about 4 hours followed by a meal with further evaluation 2 hours after eating [15]. Medications such as erythromycin (a promotility agent) may be given during the evaluation to determine if the medication can induce contraction of the stomach. Symptoms throughout the study will also be recorded to aid in interpreting the movement of the GI tract. Depending on the catheter type, the study may record for 6–24 hours [15]. The child or adolescent is expected to stay in bed until the completion of the study; therefore, they are not allowed to get up to use the toilet, walk around the room, or stand up during the study. The catheter may cause mild discomfort but does not typically cause pain. This study is often reserved for youth who are at least >10 kg due to the size of the catheter.

Colonic manometry

Colonic manometry can be considered to evaluate the colon's relaxation and contractility. This may be considered in youth with recurrent constipation or refractory constipation. Prior to placing the colonic catheter, a bowel clean-out will have to be completed. This means that a laxative solution is ingested or given through a nasogastric tube until the colon is clear of any stool; therefore, this test may require admission to the hospital 24 hours before the placement. The catheter is then placed using a colonoscope through the anus while the youth is under sedation. The position of the catheter is then verified with an X-ray. Information is usually recorded over a 6-hour period and the youth/family records the symptoms to help the provider interpret changes seen in the study [16]. Medications such as bisacodyl (a pro-contractile medication) may be given to stimulate the bowel and can cause mild abdominal cramping [16]. The catheter is removed by a technician by slowly tugging at the tube until it is out. All age groups are eligible for colonic manometry.

Anorectal manometry

Anorectal manometry is considered for symptoms of constipation. This is a shorter study than colonic manometry as it only evaluates the anal and rectal muscle coordination [17]. The test can be done with or without sedation based on the discretion of the provider and the neurodevelopmental stage of the child. Prior to testing, an enema is given about 1–2 hours prior to the test to clear stool from the anorectal canal. While lying on the side, a lubricated catheter tip is placed inside the anus. Typically, youth 6 years or older can follow instructions from a technician to perform a series of tasks including squeezing the anus, relaxing the anus, attempting to generate a push, and notifying the technician when they feel an urge to stool [17]. As the tasks are being performed, pressures are being measured to determine if there is appropriate coordination to generate a normal bowel movement [17]. Infants and youth 0–6 years old can still have the test performed but only limited information about the involuntary relaxation of the anal sphincter can be collected as they typically cannot follow commands. Therefore, this test may not be offered routinely to youth less than 6 years old. The procedure should not cause pain, but the test often varies in length to completion (30 minutes or more) based on adherence to tasks and the preciseness of pressures being evaluated on the machine. There are minor risks associated with this procedure including bleeding and irritation.

pH/impedance monitoring

pH (acid) monitoring can be coordinated to evaluate the amount of acid exposure present in the esophagus. This study is used to indicate whether acid reflux is present when there are symptoms of heartburn. Although acid reflux is common worldwide, pH monitoring is not always indicated in all clinical presentations of reflux and is up to the discretion of the clinical provider. pH monitoring is often considered in youth that are refractory to medical treatment or at risk of recurrent inflammatory changes to the esophagus. A small 2 mm-diameter tube is placed through the nose into the esophagus. The tube has sensors to detect the level of acidity between the lower end of the esophagus and the stomach. Some probes also have impedance markers throughout the tube that make it possible to evaluate non-acid reflux which is an important cause of symptoms in pediatrics. These sensors are also helpful in evaluating the extent of reflux and air transit (aerophagia and belching). The probe is left in place for about 24 hours and a diary log is given to the youth/family to record when symptoms occur in relation to activities of daily living. All acid suppression medications such as proton-pump inhibitors and H_2 antagonists are usually discontinued at least 5 days prior to the study to reduce false negative results of the testing. There are minor risks of pH probe placement including nosebleeds, congestion, and sore throat. Probe positioning needs to be confirmed with an X-ray. Families are often discharged home to complete the 24-hour test.

EndoFLIP (endoluminal functional lumen imaging probe)

EndoFLIP can be considered for difficulty swallowing, vomiting, or complications after upper GI tract surgical interventions. EndoFLIP may also be used when imaging and manometry have discordant findings to add supplemental information to these tests. EndoFLIP is a catheter with a balloon that contains 16 impedance markers and one pressure sensor [18]. The balloon is inflated typically in the esophagus across the esophago-gastric junction or at the end of the stomach (pylorus) to evaluate the ability of the tissue to stretch and accommodate the balloon [18]. This procedure creates a three-dimensional image showing the pressure, diameter, and volume of the esophagus or pylorus [18]. EndoFLIP is coordinated with upper endoscopy under sedation, which is advantageous as there is no need for immobilization by the parent or pressure to follow commands. There are minor symptoms after EndoFLIP including possible sore throat, but there should not be pain (see Table 4.3 for common motility testing indications).

Table 4.3 Common motility testing indications

Type of testing	*Time*	*Description of test*	*Common clinical indications*
pH probe/impedance probe	24 hours	Evaluation of liquid and gas in the esophagus as well as acid content	Reflux, heartburn, regurgitation, difficulty swallowing, feeding intolerance, poor weight gain, belching disorders
Esophageal manometry	30 minutes	Measures muscle/sphincter coordination of the esophagus	Difficulty swallowing, choking, recurrent lodging of food in esophagus, reflux, feeding intolerance
EndoFLIP	30 minutes	Three-dimensional study to measure the stiffness pressure, and volumes of the esophagus and pylorus	Difficulty swallowing, choking, recurrent lodging of food in the esophagus, vomiting, heartburn, abdominal pain, symptoms after surgeries of the upper GI tract
Antroduodenal manometry	6–24 hours	Measures muscle contraction/relaxation and sphincter coordination of the stomach and first portion of the small intestine	Abdominal pain, vomiting, nausea, weight loss, feeding intolerance
Colonic manometry	6–24 hours	Measures muscle contraction and relaxation of the colon	Abdominal pain, chronic constipation
Anorectal manometry	30 minutes or more	Measures the muscle relaxation, coordination, and generation of push of the rectum and anus	Constipation

Endoscopy

Endoscopic procedures are commonly used to investigate visual and microscopic changes to the tissue within the GI tract that could be diagnostic of an ongoing disease process. Both upper endoscopy and colonoscopy in infants, children, and adolescents are done under sedation to improve diagnostic outcomes for the child. Youth are required to fast 8–12 hours prior to the procedure to reduce the risk of undigested food entering the airway during the procedure. In the United States, youth may be intubated to reduce the risk of aspiration (food getting into the windpipe) and protect the airway. In preparation for a colonoscope, a bowel clean-out must be completed with the ingestion of laxatives. Youth may have symptoms of nausea, bloating, or vomiting during bowel preparation due to the volume of laxatives recommended for ingestion. The bowel regimen should be completed despite these symptoms. A complete bowel preparation is needed to clearly visualize the colon for an accurate diagnosis and reduce the risk of complications.

Endoscopes are tube-like structures with a camera at the end that can capture pictures of the inside of the GI tract (see Figure 4.3). These pictures can then be reviewed with the family at the end of the procedure. Small pieces of tissue (biopsies) are collected during endoscopy to evaluate for areas of inflammation, structural changes, or infection under a microscope (these biopsies are not painful). An upper endoscope is placed through the mouth to evaluate the esophagus, stomach, and small intestine. The colonoscope is placed through the anus to evaluate the colon and the last portion of the small intestine. Capsule endoscopy, which is a camera in the shape

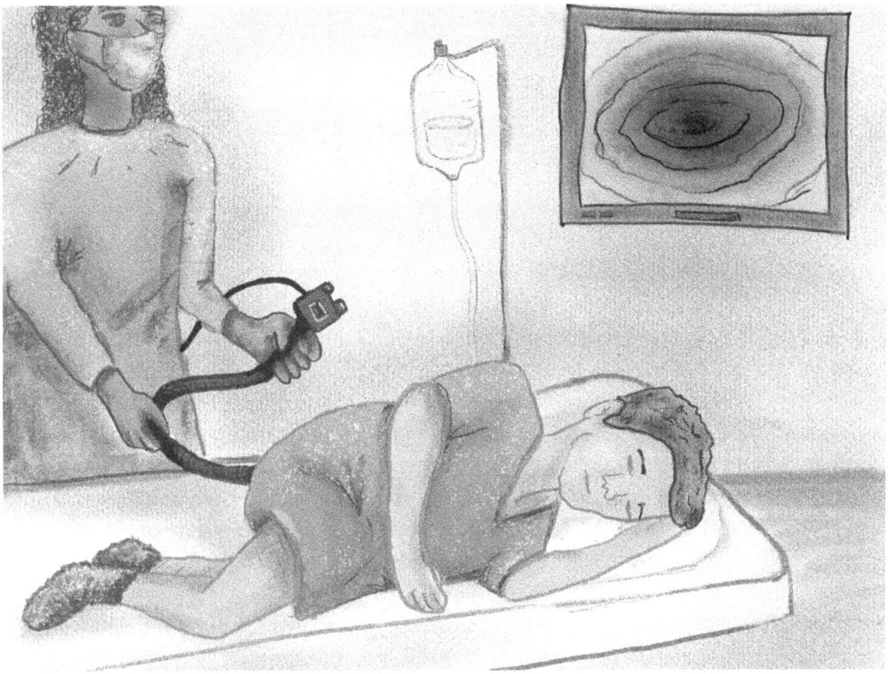

Figure 4.3 Child receiving colonoscopy (Source: Authors).

of a plastic pill, can be swallowed or endoscopically placed if not able to swallow the capsule to evaluate the deeper portions of the small bowel that cannot be reached with traditional endoscopes. Deep enteroscopy is another method (a normal endoscope with an overtube attached) to help the provider maneuver further into the small bowel. It is important to note that capsule endoscopy or deep enteroscopy may not be readily available in a variety of centers worldwide.

Families are often concerned that endoscopy is an invasive procedure with similar risks to surgery. However, both upper endoscopy and colonoscopy are tolerated well and safe. Based on adult data, there is a small risk of bleeding (0.1–0.6%), perforation (<0.04% for upper endoscopy; 1:1,000 for colonoscopy), and death (0.007%) [19]. Other potential risks include infection, general injury (tooth loss), and post-anesthesia complications [19]. Capsule endoscopy has a potential risk of obstructing the bowel from capsule retention within the bowel (1.2-2.6%) [20]. Youth may experience sore throat, and flatulence within the day after the procedure as carbon dioxide air is used to inflate the GI tract for better visualization during the procedure. These symptoms should not persist for longer than 24 hours. Capsule endoscopy is contraindicated if there is concern for a known blockage or stricture within the bowel.

The harms of overtesting

Clinical judgment by the provider's expertise remains at the forefront of determining diagnoses for GI disorders within pediatrics. Numerous guidelines, consensus statements, and protocols can guide a physician in determining what organic or structural GI disorders should be evaluated prior to diagnosing youth with a DGBI [21]. This is important to consider as organic and structural GI diseases can coexist with DGBI. However, the Rome IV criteria, which provides guidelines for the diagnosis of DGBI, allows providers to use clinical discretion rather than strict exclusion of organic GI disorders with testing prior to diagnosing DGBI [21].

Testing to investigate clinically insignificant diagnoses without clear health outcome benefits can be harmful to youth [22]. Potential harms of overtesting when not indicated include false positives or false negatives on blood, stool, or imaging tests which can lead to misdiagnosis or a false label of having a disease process for which the youth does not in fact exhibit symptoms [22]. For example, *H. pylori* can be incidentally found in youth who are asymptomatic due to bacterial colonization of the stomach. However, these youth are often asymptomatic without evidence of gastritis. Labeling youth with *H. pylori* infection when not indicated could lead to prolonged antibiotic and acid suppression courses that ultimately will lead to long-term side effects [4].

Unnecessary investigations can lead to increased physical, psychological, and financial strain on families. Testing with no clinical indication with specialized studies prevents accessibility to other youth that may need more timely access to these studies [22]. Studies consistently show that youth with anxiety are more likely to request further testing when not indicated [23]. This may ultimately put strain on the doctor–patient relationship. Especially when a DGBI is the most appropriate diagnosis for the presenting symptoms, youth and families may experience difficulty accepting the diagnosis due to a lack of positive imaging and testing findings. Difficulty accepting an appropriate diagnosis does not in and of itself provide necessary justification for further testing for the reasons discussed above. Partnership between GI mental health professionals and pediatric gastroenterologists can aid in guiding youth through these complex diagnoses and the challenges associated with diagnosis acceptance.

Pearls of wisdom

- A detailed clinical history and medical examination are enough to diagnose DGBI. Diagnostic tests can sometimes be useful in ruling out GI or systemic disorders but may not be indicated once organic structural GI and systemic disorders are ruled out.
- Diagnostic testing when not indicated does not improve clinical decision-making or health outcomes for youth.
- Mental health professionals can partner with providers to reduce fears surrounding the need for more testing when a diagnosis of functional GI disorder is determined.

Summary

There are several modalities available to evaluate youth that present with common GI symptoms. Testing with blood, stool, breath, and imaging studies can provide further information to the gastroenterologist about the type of disorder that needs to be managed. Minimally invasive procedures such as manometry testing and endoscopy may be needed to get a better idea of the movement and architecture of the GI tract, respectively. A detailed clinical history by the gastroenterologist can diagnose a variety of disease processes without advanced studies (especially in regions where access to certain studies is limited). If studies are indicated, there are minimal risks associated with procedures commonly used in gastroenterology evaluation. Mental health professionals can partner with providers to reduce fears associated with testing (see Chapter 5). However, the harm of overtesting for GI symptoms should be considered strongly by all youth due to the risk of financial, emotional, and physiological distress to the child and family.

Recommended readings

For youth and caregivers:

- McKenzie, A. (2014) *Everybody Stay Calm: How to Support Your Young Child Through Medical Tests and Procedures*. Global Publishing Group.
- Meg Foundation (2022). *Procedural Pain Resources*: https://www.megfoundationforpain.org/resources/?_type_of_pain=procedural-pain.

For mental health professionals:

- Lang E.V., Viegas J., Bleeker C., Bruhn J., & Geert-Jan van, G. (2017) Helping children cope with medical tests and interventions. *Journal of Radiology Nursing 36*(1):44–50.
- Lamparyk, K. et al. (2019). Effects of psychological preparation intervention on anxiety associated with anorectal manometry. *International Journal of Pediatrics, 2019*, 7569194.

References

1. McFerron BA, Waseem S. Chronic recurrent abdominal pain. *Pediatr Rev.* 2012;33(11):509–17.
2. World Health Organization. *WHO guidelines on drawing blood: Best practices in phlebotomy*. Geneva, Switzerland: World Health Organization; 2010.
3. Popp A, Mäki M. Changing pattern of childhood celiac disease epidemiology: Contributing factors. *Front Pediatr.* 2019;7:357.
4. Sahin Y. Celiac disease in children: A review of the literature. *World J Clin Pediatr*. 2021;10(4):53.
5. Jones NL, Koletzko S, Goodman K, Bontems P, Cadranel S, Casswall T, et al. Joint ESPGHAN/NASPGHAN guidelines for the management of *Helicobacter pylori* in children and adolescents (update 2016). *J Pediatr Gastroenterol Nutr.* 2017;64(6):991–1003.
6. Haque R. Human intestinal parasites. *J Health Popul Nutr*. 2007;25(4):387–91.
7. Ng SC, Shi HY, Hamidi N, Underwood FE, Tang W, Benchimol EI, et al. Worldwide incidence and prevalence of inflammatory bowel disease in the 21st century: A systematic review of population-based studies. *The Lancet*. 2017;390(10114):2769–78.
8. Hammer HF. Management of chronic diarrhea in primary care: The gastroenterologists' advice. *Digestive Diseases*. 2021;39(6):615–21.
9. Saad RJ, Chey WD. Breath tests for gastrointestinal disease: The real deal or just a lot of hot air? *Gastroenterology*. 2007;133(6):1763–6.
10. Lin EC. Radiation risk from medical imaging. *Mayo Clin Proc*. 2010;85(12):1142–6.
11. Revels JW, Moran SK, O'Malley R, Mansoori B, Revzin MV, Katz DS, et al. Upper gastrointestinal fluoroscopic examination: A traditional art enduring into the 21st century. *RadioGraphics*. 2022;42(5):E152–E3.
12. Farrell MB. Gastric emptying scintigraphy. *J Nucl Med Technol.* 2019;47(2):111–9.
13. Goyal M, Nagalli S. *Esophageal motility disorders. StatPearls [Internet]*. Treasure Island (FL): StatPearls Publishing; 2021.
14. Wang A, Pleskow DK, Banerjee S, Barth BA, Bhat YM, Desilets DJ, et al. Esophageal function testing. *Gastrointestinal Endosc*. 2012;76(2):231–43.
15. Patcharatrakul T, Gonlachanvit S. Technique of functional and motility test: How to perform antroduodenal manometry. *J Neurogastroenterol Motil*. 2013;19(3):395.
16. Lee YY, Erdogan A, Rao SS. How to perform and assess colonic manometry and barostat study in chronic constipation. *J Neurogastroenterol Motil*. 2014;20(4):547.
17. Lee TH, Bharucha AE. How to perform and interpret a high-resolution anorectal manometry test. *J Neurogastroenterol Motil*. 2016;22(1):46.

18. Donnan EN, Pandolfino JE. EndoFLIP in the esophagus: Assessing sphincter function, wall stiffness, and motility to guide treatment. *Gastroenterol Clin.* 2020;49(3):427–35.
19. Fisher DA, Maple JT, Ben-Menachem T, Cash BD, Decker GA, Early DS, et al. Complications of colonoscopy. *Gastrointestinal Endosc.* 2011;74(4):745–52.
20. Liao Z, Gao R, Xu C, Li Z-S. Indications and detection, completion, and retention rates of small-bowel capsule endoscopy: A systematic review. *Gastrointestinal Endosc.* 2010;71(2):280–6.
21. Hyams JS, Di Lorenzo C, Saps M, Shulman RJ, Staiano A, van Tilburg M. Childhood functional gastrointestinal disorders: Child/adolescent. *Gastroenterology.* 2016;150(6):1456–68. e2.
22. Lam JH, Pickles K, Stanaway FF, Bell KJ. Why clinicians overtest: Development of a thematic framework. *BMC Health Serv Res.* 2020;20(1):1–11.
23. van der Weijden T, van Bokhoven MA, Dinant G-J, van Hasselt CM, Grol RP. Understanding laboratory testing in diagnostic uncertainty: A qualitative study in general practice. *Br J Gen Pract.* 2002;52(485):974–80.

Chapter 5

Helping youth manage medical procedures

Delane Linkiewich, Olivia Dobson, and C. Meghan McMurtry

Chapter aims

This chapter provides an overview of the pain and fear that can be experienced related to medical procedures encountered in gastrointestinal (GI) care for pediatric populations followed by evidence-based strategies to reduce pain and fear.

Learning points

- The bidirectional relationship between pain and fear and the importance of assessing and managing both.
- Practical, evidence-based strategies to help youth (3–18 years old) cope with medical procedures.
- The important role that GI mental health professionals, other health professionals, and caregivers play in managing youths' procedural pain and fear.

Background

Medical procedures are common throughout childhood and are important for the prevention, diagnosis, measurement, and treatment of diseases, injuries, and health conditions. In addition to routine procedures, such as immunizations, youth living with GI conditions commonly undergo other medical procedures including venipunctures for blood tests, intravenous (IV) insertion to deliver analgesia, and endoscopies (see Chapter 4). Before, during, and after these procedures, youth often experience pain and fear (i.e., the feeling of being afraid or scared due to an alarm reaction in response to a perceived threat). While there are evidence-based strategies for managing pain in youth (see Handout 5.1), their pain frequently remains undertreated [1].

Acute and chronic pain

Pain is both an unpleasant sensory and emotional experience and is related to actual or potential tissue damage [2]. The two broad types of pain are acute pain, which is pain that lasts for <3 months (e.g., postoperative pain), and chronic pain, which is pain that lasts ≥3 months (e.g., chronic abdominal pain). Recurrent and/or chronic pain are common symptoms within GI conditions (e.g., Crohn's disease). Thus, when youth undergo painful medical procedures as part of their GI care, they may be experiencing acute pain in addition to chronic pain; this has relevance to how mental health professionals conceptualize their experience and improve their comfort.

DOI: 10.4324/9781003308683-6

Procedural pain and fear

Medical procedures, particularly those involving needles, are a source of fear and anxiety for many youth. Fear is a normative, present-oriented alarm reaction that is experienced when one is threatened (e.g., fear during needle insertion). Anxiety is future-oriented distress, such as worrying about an EndoFLIP scheduled in 3 days. Shaped through direct experience, information provided by others, and vicarious learning, threat, and trauma are subjective: what matters most is the youth's experience or expectations regarding their medical procedure, not how objectively invasive the procedure is to others. Consider a 5-year-old undergoing their first endoscopy and how the "medically routine" procedure would be far from their usual experience and frightening. Fear and pain often exacerbate each other such that when one experiences pain it can increase fear and vice versa; yet different interventions may be needed to appropriately address fear vs. pain. Specifically, for youth with high levels of medical-related fear or phobia, exposure-based interventions, facilitated by a GI mental health professional, are recommended (see Handout 5.2). Fear left unmanaged can interfere with the effectiveness of the strategies described below.

When pain and distress related to a medical procedure are not adequately managed, there are short- and long-term consequences. For the immediate procedure, negative sequelae include longer procedure times, risk of fainting and/or injury, use of restraint, and increased distress of everyone involved (youth, caregiver, health professional). Consequences for future procedures can include increased anxiety, increased need for analgesics, avoidance of the specific procedure, or generalized avoidance of healthcare, which can have catastrophic effects on youths' health. Thus, when caring for youth with GI conditions, it is critical to understand and manage their pain and fear related to medical procedures since they will repeatedly encounter them, and their negative experiences can become exponentially negative over time.

In addition to showing this longitudinal trajectory throughout childhood, Figure 5.1 shows that caregivers were once youths themselves. The social context of these medical procedures is paramount: caregivers who have had negative procedural experiences or caregivers who are highly anxious for other reasons may need additional support to effectively help their youth cope. These caregivers may benefit from skills training in deep breathing, mindfulness, guided imagery, and cognitive restructuring.

Assessment of pain and fear

Assessing youths' pain and fear, in a developmentally appropriate way, is essential to understanding their procedural experience and providing appropriate intervention. Health professionals should assess youths' pain and fear as part of usual care and GI mental health professionals can advocate for the use of these tools (see Table 5.1).

Strategies for coping with medical procedures and GI mental health professionals' roles (education, implementation, and advocacy)

Process/preparatory, physical, psychological, and pharmacological strategies should be used to reduce youths' procedure-related pain and fear (see Handout 5.1). These strategies are understood from a biopsychosocial perspective in that they all interact and may cut across the

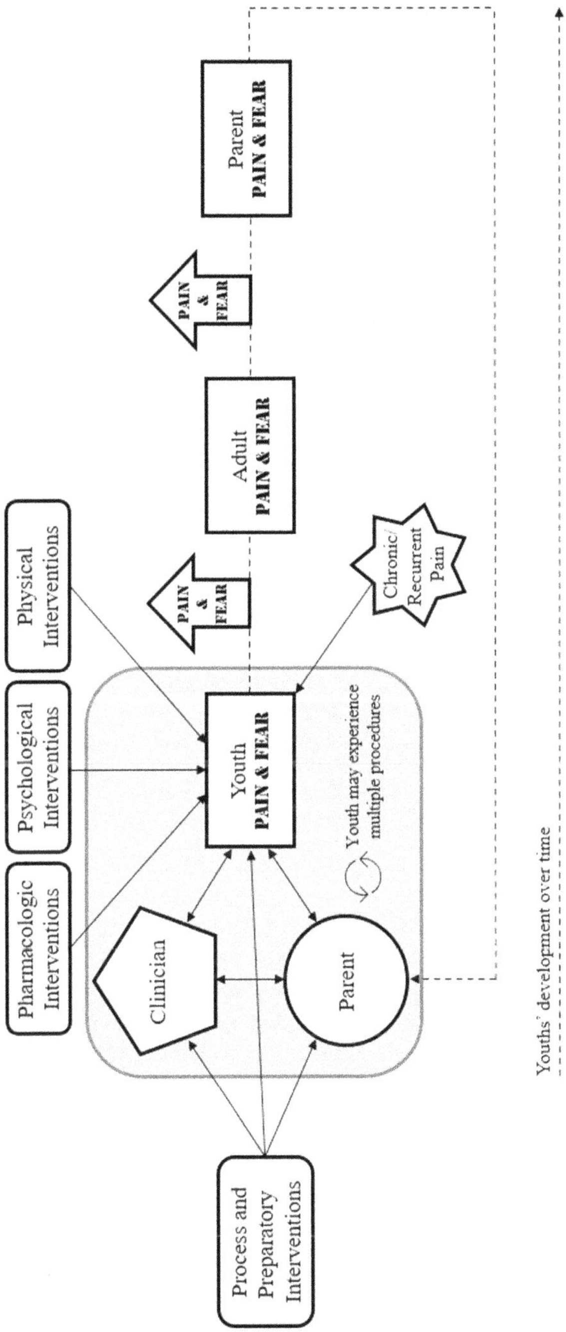

Figure 5.1 A longitudinal view of medical procedures. (Source: Adapted from McMurtry et al. [3]).

Table 5.1 Assessment of pain and fear (all measures are freely accessible)

Measure	*Report type*	*Description*	*Age*
Numerical rating scale [4]	Self-report (SR) or observer report (OR)	One item presents a scale from 0 (no pain) to 10 (most severe pain) to measure pain intensity.	7+ years for SR; all caregivers for OR
The faces pain scale-revised [5]https://www.iasp-pain.org/resources/faces-pain-scale-revised/	SR or OR	One item presents six faces ranging from no pain (neutral) to very much pain to measure pain intensity.	5+ years; all caregivers for OR
Face, legs, activity, cry, and consolability scale [6, 7]	OR (behavioral observation of pain and distress)	Five items assess different pain behaviors (e.g., squirming) on a scale from 0 to 2 with a summed score of items ranging from 0 (relaxed and comfortable) to 10 (7–10 being severe pain, discomfort, or both).	All including those with cognitive impairments
Children's fear scale [8]https://pphc.uoguelph.ca/childrens-fear-scale/	SR, caregiver, and/or OR	One item presents five faces ranging from no fear (neutral) to extreme fear to measure fear during medical procedures.	5 years+ for SR; all caregivers for OR
Scary scale [9]	SR	One item presenting six faces ranging from no fear at all to very afraid to measure fear in hospital settings.	7–12 years

aforementioned categories. The CARD™ system (https://www.aboutkidshealth.ca/card) is a framework for delivering patient-centered care, which organizes these strategies; CARD™ was developed in the context of school-based immunizations but has successfully been used in other contexts and can be a helpful resource for caregivers.

These strategies should be bundled, taking a multi-method and developmentally appropriate approach, to optimize youths' comfort and experience. GI mental health professionals may be involved in the direct application of some strategies (e.g., hypnosis), preparing/training youth and caregivers in using strategies, and/or advocating for the use of all strategies listed below to help prevent negative medical experiences for youth. While Handout 5.1 outlines who is responsible for using each strategy, it is important for GI mental health professionals to be aware of all the strategies. Many of the recommendations below are informed by evidence for coping with pediatric needle-related pain and fear as this literature is well developed. Furthermore, needle procedures, like IV insertions, are often youths' largest fear related to GI procedures, such as endoscopies [10]. This chapter focuses on strategies that are suitable for youth aged 3–18 years old and are likely applicable to a variety of painful procedures, including GI procedures.

Process and preparatory strategies

Youth education

Providing youth, 3 years and older, with education about what to expect for their procedure can reduce anxiety, fear, and uncertainty and improve post-procedural outcomes [10–15]. The timing, content, and format (e.g., oral or written summaries, instructional videos (e.g., example instructional video from Children's Wisconsin: https://childrenswi.org/medical-care/gastroenterology-liver-and-nutrition-program/tests-and-treatments/endoscopy/endoscopy-videos), hospital tours, and role-play) of preparation should consider the youth's developmental level and learning needs [16]. Youth benefit from learning about why the procedure is necessary, the procedure itself (e.g., how long it will take), sensory information (e.g., how the procedure feels), and the medical tools used [13–15, 17]. Giving the youth new and potentially distressing information immediately before the procedure should be avoided. Preparatory information should be provided using neutral/non-emotive language [14, 16]. Youth should also learn about coping strategies, be offered choices to feel more in control (e.g., what toy to bring, to watch or look away), and create and practice positive self-statements (see Handout 5.3) [13–15, 18]. GI mental health professionals, caregivers, and other members of the care team can provide youth education/preparation; notably, youth may want a limited number of people to be aware of the GI procedure and therefore may want to keep discussions about their procedure private [18]. A child life specialist can assist in providing families with information beforehand and utilizing coping techniques on the day of the procedure [10].

Caregiver education

Caregivers should be informed about medical procedures as they are often the primary question-answerer and conveyer of information to their child. Thus, caregivers benefit from learning about what to expect, coping strategies, and helpful ways to communicate with their child (see Handout 5.3) [14, 15]. Caregivers who receive procedural information and education on coping skills prior to their child's medical procedure display more coping-promoting and fewer distress-promoting behaviors during their child's procedure [15]. While caregiver education can be provided on the day of the procedure, caregivers can be encouraged to contact the hospital/clinic beforehand since it is helpful to ask questions and gather information in order to plan [10]. GI mental health professionals can support caregivers in generating and rehearsing questions they or their child may have regarding the procedure (see Handout 5.4).

GI mental health professional education

GI mental health professionals should be knowledgeable about environmental, physical, psychological, and basic pharmacological pain management, as well as coping strategies to teach youth and their families. They can also advocate for, and support caregivers in advocating for, practices that support youth coping including the presence of a calm support person such as a caregiver [14, 15]. The physical environment is important to youth coping. Youth living with GI conditions may associate clinical settings with negative memories from past experiences.

Unnecessary cues and situations that can heighten distress should be avoided, including a lack of privacy, crowded waiting areas, prolonged standing, uncomfortable temperatures, and hearing others in distress [19–21]. Making the environment developmentally friendly, such as having colorful décor and art, toys available, and information at youths' eye level, may also help ease distress [15]. For toddlers and children, transporting them to the procedure in a fun form of transportation (e.g., toy car) could help reduce their anticipatory anxiety [22]. GI mental health professionals can also encourage families to prepare for making the environment as comfortable as possible for their child, such as bringing headphones to buffer anxiety-provoking noises or dressing the child in layers to adjust clothing for different temperatures.

Physical strategies

Positioning

Positioning can optimize the youth's comfort and sense of control [14, 15]. For example, during a needle procedure, sitting upright or on a caregiver's lap is suggested for youth 3 years and older [14, 15]. Restraining/holding the youth down should be avoided as it can increase the youth's fear and be traumatic [14, 15]. Caregivers might need further psychoeducation from GI mental health professionals about why restraint should be avoided. The "Buzzy" device combines physical strategies (external cold and vibration) with distraction and reduces needle-related pain and anxiety in youth [23, 24].

Muscle tension

For youth 7 years and older who are at risk of feeling dizzy or fainting during medical procedures, muscle tension techniques (i.e., repetitive tensing and releasing of muscle groups) can be helpful. Muscle tension techniques can be taught to youth and caregivers by GI mental health professionals and practiced prior to a procedure (see https://pphc.uoguelph.ca/needle-fear-resources/). Younger children may need coaching/prompting to use this strategy.

Psychological strategies

Procedure-related communication

Caregivers, GI mental health professionals, and other healthcare providers should avoid simplistic, uninformative, and/or repetitive reassurance, apologizing, false suggestion, and minimizing youths' feelings (see Handout 5.3 for examples) [14, 15]. GI mental health professionals can provide space for youth to express their feelings about their procedure and help them to develop positive self-coping statements to use during their procedure (see Handouts 5.1 and 5.3). Communication can also be used by members of the care team to prompt youths' use of coping strategies and positive self-statements.

Distraction

For youth of all ages, distraction should be used to reduce pain and distress by directing the youth's attention away from the pain and fear-inducing stimuli (e.g., needle) towards something more engaging or enjoyable [14, 15, 25]. Distraction may take place before (e.g., in the waiting room), during (if the youth is not currently sedated), or after the procedure. Distraction can take many forms and should be appropriate for the youth's age and preferences/interests. For example, verbal distraction is recommended for youth 3 years and older, such as talk unrelated to the procedure or jokes/humorous statements [14, 15]. Videos, toys, music, and squeezing a soft ball can also distract youth of all ages from a painful procedure [14, 26, 27] and has been shown to effectively reduce youths' pain during a colonoscopy [28]. Caregivers can be encouraged to bring preferred distraction items from home [10]. For neurodiverse or younger youth, caregivers may need to assist with selecting a distractor and facilitate the distraction, such as co-watching a video and making comments about it.

Hypnosis

Hypnosis is a strategy that can be administered by trained GI mental health professionals, which involves deep relaxation and imagery to alter youths' cognitive state to be more suggestible; for example, the "magic glove" technique [29] encourages youth to imagine that they are wearing a protective glove that reduces their pain sensitivity. Hypnosis can minimize both anticipatory anxiety and pain during the procedure [15, 25, 29], although evidence in GI procedures is sparse. One study found that hypnosis combined with other analgesic agents helped to facilitate endoscopy for children 6 years and older [30]. Youth can also be taught to use hypnotic imagery, such as imagining being in their favorite place, whereas older youth may wish to learn and use self-guided hypnotic approaches [21].

Memory reframing

Youth with GI challenges, especially if chronic, have likely built a repertoire of painful and distressing memories associated with their past symptoms and procedures. For example, a youth may recall a brief needle procedure lasting for hours. Youth can recall more severe pain and distress than they previously reported, which can ultimately influence their future pain experiences [31]. Although more research specific to GI procedures is needed, memory reframing by talking/reminiscing about painful experiences in a positive and accurate way can help youth develop more accurate and positive memories and relieve anticipatory anxiety leading up to future procedures (see https://www.peakresearchlab.com/_files/ugd/79aa9d_e0fd1aeb50c74c24ba08aaf238befd00.pdf for more information) [31–33]. Caregivers, GI mental health professionals, and other healthcare providers can learn to implement memory reframing (see Handout 5.3).

Pharmacological strategies

Topical anesthetics

Topical anesthetics (TAs) effectively reduce pain for youth undergoing needle procedures. TAs are creams, gels, or patches (e.g., EMLA, Maxilene) that are applied to the skin and numb the area of needle insertion [15]. When TAs are used during IV insertions, they have the potential to decrease later GI-procedure-related distress [11]. Since TAs have different manners of application, activation onsets, and duration of effect, select the optimal method based on the procedure and youths' needs. GI mental health professionals can inform caregivers about and advocate for the use of TAs by informing other healthcare providers of the benefits of reducing youths' pain and fear.

Sedation/general anesthesia

Youth with GI conditions often undergo medical procedures that require sedation or general anesthesia (e.g., endoscopy). Sedation and general anesthesia are often administered via IV, which may be painful or fear-inducing. If administered via inhalation, even if not painful, the masks used can be fear-inducing for youth. Therefore, GI mental health professionals can prepare youth for what to expect if they receive sedation and encourage them to use coping strategies, like distraction, if they are distressed about this. GI mental health professionals can also help to prepare families by encouraging them to ask questions about the process (see Handout 5.4).

Pearls of wisdom

- Medical procedures have the potential to be traumatic, and trauma is in the "eye of the beholder". There are a host of evidence-based coping strategies available to help, and if youth are highly fearful of medical procedures, then exposure-based intervention is recommended.
- The more information that the caregiver and youth have about what to expect going into the procedure, the better the youth will cope.
- It is understandable for caregivers and health professionals to gravitate towards reassuring the youth undergoing a painful procedure. Instead, use neutral language and praise-focused statements.

Summary

Youth with GI conditions commonly undergo medical procedures that can be associated with pain and fear, which can escalate each other. Fortunately, there are many strategies (i.e., process/preparatory/education, physical, psychological, pharmacological) to reduce pain and fear in youth undergoing painful medical procedures. Ultimately, everyone, including GI mental health professionals and caregivers, plays a role in advocating for and ensuring that youths' pain and fear are managed through using a combination of strategies: process and preparatory, psychological, and physical. Proper assessment and management of youths' pain and fear before, during, and after their medical procedures promote comfortable person and family-centered healthcare. In turn, youth and families can feel confident in seeking care, and youth are empowered to engage in their healthcare in a developmentally appropriate manner.

Recommended readings

For youth and caregivers:

- Info About Kids – Nervous About Needles?: http://infoaboutkids.org/blog/nervous-about-needles/.
- What to do when your child is highly fearful of medical procedures: https://theconversation.com/if-your-child-is-afraid-of-or-refusing-a-medical-procedure-heres-how-to-help-170923.

For mental health professionals:

- HELP eliminate pain in kids and adults: https://phm.utoronto.ca/helpinkids/publications1.html
- Trottier, E.D. et al. (2019). Managing pain and distress in children undergoing brief diagnostic and therapeutic procedures: https://www.cps.ca/en/documents/position/managing-pain-and-distress.

References

1. Birnie KA, Chambers CT, Fernandez CV, Forgeron PA, Latimer MA, McGrath PJ, et al. Hospitalized children continue to report undertreated and preventable pain. *Pain Res Manag.* 2014;19(4):198–204.

2. Raja SN, Carr DB, Cohen M, Finnerup NB, Flor H, Gibson S, et al. The revised international association for the study of pain definition of pain: Concepts, challenges, and compromises. *Pain.* 2020;161(9):1976–82.
3. McMurtry CM, Pillai Riddell R, Taddio A, Racine N, Asmundson GJ, Noel M, et al. Far from "just a poke": Common painful needle procedures and the development of needle fear. *Clin J Pain.* 2015;31(10 Suppl):S3–11.
4. von Baeyer CL. Numerical rating scale for self-report of pain intensity in children and adolescents: Recent progress and further questions. *Eur J Pain.* 2009;13(10):1005–7.
5. Hicks CL, von Baeyer CL, Spafford PA, van Korlaar I, Goodenough B. The faces pain scale–revised: Toward a common metric in pediatric pain measurement. *Pain.* 2001;93(2):173–83.
6. Malviya S, Voepel-Lewis T, Burke C, Merkel S, Tait AR. The revised FLACC observational pain tool: Improved reliability and validity for pain assessment in children with cognitive impairment. *Paediatr Anaesth.* 2006;16(3):258–65.
7. Merkel S, Voepel-Lewis T, Malviya S. Pain control: Pain assessment in infants and young children: The FLACC scale. *Am J Nurs.* 2002;102(10):55–8.
8. McMurtry CM, Noel M, Chambers CT, McGrath PJ. Children's fear during procedural pain: Preliminary investigation of the children's fear scale. *Health Psychol.* 2011;30(6):780–8.
9. Thurillet S, Bahans C, Wood C, Bougnard S, Labrunie A, Messager V, et al. Psychometric properties of a self-assessment fear scale in children aged 4 to 12 years. Scary scale. *J Pediatr Nurs.* 2022;65:108–15.
10. Heard L. Taking care of the little things: Preparation of the pediatric endoscopy patient. *Gastroenterol Nurs.* 2008;31(2):108–12.
11. Lewis Claar R, Walker LS, Barnard JA. Children's knowledge, anticipatory anxiety, procedural distress, and recall of esophagogastroduodenoscopy. *J Pediatr Gastroenterol Nutr.* 2002;34(1):68–72.
12. Tanaka K, Oikawa N, Terao R, Negishi Y, Fujii T, Kudo T, et al. Evaluations of psychological preparation for children undergoing endoscopy. *J Pediatr Gastroenterol Nutr.* 2011;52(2):227–9.
13. Bray L, Appleton V, Sharpe A. The information needs of children having clinical procedures in hospital: Will it hurt? Will I feel scared? What can I do to stay calm? *Child Care Health Dev.* 2019;45(5):737–43.
14. Taddio A, McMurtry CM, Shah V, Riddell RP, Chambers CT, Noel M, et al. Reducing pain during vaccine injections: Clinical practice guideline. *CMAJ.* 2015;187(13):975–82.
15. Trottier ED, Doré-Bergeron MJ, Chauvin-Kimoff L, Baerg K, Ali S. Managing pain and distress in children undergoing brief diagnostic and therapeutic procedures. *Paediatr Child Health.* 2019;24(8):509–21.
16. Jaaniste T, Hayes B, Von Baeyer CL. Providing children with information about forthcoming medical procedures: A review and synthesis. *Clin Psychol.* 2007;14(2):124.
17. Gordon BK, Jaaniste T, Bartlett K, Perrin M, Jackson A, Sandstrom A, et al. Child and parental surveys about pre-hospitalization information provision. *Child Care Health Dev.* 2011;37(5):727–33.
18. Vejzovic V, Wennick A, Idvall E, Bramhagen AC. A private affair: Children's experiences prior to colonoscopy. *J Clin Nurs.* 2015;24(7–8):1038–47.
19. Duff AJ. Incorporating psychological approaches into routine paediatric venepuncture. *Arch Dis Child.* 2003;88(10):931–7.
20. Gold MS, MacDonald NE, McMurtry CM, Balakrishnan MR, Heininger U, Menning L, et al. Immunization stress-related response–redefining immunization anxiety-related reaction as an adverse event following immunization. *Vaccine.* 2020;38(14):3015–20.
21. Lang EV, Viegas J, Bleeker C, Bruhn J, Geert-Jan van G. Helping children cope with medical tests and interventions. *J Radiol Nurs.* 2017;36(1):44–50.
22. Liu PP, Sun Y, Wu C, Xu WH, Zhang RD, Zheng JJ, et al. The effectiveness of transport in a toy car for reducing preoperative anxiety in preschool children: A randomised controlled prospective trial. *Br J Anaesth.* 2018;121(2):438–44.

23. Canbulat N, Ayhan F, Inal S. Effectiveness of external cold and vibration for procedural pain relief during peripheral intravenous cannulation in pediatric patients. *Pain Manag Nurs.* 2015;16(1):33–9.
24. Moadad N, Kozman K, Shahine R, Ohanian S, Badr LK. Distraction using the BUZZY for children during an IV insertion. *J Pediatr Nurs.* 2016;31(1):64–72.
25. Birnie KA, Noel M, Chambers CT, Uman LS, Parker JA. Psychological interventions for needle-related procedural pain and distress in children and adolescents. *Cochrane Database Syst Rev.* 2018;10(10): 1–162 https://www.ncbi.nlm.nih.gov/pmc/articles/PMC6517234/pdf/CD005179.pdf.
26. Sadeghi T, Mohammadi N, Shamshiri M, Bagherzadeh R, Hossinkhani N. Effect of distraction on children's pain during intravenous catheter insertion. *J Spec Pediatr Nurs.* 2013;18(2):109–14.
27. Cohen LL, Cousins LA, Martin SR. *Procedural pain distraction: Oxford textbook of paediatric pain.* 1st ed. Oxford: Oxford University Press; 2013. p. 519–30.
28. Kiani MA, Heydarian F, Feyzabadi Z, Saeidi M, Ali A, Hebrani P. Effect of music and toys on reducing pain during colonoscopy and acceptance of colonoscopy by children. *Electronic Physician.* 2019;11(4):7652–9.
29. Kuttner L. Pediatric hypnosis: Pre-, peri-, and post-anesthesia. *Paediatr Anaesth.* 2012;22(6):573–7.
30. Tran LC, Coopman S, Rivallain C, Aumar M, Guimber D, Nicolas A, et al. Use of hypnosis in paediatric gastrointestinal endoscopy: A pilot study. *Front Pediatr.* 2021;9:719626.
31. Pavlova M, Lund T, Nania C, Kennedy M, Graham S, Noel M. Reframe the pain: A randomized controlled trial of a parent-led memory-reframing intervention. *J Pain.* 2022;23(2):263–75.
32. Pavlova M, Orr SL, Noel M. Parent–child reminiscing about past pain as a preparatory technique in the context of children's pain: A narrative review and call for future research. *Child.* 2020;7(9):130.
33. Noel M, McMurtry CM, Pavlova M, Taddio A. Brief clinical report: A systematic review and meta-analysis of pain memory-reframing interventions for children's needle procedures. *Pain Pract.* 2018;18(1):123–9.

Chapter 6

Case conceptualization and assessment

Michele H. Maddux and Amanda D. Deacy

Chapter aims

The aim of this chapter is to provide an evidence-based guide to psychosocial assessment and case conceptualization of youth living with gastrointestinal (GI) conditions. The chapter will highlight important domains of functioning and validated measures and screeners to consider when developing an assessment strategy for these youth.

Learning points

- Case conceptualization should consider data from a medical examination, clinical interview, screening measures, and behavioral observation.
- Use of validated GI-specific assessment measures is recommended for initial assessment and progress monitoring of youth living with a GI condition.
- Thoughtful interpretation of assessment findings is key to prioritizing psychosocial treatment targets and to knowing when (and to whom) to refer youth living with a GI condition.

Background

Pediatric GI disorders include a range of diagnosed conditions that vary in terms of the area(s) of the digestive tract affected, the age of symptom onset and course, relevant psychosocial factors, and options for intervention. Youth with GI disorders are shown to be at a greater risk of psychopathology, poor health-related quality of life, as well as poor social, family, and school functioning [1]. As such, pediatric GI disorders are collectively, and most effectively, conceptualized and treated from a biopsychosocial perspective [2, 3].

Biopsychosocial model

Biological factors typically implicated in GI symptom presentation include gut motility, inflammation, visceral hyperalgesia or altered sensory processing, and gut microbiota (see Chapter 2 for more in-depth information regarding these concepts). Psychological factors in need of consideration include sleep, emotional distress, coping styles, and attention and cognition as they relate to symptoms (e.g., pain catastrophizing). Social factors are equally plentiful and impactful. The environment of youth living with a GI condition, unlike their adult counterparts, is structured and maintained, in large part, by parents, teachers, and extended adult family members, as well as by neighborhoods, health systems, and institutions like schools, sports teams,

DOI: 10.4324/9781003308683-7

clubs, and religious organizations. For each individual youth, the biological, psychological, and social systems interact in a complex way via the brain–gut axis (see Chapter 2) to give rise to, and maintain, GI symptoms. Importantly, while the general contributions of factors in each of these domains for pediatric GI disorders are well accepted, the *relative* contribution of each is best determined at the level of the individual youth [3]. Finally, it is also necessary to distinguish at the level of the individual, the role of the above factors as antecedents, triggers, maintaining or protective factors in each unique case.

Assessment best practices

Complex problems require complex approaches and solutions. Pediatric GI conditions are no exception. What follows is a detailing of an evidence-based approach to assessment that takes into account the myriad of biological, psychological, and social factors presumed to be implicated in each child's unique GI symptom presentation.

Medical examination (and ongoing care)

Comprehensive psychosocial care of the youth living with a GI condition requires that they have undergone an appropriate medical evaluation and testing, as needed, and that they continue to receive necessary medical surveillance and follow-up. Said differently, regardless of GI diagnosis, true biopsychosocial care requires that the "bio" is not overlooked in favor of an exclusive focus on psychosocial factors, even in the case of so-called "functional" pediatric GI disorders or disorders of gut–brain interaction (DGBI). Ideally, the treating physician and pediatric GI mental health professional for youth remain in close communication throughout a youth's evaluation and treatment course, reciprocally sharing findings and impressions along the way (see Chapter 7 for a description of integrative care and how to approach it).

Clinical interview

A mainstay of pediatric psychology assessment practice is the clinical interview. From the outset of the interview, it is important that a pediatric GI mental health professional establishes themselves as a vital part of a youth's healthcare team and one that is working in partnership with, not separate from, the youth's GI medical provider. The GI mental health professional can be introduced as:

> *a mental health professional with specialty training in childhood GI disorders, who helps youth and their families better understand how their emotions, beliefs, and behaviors can impact their GI condition, and vice versa, and is focused on improving the daily function and quality of life of such youth.*

The mental health professional will need to demonstrate knowledge of the youth's medical condition, as well as the variety of ways in which it can impact a youth's individual and family quality of life. The mental health professional is also encouraged to give concrete examples of the ways in which they can be helpful to the youth and family. For example, by supporting them in their adjustment to a new diagnosis, providing strategies to make taking medications easier, offering advice to parents struggling to respond to frequent symptom complaints, and/or teaching cognitive skills to youth to help manage worried thoughts related to their GI diagnosis or any other concerns.

The clinical interview must be tailored to the age and developmental level of the youth, with care given to avoiding medical terms or jargon that might be difficult to understand. For example, while terms such as "stomach" or "abdomen" might be appropriate in conversations with older children and adolescents, terms such as "belly" or "tummy" may be more easily understood by toddlers and younger children (see Table 6.1 for additional examples). The GI mental health professional should also take the time to ask parents/caregivers whether certain terms related to GI symptoms or treatments are used at home and incorporate these into the clinical interview, as appropriate.

Table 6.1 Language adaptations by age and developmental level

Toddler and child	*Adolescent*
Belly or tummy	Stomach or abdomen
Poop	Stool or bowel movement
Sour burps	Reflux, regurgitation
Throw up	Vomit
Feeling like you might throw up	Nausea
Hurt or "ouchy"	Pain
Potty	Toilet
Medicine	Medication

Mental health professionals are encouraged to refer parents and caregivers to educational materials designed for youth based on their age/developmental level. For example, the Crohn's and Colitis Foundation's *IBD Activity Book©* or comic book, *Pete Learns All About Crohn's and Colitis©*, can help children better understand their inflammatory bowel disease (IBD) and treatment. Finally, visual guides, diagrams, or videos, such as of the digestive tract, can also be instrumental to help youth better locate and understand their GI anatomy and symptoms.

Uniquely, pediatric practice requires an understanding of the value and appropriateness of speaking with parents alone, children alone, and with parents and children together. This is typically based on the age or developmental level of the youth, although other important factors should be considered (e.g., nature of content to be discussed, youth's comfort/willingness to discuss certain topics in the presence of a caregiver). When possible, information collected from parents or other primary caregivers should be used in combination with youth report to most accurately capture a child's psychosocial context and to provide the most valid estimates of a child's functioning. Often, clinical interviews are initiated with parents and children together, allowing the pair to offer a shared version of the medical and psychosocial history (and to allow for parents to fill in historical gaps, especially in the case of younger children). An astute health professional will make note of important similarities and inconsistencies in each one's report and follow up with each party individually, as needed.

Pediatric clinicians may choose to meet with parents alone to gather sensitive family history, potentially embarrassing details of a child's GI symptoms (e.g., stooling accidents), and/or obtain a candid view of a child's functioning. Likewise, a mental health professional should consider allowing time during the interview to be spent with the child alone to assess the child's ability to communicate independently of their parents, as well as to provide an opportunity for the child to speak openly about difficult or private topics. This is especially important as children become pre-teens and teens. Establishing confidentiality of the therapeutic relationship from the start, during the initial clinical interview, can have profound and long-lasting effects.

Broadly speaking, topics to be covered in a clinical interview include disease (or diagnosis) knowledge, social functioning, school, family, and emotional and physical functioning. Likewise, health and lifestyle behaviors such as sleep, nutrition, exercise, and treatment regimen adherence should also be assessed. Finally, a comprehensive assessment of the youth living with a GI condition also must address relevant social determinants of health (SDOH), which refer to the social circumstances within, or under, which people live and work, i.e., economic stability, education, social and community context, health and healthcare, and neighborhood environment [4]. SDOH have received national recognition from the American Academy of Pediatrics and are powerful influences on health and development, as well as significant predictors of healthcare access, healthcare utilization, and follow-through on medical recommendations [5, 6]. These issues can, and should, be routinely assessed via a clinical interview and/or validated screeners or brief checklists.

While topics such as family and emotional functioning and sleep are likely to be very familiar to most clinical child mental health professionals, becoming facile with the pathophysiology of, and communicating about, specific pediatric GI conditions is essential in conducting a successful interview. This knowledge is likely to engender trust in youth and families and to improve health professionals' fluency in communicating the reciprocal relationships among the relevant factors of the biopsychosocial model. Also critical to the quality of the clinical interview with youth living with a GI condition and their families, interviewers are urged to use open-ended questions, employ active listening, and display empathy (see Handout 6.1 for sample-intake interview questions [7]).

Unlike the role of a mental health provider conducting a traditional clinical child assessment, the role of the pediatric GI mental health professional is *not* to necessarily assign a mental health diagnosis or provide services to youth to whom a mental health diagnosis has been assigned. For example, in the United States coding and billing practices are available that reflect the provision of psychological services (assessment and intervention) for youth with physical health issues who do *not* have a mental health diagnosis. Compared to mental health diagnostic codes, health and behavior (H&B) current procedural terminology (CPT) codes require a physical health diagnosis but not a mental health diagnosis and apply to psychological services that address biopsychosocial factors affecting the prevention, treatment, or management of physical health. H&B services address an assortment of physical health issues, including patient adherence to medical treatment, symptom management, health-promoting behaviors, health-related risk-taking behaviors, and overall adjustment to physical illness.

H&B CPT codes that can be used by pediatric GI mental health professionals include 96150 (health and behavior assessment – initial), 96152 (health and behavior intervention – individual), and 96154 (health and behavior intervention – family with patient). The specific codes for assessment and psychosocial intervention do vary by state and by institution; as such, GI pediatric mental health professionals are advised to speak with their respective coding and billing departments about the recommended coding and billing options and to be prepared to educate their coding and billing departments about billing practices that apply to their practice. Similar processes may or may not exist in other countries, and mental health providers are encouraged to obtain local information about billing and coding in their respective countries for psychogastroenterology care.

Validated measures and screeners

Paper-and-pencil or electronically administered measures and screeners are yet another important aspect of assessment best practice in pediatric GI practice and are described in greater detail below. Notably, pediatric specialty programs are integrating validated tools and screeners, as well as routine behavioral assessments, into standard practice as a method for monitoring treatment progress over time, as well as to demonstrate fiscal responsibility for employing an integrated care model [8].

Behavioral observation

Behavioral observations supply yet another stream of valuable assessment information. Through careful observation of the youth living with a GI condition, the practitioner can glean useful information about youths' overt symptom behaviors (e.g., facial grimacing, holding one's abdomen), their type and frequency, as well as caregivers' reactions to the display of symptoms. This is especially pertinent for infants, toddlers, and younger children who lack the communication skills to fully convey the presence or location of symptoms. Generally speaking, parent behavior thought to maintain pediatric illness behaviors can be classified as either the provision of attention or privileges or the release from responsibility [9].

Research has shown that both are important to understand as a part of a youth's social context with release from responsibility (i.e., releasing a child from chores, homework, or having to go to school) likely being the most problematic [10]. The quality of the parent–child relationship can also be observed during a youth–parent interaction, and it provides yet another bit of important data and potential treatment target. As one example, if parents and caregivers are observed to respond to youth reports of pain or other physical symptoms via reassurance, illness encouragement, or pain catastrophizing, the pediatric GI mental health professional can subsequently provide psychoeducation on the link between such parenting behaviors and increased symptoms and distress, and then provide coaching on alternative responses that promote wellness and recovery. See Chapter 8 for more information relating to the parent–child relationship in pediatric GI disorders and how to work with caregivers.

Case conceptualization

It is important to note that while many families recognize the impact of psychosocial factors on their child's GI health and functioning, others are wary of this approach and misperceive that consideration of a psychological perspective on their child's symptoms somehow discredits or minimizes the legitimacy of their physical complaints. For this reason, it is imperative for pediatric GI mental health professionals to educate families on the interplay of biological, psychological, and social factors in the development and maintenance of symptoms in pediatric GI disorders.

It is equally important to evaluate and address any misconceptions, concerns, or uncertainty held by families as these can become significant barriers to the youth's and family's willingness to engage in treatment with a pediatric GI mental health professional. In fact, prior research has shown that providing education on the biopsychosocial model of care (see Chapter 2 for sample dialogue), the role of the pediatric GI mental health professional as a member of the medical team, and how screening data are used to promote care, helps families become more receptive and decreases the perceived threat of having a pediatric GI mental health professional involved in their treatment plan [11].

Education on the biopsychosocial model of care for pediatric GI conditions should take place at the initial appointment as it serves as a framework for the ongoing care of the youth living with a GI condition and their family. The figure contained within Handout 6.2 has previously been published by Reed-Knight and colleagues (2017) as a visual guide to orient youths and families to the multiple factors involved in the development and maintenance of pediatric chronic GI disorders, and the importance of considering these factors in case conceptualization [2].

Validated measures and screeners

While many well-established assessment measures are available for youth with GI disorders, it is beyond the scope of the current chapter to review all of them. Instead, this chapter will summarize what is available for assessing pediatric GI disease severity and activity, diagnostic classification, health-related quality of life, and parental response to symptoms. Standardized measures are also available to assess SDOH, as well as domains such as sleep, treatment adherence, and functional disability and impairment.

The pediatric GI mental health professional must, however, exercise caution when interpreting assessment findings, particularly for measures that are not specifically designed for youth with chronic medical needs but that nonetheless provide clinically useful information. As one example, a measure of depressive symptoms (e.g., patient health questionnaire-9 [PHQ-9]) may show poor appetite, fatigue, or sleep disruptions caused by symptoms of the GI disorder rather than an underlying depression. As such, assessment measures should not be interpreted in isolation and instead be considered in combination with a clinical interview, observations, and medical examination.

A summary of validated measures was previously published by the Division 54 Pediatric Gastroenterology Special Interest Group (SIG) – Assessment Working Group of the American Psychological Association (see Handout 6.3) [12]. The summary table includes assessment measures that have been specifically developed for pediatric GI populations, measures that have been validated in pediatric GI populations, as well as measures whose content is broadly applicable (e.g., quality of life, treatment adherence, and collateral emotional symptoms) to youths presenting with a range of GI symptoms and conditions.

In the past 3 years, psychological practitioners have been at the forefront of telemedicine expansion in order to ensure access for patients and families to needed mental health services. This has required adaptations across the continuum of care – from scheduling to service delivery to documentation. Psychologists have been especially critical to the development and implementation of workflow processes, whereby assessment measures can be sent to families and subsequently reviewed by providers before, or at, the point of care. Several electronic health record (EHR) systems have built-in capabilities to push assessments out to patients and families before, or at a visit, and save patient responses automatically within a patient's chart. Research electronic data capture (REDCap), a secure web application for building and managing online surveys and databases, is another tool that can be used to push out screeners and questionnaires to families, with options to integrate responses into the EHR [13].

Pediatric psychologists must practice caution, however, to ensure that urgent patient needs that are endorsed via telemedicine or via completed/submitted measures are addressed in a timely manner. During the clinical interview, this can be accomplished by confirming with the family that the phone number and address listed in the electronic medical record match their current location, confirming that legal guardians are present, and having a plan in case urgent concerns arise and the family must access emergent services (e.g., provider pager, suicide hotline).

Such caution must also be applied to any electronically administered assessments, screeners, or questionnaires. As part of the electronic communication, providers can include a disclaimer informing patients that responses will not be reviewed until the day of the appointment and also directing families to appropriate emergency services including emergency telephone numbers (e.g., 911), local hospital emergency departments, and/or an on-call provider who can be reached outside normal business hours.

Implications of assessment findings

When tasked with using assessment findings to identify treatment targets and guide clinical intervention, the pediatric GI mental health professional must determine a starting place that prioritizes the needs of the youth, family, and/or care team. This can be done by selecting behaviors that are identified as most problematic or disturbing to others, selecting behaviors that are easiest to change, or selecting "keystone" behaviors – that is, "behaviors that produce response generalization, such that altering the keystone behavior would alter or produce desirable change in other target behaviors" [14, p. 72]. As one example, a pediatric GI mental health professional might choose to address a youth's treatment non-adherence given that poor adherence is likely to result in worsening health and subsequent declines in the youth's daily functioning and/or quality of life. As another example, a pediatric GI mental health professional might start by addressing parental responses to a child's pain (e.g., illness encouragement, catastrophizing), since this is intended to shift the focus from disability to wellness and translate into more positive coping behaviors in the child.

The pediatric GI mental health professional must also consider the ways in which GI disorders and mental health symptoms might overlap in their presentation. Anxiety and depression, for example, can manifest themselves via significant changes in weight or appetite, fatigue or loss of energy, sleep disturbances, changes in activity level, abdominal pain, diarrhea, and vomiting; all of which are symptom presentations commonly seen in many pediatric GI disorders. As such, the evaluation of assessment findings requires thoughtful consideration of the timing and onset of symptoms (e.g., Were symptoms present before the GI diagnosis was made?), symptom triggers and antecedents, and disease activity (via consultation with the youth's GI care team), to determine the likely underlying cause and mechanism of the symptoms.

Consideration must also be given to referral and/or collaboration with other pediatric specialists. In the case of the child/adolescent with a GI disorder, collaboration with social work, psychiatry, physical therapy (PT), occupation therapy (OT), and/or biofeedback specialists can be an integral component of the child's treatment. Social workers, for example, should be incorporated into the youth's care to address SDOH and any related barriers to healthcare access (e.g., financial, transportation) or guardianship needs in the context of medication decision-making. Another potential collaboration/referral for the pediatric GI mental health professional and GI medical team to consider is with psychiatry.

Depending on the child's GI diagnosis, psychopharmacology (e.g., antidepressants) may be sought to improve bowel regularity, colonic motility, and/or visceral hyperalgesia [15–17]. A referral to psychiatry may also be appropriate under the following conditions: (1) clear evidence of widespread anxiety/mood disturbance beyond that expected in the context of chronic physical symptoms, (2) concerns for the child's safety, (3) noticeable changes in behaviors (e.g., decreasing grades in school, social isolation/withdrawal, loss of interest in normal activities), (4) evidence of major mental illness, (5) the presence of anxiety/mood symptoms that prohibit participation in psychological therapy, and/or (6) clear evidence of a link between GI symptoms and mental health symptoms (especially anxiety).

Collaboration with teachers and other school personnel is also essential, especially in light of research that shows greater school absenteeism and poorer school functioning among youth with various GI disorders [18], and the link between school absences and increased educational risk [19]. Such collaboration should, at a minimum, include education to school personnel on the child's GI diagnosis (if the family is agreeable) and how it may impact the student's attendance or academic performance, as well as any needed school-based accommodations to ensure the student's success at school. Finally, additional collaboration/referral of high relevance to pediatric GI disorders might include PT/OT to address deconditioning and desensitization for pain and biofeedback-assisted relaxation therapy (BART) for general stress and pain management.

Pearls of wisdom

- It is essential for pediatric GI mental health professionals to educate themselves on the physiology of the GI tract and, specifically, the GI conditions of the youths they serve. Being able to communicate this knowledge using patient-friendly language is essential to quality whole-person care and to distinguishing oneself as an invaluable member of an interdisciplinary team.
- In the initial phase of care, pediatric GI mental health professionals should take the time to orient and educate youth living with a GI condition and families on the brain–gut connection to increase engagement and decrease defensiveness and perceived stigma.
- Addressing sleep, difficulty with mood and anxiety, treatment adherence, and school and social functioning is especially important for children with GI conditions.

Summary

Understanding the role of biological, psychological, and social factors in the presentation of pediatric GI conditions is critical to achieving good outcomes. To do this, pediatric GI mental health professionals must establish themselves as an indispensable part of the care team through demonstration to families of their knowledge of the youth's GI disease. Pediatric GI mental health professionals must approach psychological topics directly and with care, appreciating that families' adoption of a biopsychosocial conceptualization is key to improving both disease-specific and psychosocial impairment. Finally, pediatric GI mental health professionals should make use of the variety of broad, and disease-specific, standardized measures available to evaluate a child's psychosocial functioning (e.g., sleep, mood and anxiety, academic and social functioning), taking care to adapt the measures for use in telemedicine and electronic communication as allowed. Compilation and monitoring of all this data are essential for a complete understanding of a youth living with a GI condition's baseline functioning and improvement over the course of treatment.

Recommended readings

For youth and caregivers:

- Deacy AD, Huston P. *Cognitive-Behavioral Therapy*: https://gikids.org/digestive-topics/cognitive-behavioral-therapy/.
- ImproveCareNow (ICN) Collaborative Network, Social Workers and Psychologists Group (SWAP). *Finding a Mental Health Provider for your Child or Teen with IBD*: https://www.improvecarenow.org/finding_a_mental_health_provider_for_your_child_and_teen_with_ibd.

For mental health professionals:

- Maddux MH, Deacy AD, Colombo J. Organic GI Disorders. In Carter B, Kullgren K, editors. (2020). *Clinical Handbook of Pediatric Psychological Consultation in Medical Settings*. Cham, Switzerland: Springer Nature Switzerland AG.
- Reed-Knight B, Maddux MH, Deacy AD, Lamparyk K, Stone AL, Mackner L. (2017). Brain-Gut Interactions and Maintenance Factors in Pediatric Gastroenterological Disorders: Recommendations for Clinical Care. *Clinical Practice in Pediatric Psychology*, 5(1), 93–105.

References

1. Mackner LM, Greenley RN, Szigethy E, Herzer M, Deer K, Hommel KA. Psychosocial issues in pediatric inflammatory bowel disease: Report of the North American Society for pediatric gastroenterology, hepatology, and nutrition. *J Pediatr Gastroenterol Nutr*. 2013;56(4):449–58.
2. Reed-Knight B, Maddux MH, Deacy AD, Lamparyk K, Stone AL, Mackner L. Brain-gut interactions and maintenance factors in pediatric gastroenterological disorders: Recommendations for clinical care from the division 54 pediatric gastroenterology special interest group. *Clin Pract Pediatr Psychol*. 2017;5(1):93–105.
3. Verrill Schurman J, Drews Deacy A, Friesen CA. Recurrent abdominal pain. In: Stevens BJ, Hathway G, Zempsky WT, Stevens BJ, Hathway G, Zempsky WT, editors. Oxford Textbook of Pediatric Pain: Oxford University Press; 2021.
4. Office of Disease Prevention and Health Promotion. Social determinants of health. 2014. Available at: https://www.healthypeople.gov/2020/topics-objectives/topic/social-determinants-of-health. Accessed August 23, 2022.
5. Billioux AK, Verlander SA, Alley D. Standardized screening for health-related social needs in clinical settings: The accountable health communities screening tool. *NAM Perspectives*. 2017. Discussion Paper, National Academy of Medicine, Washington, DC.
6. Hardy R, Boch S, Keedy H, Chisolm D. Social determinants of health needs and pediatric health care use. *J Pediatr*. 2021;238:275–81 e1.
7. Maddux MH, Deacy AD, Colombo J. Organic GI disorders. In Carter B, Kullgren K, editors. *Clinical Handbook of Pediatric Psychological Consultation in Medical Settings*. Cham, Switzerland: Springer Nature Switzerland AG;2020:195–210.
8. Schurman JV, Friesen CA. Leveraging institutional support to build an integrated multidisciplinary care model in pediatric inflammatory bowel disease. *Children (Basel)*. 2021;8(4):286.
9. Walker LS, Claar RL, Garber J. Social consequences of children's pain: When do they encourage symptom maintenance? *J Pediatr Psychol*. 2002;27(8):689–98.
10. Schurman JV, Hunter HL, Danda CE, Friesen CA, Hyman PE, Cocjin JT. Parental illness encouragement behavior among children with functional gastrointestinal disorders: A factor analysis with implications for research and clinical practice. *J Clin Psychol Med Settings*. 2013;20(2):255–61.
11. Maddux MH, Bass JA, Geraghty-Sirridge C, Carpenter E, Christenson K. Assessing psychosocial functioning among youth with inflammatory bowel disease: An interdisciplinary clinic approach. *Clin Pract Pediatr Psychol*. 2013;1(4):333–43.
12. Maddux MH, Deacy AD, Lukens C. Society of pediatric psychology (APA division 54). Assessment resource sheet: Pediatric gastroenterology. 2014. https://pedpsych.org/evidence_based_asses/pediatric_gastroenterology/
13. The Promise of Electronic Health Records: Are We There Yet? Rockville, MD: Agency for Healthcare Research and Quality;2019. https://www.ahrq.gov/news/blog/ahrqviews/promise-of-electronic-health-records.html

14. Rapoff MA. *Adherence to pediatric medical regimens*. 2nd ed. New York: Springer Science+Business Media, LLC;2010.
15. Bonilla S, Nurko S. Focus on the use of antidepressants to treat pediatric functional abdominal pain: Current perspectives. *Clin Exp Gastroenterol.* 2018;11:365–72.
16. Saps M, Youssef N, Miranda A, Nurko S, Hyman P, Cocjin J, et al. Multicenter, randomized, placebo-controlled trial of amitriptyline in children with functional gastrointestinal disorders. *Gastroenterology*. 2009;137(4):1261–9.
17. Lebel AA. Pharmacology. *J Pediatr Gastroenterol Nutr*. 2008;47(5):703–5.
18. Mackner LM, Bickmeier RM, Crandall WV. Academic achievement, attendance, and school-related quality of life in pediatric inflammatory bowel disease. *J Dev Behav Pediatr*. 2012;33(2):106–11.
19. Hancock KJ, Shepherd CCJ, Lawrence D, Zubrick SR. Student attendance and educational outcomes: Every day counts. Report for the Department of Education, Employment and Workplace Relations, Canberra;2013.

Chapter 7

Collaborative, multidisciplinary treatment

Jennifer Verrill Schurman and Craig A. Friesen

Chapter aims

This chapter will provide a "how to" guide for treating youth with gastrointestinal (GI) conditions using a multidisciplinary approach, including identifying key team members, selecting a collaborative model, working with community partners, and using metrics to demonstrate the value of mental health services as a component of holistic pediatric GI care.

Learning points

- Program planning should begin with the youths' needs across the biopsychosocial spectrum.
- Define the ideal state before considering what is currently possible.
- Selecting the right people is as important as selecting the necessary roles.
- Get administrative "buy-in" early and agree on success metrics.

Western medicine has long embraced a biomedical perspective that separates the mind and body when understanding and treating illness or disease. In practical terms, this drives physicians to search for organic causes initially and refer to a mental health professional only if no organic cause can satisfactorily account for a youth's physical symptoms. Likewise, mental health professionals often ask physicians to rule out organic causes before psychological or behavioral treatment can take place. This dualistic model is often played out in clinical practice but is at odds with mounting evidence suggesting that biological and psychosocial factors are mutually determinant, and often interactive, in many common pediatric GI conditions. A biopsychosocial model has gained momentum in recent years as the prevailing conceptualization for many common pediatric GI concerns (see Chapter 2). This biopsychosocial model provides the foundation for shifting toward a more collaborative, multidisciplinary approach to care. However, while intellectually appealing, integration among specialties can be difficult to achieve in practice. This chapter will focus specifically on the "how to" of launching and evolving a multidisciplinary approach to care across pediatric GI conditions based on four distinct but related phases. See Figure 7.1 for a conceptual overview and process map of each phase.

Phase 1: Identifying the "Ideal state"

When considering a shift from traditional single-discipline practice to multidisciplinary care, there is often a tendency to think in terms of logistics first, in other words: "What is possible?" This question should be set aside early in the process to instead begin with "what is ideal?"

DOI: 10.4324/9781003308683-8

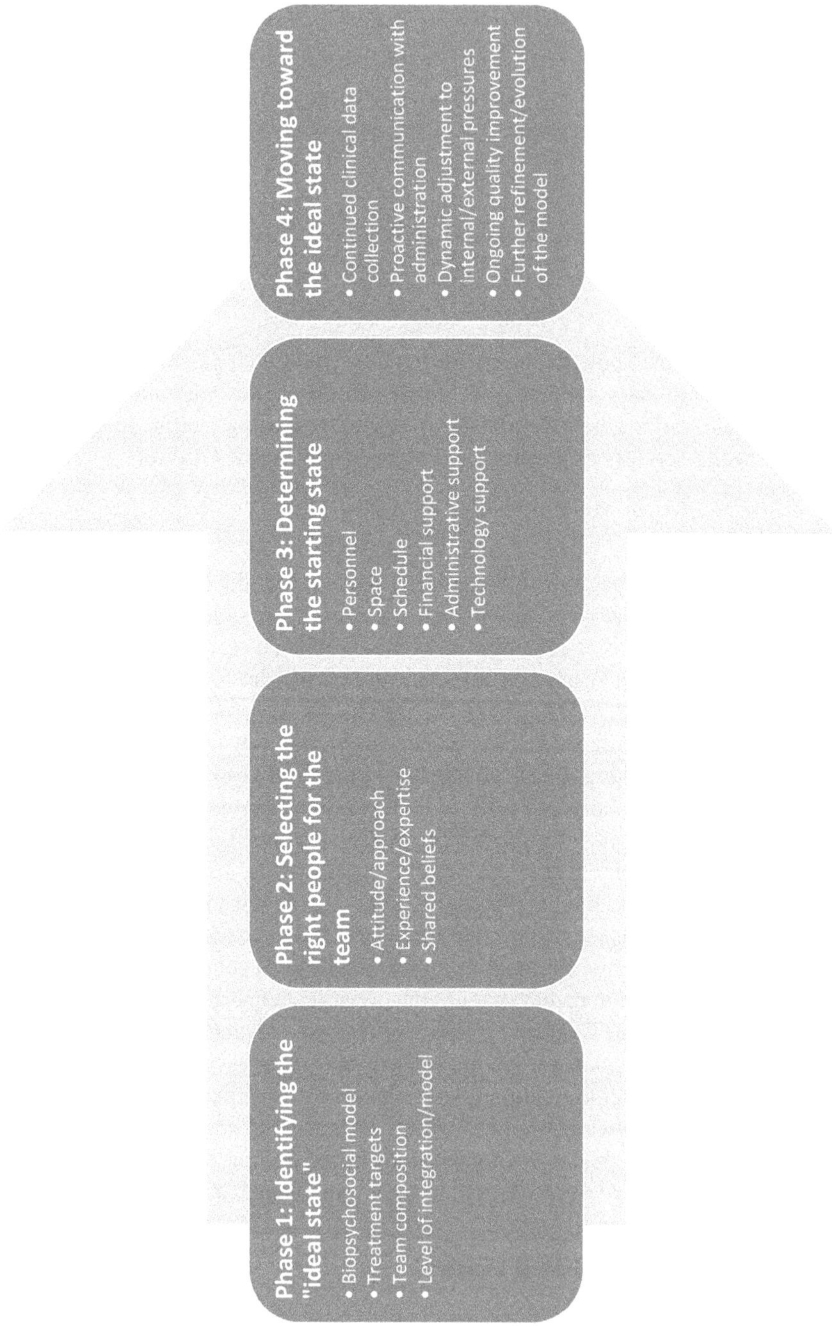

Figure 7.1 Process map with key elements to consider within each phase (Source: Authors).

While it is likely that initial plans will be modified by the local context (e.g., available personnel, funding, space), identifying the optimum structure provides an endpoint for long-term planning and a roadmap for movement from what is currently possible to what is ideal. Vital to keep at the forefront in this phase is the understanding that when mental health professionals take on youth with GI conditions, it comes with the responsibility to identify and treat relevant factors that can affect outcomes.

Outcomes should include physical symptoms, of course, but also can include quality of life and functional disability, among others. In this phase, mental health professionals need to review the existing evidence to identify relevant outcomes, as well as the array of biological, psychological, and social factors shown to affect these outcomes in the target population. The initial goal is to develop a biopsychosocial model-informed conceptualization of the patient population in as much detail as possible, including making note of which potential contributing factors are modifiable. By undertaking this approach, mental health professionals can then identify a care model and team composition that is optimally designed to match youth needs. For example, while a youth's emotional state, sleep, and living conditions may be modifiable, genetic factors are not.

Sample questions to ask during this phase include, but are not limited to:

- What are the key biological, psychological, and social factors affecting outcomes in this patient population?
- Which of these are modifiable?
- What roles/expertise is needed to assess these factors?
- Does this patient population have significant or unique psychosocial needs?
- How is this condition impacted by social determinants of health (SDOH)?
- What treatment modalities are available to address these factors?
- What roles/expertise is needed to deliver these treatments?

Answering the above questions will result in a comprehensive list of roles to consider in constructing a multidisciplinary team. It can then be determined which roles are key (i.e., need to be involved in the care of every patient) and which are ad hoc (i.e., need to be involved in the care of select, but not every, patient). For most (and likely all) chronic conditions, emotions, anxiety, and depression have a significant impact on outcomes. Additionally, treatment adherence, coping, and resilience should be universal considerations. Thus, when addressing a chronic health condition within a biopsychosocial framework, the physician and mental health professional are likely always key players.

Nursing should also be added to this list, as nurses are typically the primary point of contact between visits and are thus well situated to develop ongoing youth/family relationships. When integrated fully into the clinical team, nurses have frequent opportunities to reinforce the treatment plan, help realign youth/families with the team, and provide insights back to other key team members with regard to changes in a youth's condition, barriers, and resources in real time. Given the importance of SDOH, the other constant should be social work, which is always at least an ad hoc role [1]. It is important that an SDOH evaluation (see Chapter 6) be included in every initial assessment and revisited periodically throughout treatment, as the context of care may change over time. This does not, however, necessarily require a physical presence at each visit. For example, SDOH assessment may be completed through a screening questionnaire at the initial visit (and possibly quarterly or annually thereafter), which can trigger a face-to-face evaluation with social workers and subsequently drive specific interventions.

With the above exceptions, who is key and who is ad hoc can vary by condition, as well as between assessment and treatment phases. For example, an entire feeding team (e.g., physician, GI mental health professional, occupational therapist, speech pathologist, and dietician) may be necessary for the initial evaluation of youth with feeding difficulties. However, the dietician may become an ad hoc member during treatment for youth who have adequate nourishment and are determined to have swallowing dysfunction as the primary cause of poor feeding. Similarly, for youth with a disorder of gut–brain interaction, a physical therapist may be needed to help return a child to normal functioning, but only when functional disability is more extreme. Ultimately, how universal versus selective a factor is within a specific patient population should drive decision-making about specific roles being deemed key versus ad hoc (see Table 7.1 for additional examples). It is important to note that there is no one right answer to who should be deemed key versus ad hoc; this may vary center-by-center based on how they define the critical factors for any given patient population. This also may be dynamic in that conceptualization and treatments continue to emerge and evolve over time, which may lead to changes in who is viewed as key versus ad hoc.

Table 7.1 Sample roles by patient population (assessment phase)

Condition	*Key (in addition to medical provider, GI mental health professional, nursing, and social work)*	*Ad hoc*
Inflammatory bowel disease		Dietician, pharmacist
Feeding problems	Occupational therapist, speech therapist, dietician	
Abdominal pain		Dietician, physical therapist
Eosinophilic esophagitis	Dietician, allergist	
Liver disease		Transplant surgeon, dietician, pharmacist
Celiac disease	Dietician	
Intestinal rehabilitation	Dietician, pharmacist	Surgeon
Polyposis	Genetic counselor	Surgeon

Ad hoc members also may include community providers. Certainly, the youths' primary care provider should be viewed as a team member. They often have important insights into family dynamics and are ideally situated to coordinate care for youth with multiple medical or psychological conditions. School personnel may become ad hoc team members when accommodations and/or other support is needed within the school environment to support improvements in health and/or functioning. Community child mental health professionals also may become ad hoc members when more significant and/or long-standing mental health concerns are identified.

The primary role of the GI pediatric mental health professional on the care team will be to assess youth within the multidisciplinary program and formulate a consolidated plan to address the presenting health concerns with other team members. Trained to focus on the assessment and treatment of child health issues, GI pediatric mental health professionals also may provide brief intervention on subclinical issues that are thought to be impacting the identified health condition, but do not necessarily rise to the level of a specific child mental health disorder. Partnering with a child clinical mental health professional in the community can increase access to specialists in specific child mental health disorders and allow the GI pediatric mental health professional to continue providing support specific to the health concern (see Table 7.2 for the explanation of role definition, as well as strategies for role alignment and coordination of care). For example, a GI pediatric mental health professional may provide school intervention and/or brief relaxation training to youth with subclinical anxiety issues thought to be impacting their GI condition, which may be missed if sent out to a child mental health professional used to dealing with diagnosable mental health concerns.

The same GI pediatric mental health professional may refer youth with suspected social phobia or obsessive-compulsive disorder to a child mental health professional in the community, as mental health treatment is likely to require a different level of expertise and perhaps even a time commitment beyond treatment for their health concerns. Time and travel burden also may dictate the involvement of a community-based psychologist, although this has become less of a deciding factor with the increased availability and feasibility of telehealth. Identifying the right GI mental health professional to provide treatment for an issue is key in both utilizing the unique expertise and managing the volume demands of each. In the end, it is important for the care team and any community providers to maintain good communication and coordination of care throughout the youth's treatment for their health concern.

Once team composition is drafted, the next critical decision is the model of care. However, it is important to remember that terminology associated with various care models is not well understood and can lead to confusion around and drift from the original intention of the model when resource pressure occurs. Indeed, the term "multidisciplinary" has commonly been used to refer to any multispecialty group, without regard for relationship among the group members. An in-depth discussion of the different levels of multispecialty collaboration that may be found in clinical practice – unidisciplinary, multidisciplinary, interdisciplinary, and transdisciplinary – is beyond the scope of this chapter and can be found elsewhere [2, 3]. However, a brief discussion appears warranted given that more precise and specific terminology can help guide decision-making around team function and communication in both the short and long terms.

Truly unidisciplinary care, in which a provider works in complete isolation from other disciplines, is relatively rare in today's technologically connected healthcare system. However, multidisciplinary teams may be set up in a way that is functionally unidisciplinary, with a relative separation of disciplines in practice. This is a common practice in healthcare, in which one provider sends a patient to another provider for a specific service, and communication between the two providers is limited (e.g., send occasional visit documentation or initial treatment plan) to non-existent. Communication is generally worse when providers are removed from one another in physical and/or technological proximity (e.g., sending a patient out to a community-based provider without access to the same medical record). However, even providers within the same healthcare system, including those who are co-located, can remain conceptually separated. The risk in these functionally unidisciplinary models is that interconnectedness between various factors within the biopsychosocial model may be lost, and care can become fragmented and inefficient/ineffective as a result.

In contrast, interdisciplinary care, also referred to as integrated multidisciplinary care, involves providers from different disciplines jointly addressing biopsychosocial factors, as well as their interactions, from a shared perspective. Conceptually, interdisciplinary care allows two or more disciplines to generate ideas about treatment, assessment, and etiology that are

Table 7.2 Role definition and communication strategies for integration of psychology into GI care

	Focus of assessment	*Focus of treatment*	*Treatment scope/ duration*
GI pediatric mental health professional	• Psychosocial factors that may influence GI symptom presentation, maintenance, and recurrence, as well as treatment adherence and response • Proactive/early intervention • Population level • Subclinical issues	Intervention relevant to symptom management and/or treatment (not limited to): • Stress management • Relaxation training • Treatment adherence • School intervention • Lifestyle intervention • Sleep hygiene • Diet reintroduction • Parental support • Family functioning	• Targeted • Limited timeframe (e.g., 4–6 sessions) • Short term • Typically as long as the duration of GI symptoms or involvement with team/clinic • Higher volume, faster turnover needed to touch all youth
Child mental health professional	• Diagnosable mental health conditions • Reactive • Individual level • Clinically significant issues	Intervention relevant to identified mental health conditions (not limited to): • Anxiety disorders • Depressive disorders • Externalizing disorders • Developmental disorders • Eating disorders	• Comprehensive • Undefined timeframe • Short- to long-term • Typically as long as the duration of need for treatment of mental health condition and maintenance of gains over time • Lower volume, longer relationships needed for more significant mental health issues
Strategies for communication	• Discussion of differences in training, roles, and focus areas of GI pediatric versus child mental health professionals (and often versus psychiatrist) with family. • Provision of standard letter for family to share with clinical child psychologist outlining pediatric psychology role in treatment and considerations for ongoing individual/family therapy with clinical child psychologist for treatment planning. • Direct (and potentially ongoing) communication between providers by phone to ensure coordination of care and alignment of roles/perspectives moving forward.		

impossible to generate from one discipline acting independently. An interdisciplinary model is intentionally set up to enhance communication (e.g., take joint histories, engage in routine case conferences) and shared decision-making (e.g., meet together with families in clinic, collaborate on treatment plans) at key points and/or on an ongoing basis. Important to note is that the patient experience often is enhanced by being able to see relevant providers in a single visit and know their care team is aligned [4]. This helps prioritize recommendations, as the whole team is aware of each other's recommendations, and allows the team to clearly communicate the most important and/or timely ones to the family. In this way, the odds are reduced by overwhelming the youth/family with a vast array of recommendations or inadvertently encouraging them to pick the easiest (as opposed to the most important) among them. Thus, the value to the patient is enhanced.

Of course, multidisciplinary care exists along a continuum, from complete separation to complete integration of disciplines/providers. The key for any new multidisciplinary program is to choose a model that best meets the needs of the patient population and enhances outcomes across all key areas. Further, this phase should be undertaken with the goal of not only optimizing outcomes but enhancing value from the patient's perspective. In general, for those looking to shift into multidisciplinary care, higher levels of integration, at least among core team members, will be the ideal state. The need for communication and shared decision-making for each role with other team members at key points and/or throughout treatment should be carefully considered and prioritized above convenience or other pragmatic concerns when defining the ideal state (see Table 7.3 for examples of communication strategies to consider in advancing toward more integrated care).

Table 7.3 Key strategies to enhance communication and collaboration in multidisciplinary care

Target team member	*Strategies to consider*
Key	• See patients together, routinely or at key points. • Pre-visit plan together and jointly decide on recommendation priorities. • Engage in joint documentation for discharge summary and other patient/family support materials (separate documents for billing). • Schedule frequent standing case conferences to discuss current patients. • Copy key personnel on all communication with families.
Ad hoc	• Discuss patient referrals and collaborative goals. • Invite to participate in select case conferences. • Schedule joint visits, as indicated.
Ad hoc/community	• Utilize a standard referral form for intake that has space for referring provider goals and insights. • Develop reference materials/handouts to help explain the patient's condition and treatment plan to community providers. • Develop templated letters to send with youth/family for initial contact (e.g., therapy targets, school accommodations). • Proactively seek release of information (ROI) for community partners up front to support follow-up communication/coordination.

Phase 2: Selecting the right people for your team

Once decisions relating to the ideal model and team composition are made, the next step is to select the right people to fill those roles. Determining the right people not only involves assessing expertise for patient assessment and treatment of contributing factors, but selecting people driven by shared beliefs. This must include shared beliefs regarding the necessity and value of multidisciplinary team care, as well as shared beliefs regarding how team members interact. Initially, team members need to respect boundaries, deferring recommendations to the team member with the credentials and expertise in the specific aspect of care. However, with time, high-functioning teams will begin to blur these boundaries, with team members feeling comfortable offering thoughts across disciplinary lines and couching recommendations from their discipline in terms of their interconnectedness with other areas. This productive blurring of professional boundaries that can occur in teams over time is typically referred to as transdisciplinary care and requires a high degree of trust among team members.

For both key and ad hoc roles, attitude is critical. The goal is to assemble a team whose members are collaborative, non-defensive, and open to learning. This is best determined by making plans for a hard reset or cultural shift to a new model where there is agreement on the ideal state. Change can be difficult for anyone, as there is a pull toward the status quo; thus, while not impossible, altering the model dramatically while keeping some or all team members with experience in the "old" model can be a much more difficult and painful process. Thoughtful reflection and mutual understanding should occur early, along with agreement that this will be an iterative process with the model evolving over time. Whether potential team members are the right people will become apparent if they agree to a model, collaborate well, and are enthusiastic and energized by the process. For the long-term health and functioning of the team, which subsequently benefits the patients, this phase is as important as the initial identification of team roles and models of care.

It should be noted that, at times, the right individuals may not be available. For example, professional specialization in pediatric psychology broadly, and GI subspecialization in pediatric psychology specifically, has become more plentiful in urban centers in the United States of America (USA) over the past 20 years, but remains limited in rural geographic locations within the USA. More globally, while there is a growing interest in and training opportunities for GI-focused mental health, in reality these opportunities are lacking. Several factors contribute to this disparity in the availability of GI-trained pediatric mental health professionals, including differences in perceived value at a cultural level, access to professional education, and availability of financial support/reimbursement.

This may also be true for other professionals (e.g., pharmacy, nutrition support). When a specific type of provider is unavailable, this creates an important limitation to be considered in the starting state as discussed later. In these cases, you may need to determine whether other members of your team can pick up some or all of the duties of a missing key or ad hoc role in the short term (e.g., physician also providing limited nutrition support; social worker providing some psychosocial assessment and triage). However, when such gaps are identified, this also should be viewed as an opportunity for advocacy over the long term to increase the pool of appropriate professionals available to support your team as you continue to evolve toward your ideal state. This type of advocacy can be seen in Mikocka-Walus et al. [5], in which a group of Australian GI-focused experts called for increased support and integration of psychology in the treatment of their patients with GI conditions. Without such systemically focused advocacy, the continued movement toward this ideal multidisciplinary approach will be made more difficult.

Phase 3: Determining the starting state

Once the care model is built and team members are selected, the question of "what is currently possible?" must be addressed. This is the phase in which to take stock of existing resources, including things such as available personnel, funding, support, and space, and articulate gaps between the current and ideal state.

Specific questions to ask include, but are not limited to, the following:

- Are there specific people that can be identified to fill all the team roles (both key and ad hoc)?
- Do these team members have sufficient time to allot to this program or do they have competing demands?
- Are there ways to "buy out" and free up sufficient time for team members?
- How will billing work across the team?
- Who gets credit for the revenue brought in?
- How will individual and/or joint documentation be set up to ensure optimal appropriate billing for team members?
- Where can the multidisciplinary clinic be run?
- How should patients be scheduled? How will non-attendance be measured and addressed?
- How can the joint schedule be reflected across multiple individual schedules?
- What procedure will be needed to deal with one or more key team members being unavailable due to illness, vacation, or other out-of-office time?
- What kind of clinical data (e.g., symptoms, medical tests, school attendance, quality of life, sleep, interventions provided, coping) needs to be collected?
- When, where, and how is this clinical data best collected?
- What kind of technology/administrative support is needed for clinical data collection?
- What other kind of administrative support is needed for the multidisciplinary clinic?
- Where will the administrative support come from (especially if pulling key team members from across divisions)?

Once the current state has been assessed and available needs/resources identified, a list of priorities should be developed; at one end, critical missing pieces that need to be addressed urgently (before embarking on seeing youth with GI conditions), to the other end, items that can be gradually incorporated over time (to increasingly support alignment with the ideal state). Advocating with administrative leaders to fill the urgent gaps then becomes the next logical step. While it may be readily apparent to clinicians (from both experience and knowledge of the literature) that integrated multidisciplinary care addressing all relevant disease factors provides optimal outcomes, this is not always apparent to non-clinicians. This includes administrators who make decisions regarding resource allocation. It is important to educate administrators on the current literature, best practices, and local patient needs while also addressing financial implications of the proposed program. This will also likely require providing a case for always including the medical provider and GI mental health professional as key members of every team. This can begin with generalities, but then become condition-specific and move from broad-based information to local context and logistics (see Table 7.4 for a list of recommended talking points to include when presenting to administrative leaders).

Table 7.4 Recommended talking points with administrative leaders

Topic	*Rationale*	*Specific points to consider/cover*
General statement	Broad context	• Sample script: "It has been demonstrated that pediatric gastroenterologist/pediatric psychologist integrated care improves patient/family satisfaction, enhances adherence to recommendations (both medical and psychological), and results in an increase in psychology referrals with a shorter lag time, as well as a significant increase in the rate of follow through with mental/behavioral health treatment" [4, 6].
Literature summary	Why should anyone care?	• Numbers affected by health condition worldwide. • Cost of condition and care (to families, healthcare systems, societies). • Cost off-set (where available) of the type of care you propose to provide vs. care-as-usual.
Data from local context	Why should we care here?	• Population size treated locally/regionally. • Frequency of relevant factors (e.g., psychological, social, functional). • Current cost to care for these patients (e.g., capitated care patients, access for other patient groups, hospital bed days/ emergency room visits).
Detailed plan for ideal care model	What can we do about it?	• The biopsychosocial factors identified as key in target patient population, as basis for: • The intended care model. • The clinical data to be collected. • Assessment and treatment options offered. • Relevant key and ad hoc team members with justification of time.
Business plan	How can we make it viable?	• Catchment area and anticipated referral base. • Assessment of total cost and expected revenue (including downstream procedures, tests, and interventions). • Consideration of different payment models (e.g., fee for service, capitated, and bundled payment) and impact on overall finances. • Plan for growth dependent on meeting specified benchmarks.

The literature summary utilizes the material already accumulated when planning the multidisciplinary team. For example, describing how often psychological factors are present in the population with the specific condition, the impact these factors have on outcomes, and how treatment of these factors affects outcomes (including symptoms, quality of life, and disability) and overall costs of care (for an inflammatory bowel disease-specific example, see Schurman and Friesen [7]). The literature is robust with reports on psychologic comorbidity in pediatric GI diseases, including – but certainly not limited to – chronic abdominal pain, inflammatory bowel disease, eosinophilic esophagitis, celiac disease, and feeding disorders [8–12]. Likewise, there is ample literature reporting on the benefits of multidisciplinary care across multiple pediatric GI conditions [13–18].

While examining the literature provides a basis for multidisciplinary care, collecting local data is essential. This can be accomplished by screening for psychological dysfunction, SDOH, and other factors which are relevant to each proposed team member. Clinical data can help to provide a quick assessment of the array of potentially modifiable factors deemed important to your patient population for an individual patient, identify and document changes over time on these factors and key outcomes in response to treatment, and – if done in advance of visits – shift actual time spent during the clinic visit away from basic assessment toward meaningful face-to-face discussion with the youth/family, further increasing value. On a global level, clinical data combined across patients also can provide an opportunity for program-level quality improvement work and, with appropriate ethical review/approval, retrospective chart reviews to be published that can help move knowledge forward and propel national reputation (another currency frequently understood by administrators). When combined with information on hospital days, emergency room visits, and other cost-of-care indicators (e.g., messages/phone calls, procedures, tests), clinical data can provide useful information that can amplify the urgency of change, particularly in capitated care scenarios and/or in the face of significant access challenges. The goal in this step is to bring the issue "home" to administrators who manage budgets, patient complaints, and care access issues, providing them with a reason to change the status quo and build a solid foundation for presenting your ideal state and business plan (see Handout 7.1 for a sample strategic plan for program development or expansion).

It is important to provide administrators with a detailed plan for the proposed program, both theoretical and practical. This not only increases credibility and demonstrates thoughtful, careful planning, but also allows for more accurate financial planning. It is important to team up with business partners within the institution to provide data that breeds confidence in administrators regarding business projections. It is also very important for the clinical team to be active partners in financial planning to ensure that financial analysis is not built on faulty assumptions but based on the experience and plans of the clinical team.

Lastly, it is critical to convince administrative decision-makers to assess program finances as a whole (total revenue-total costs), rather than examining individual team members separately as this can lead to, at least, partial dismantling of the team. For example, administration could decide that one team member could be more productive seeing patients independently rather than as part of team care, thus hampering team communication and the family's understanding of how all the factors interact in the youth's condition and care plan. When individual-level finances are the sole basis for productivity evaluation, programs will be at risk for accepting a lower standard of care, decreased value from a youth/family perspective, and diminished outcomes.

The primary goal in this phase should be to effectively sell your vision to, and secure buy-in from, relevant administrative decision-makers. Agreement in principle is a necessary first step that allows a clinical team to advocate with administrators to get the most support possible for your starting state and define parameters (e.g., financial, clinical outcomes) that need to be met to support a continued transition toward the ideal state. It is important to note that a program may not be fully funded at the onset and, in fact, this would be expected. Some of these situations will be more immediately fixable than others. For example, the right person with the right skills may not be available to fill a specific role on the team, requiring additional time for a search and hiring process. In other situations, the resources requested may not be readily available, or administrators may want an initial demonstration of success by hitting specified parameters before committing these resources.

Proactive discussions about what is critical now and what will be needed in the future will help ensure a clear path forward and trust among the parties involved. Although it may be tempting to ask for less than you need, presenting a trimmed version of the ideal to get a "foot in the door" is not recommended as it can serve to erode trust and make future requests more difficult. In the end, if what is initially supported omits key components of care, severely limiting the impact of the new program on patient outcomes and value, the team will need to decide whether to move ahead, wait until they can procure additional resources, or even circle back around to the question of buy-in and what administration would need to see in order to commit resources more closely aligned to the ideal care model.

The above, of course, is predicated on key team members being housed within the same healthcare system. When key team members are at different institutions or in independent practice, the movement toward collaborative interdisciplinary care can be even more challenging, if not impossible. The goal in these situations may be different. The best approach will likely be to focus on low-cost strategies for increasing communication and collaboration around individual patients (e.g., phone/video case conferences, asynchronous clinic visits with joint treatment planning), as a starting point once potential team members with the right attitude and skills are identified (e.g., through networking at relevant conferences, offering to provide free education over the lunch hour to meet local providers, following up with discussion on referred youth). If further care integration is deemed necessary, the best pathway may be to have one team member champion the business plan to administration at their own institution/practice, with the goal of consolidating key team members within a single system to better support movement toward the ideal state. Without this consolidation, alignment of resources with vision cannot truly occur and competing demands will persist.

Phase 4: Moving toward the ideal state

Once a viable starting state is identified, and a multidisciplinary program is piloted, it is critical to remember that progress toward the ideal state is dynamic. Issues both within and outside of the local healthcare context (e.g., staff loss, economic recession, billing updates, administrative personnel changes) can result in temporary setbacks and require revisiting your business plan with administrative decision-makers. Temporary adjustments may be needed to weather these expected moments of restriction in resources. Continued communication with administration at regular intervals remains important: to sustain buy-in, deal efficiently with any setbacks, and continue the momentum toward the ideal state. Proactively reporting data collected on agreed-upon parameters can increase confidence in the model, helping administrators to see that what is created is working better than what was there before and that they are not putting the institution at financial risk. Reporting of data also can serve to trigger further resource allocation if parameters are clearly set and agreed upon in advance.

Long-term engagement of the clinical team can also be critical in moving toward the ideal state. Clinical data can be used to learn what works, identify where challenges exist, and serve as the foundation for continuous quality improvement efforts. While the ideal state initially will be based on the available literature, the shared experience of the team, combined with clinical data, can help to further refine what is considered the ideal state over time. Revisiting the clinical care model as a team approximately every 5–7 years appears helpful in extracting lessons learned, and deciding what to keep, modify, or trim to move closer to ideal care. This review should include all elements of the care model, from composition and timing of visits to the clinical data captured and used for individual patient and program monitoring, with a focus on improving both efficiency (e.g., scheduling, documentation, templated resources, scripted language) and effectiveness (e.g., clinical data collection changes, assessment/treatment offerings, timing/order of interventions). These moments of reflection and realignment, if done thoughtfully and with respect for all voices, can serve to energize and empower team members, while also amplifying value to the youth and family. In this way, a program's ideal state may continue to evolve with the increased lived experience and shared expertise of the integrated multidisciplinary team.

Pearls of wisdom

- It is critical to get the right people on board even if you have to wait, as shared vision and collaborative spirit among all team members are key to success.
- A hard reset with new players is going to be easier to accomplish than trying to shift an existing culture with the same staff.
- Selling your shared vision, coming to agreement on your business plan, and maintaining ongoing communication with administration related to your program benchmarks are critical in supporting transition from the current to the ideal state.

Summary

The biopsychosocial model provides a theoretical foundation for shifting toward a more collaborative, multidisciplinary approach to care in pediatric GI conditions. However, such integration in clinical practice is not without challenges and leads many providers to embrace a functionally unidisciplinary or dualistic approach to care. Launching a truly integrated multidisciplinary program requires more than adding resources to an existing standard of care. As outlined in this chapter, a truly integrated multidisciplinary program requires: (1) a cultural shift and fundamental rethinking from the ground up – putting the patient, their condition, and the modifiable factors that have the potential to influence health outcomes at the center of the care model, (2) putting people with the right skills and the right attitude together in a team and empowering them to work together rather than in parallel, (3) selling a vision of possibility to administrative partners while accepting accountability for outcomes and finances, and (4) maintaining engagement and investment of all parties to evolve from a starting point toward the ideal. Ultimately, it takes vision and planning, as well as patience and persistence, to make the ideal of integrated multidisciplinary care for pediatric GI conditions a sustainable reality.

Recommended readings

For youth and caregivers:

- Caring for the whole child: physical, mental, emotional, and social aspects can all play a role in abdominal pain, constipation, and other common GI concerns. Often there are biological factors (like inflammation, hypersensitivity, and gut flora), psychological factors (like mood, anxiety, and sleep problems), and social factors (like relationships with family members and peers or problems at school) that contribute to the problem. Treating just one area at a time may not be effective, but when we take a combined approach to care, the majority of families report significant improvement in their child's condition (text published at: https://www.childrensmercy.org/departments-and-clinics/gastroenterology/ Copyright Schurman and Friesen).

For mental health professionals:

- Reed, B., Buzenski, J, van Tilburg, M.A.L. (2020). Implementing psychological therapies for gastrointestinal disorders in pediatrics. *Expert Review of Gastroenterol & Hepatology, 14*(11): 1061–1067.
- Lamparyk, K., Debeljak, A., Aylward, L., & Mahajan, L. (2018). Impact of integrated care in a pediatric gastroenterology clinic on psychology utilization. *Clinical Practice in Pediatric Psychology, 6*(1), 51–60.

- Schurman, J. V., & Friesen, C. A. (2010). Integrative treatment approaches: Family satisfaction with a multidisciplinary paediatric Abdominal Pain Clinic. *International Journal of Integrated Care, 10*, 1–9.

References

1. Daniel H, Bornstein SS, Kane GC, Health and Public Policy Committee of the American College of Physicians. Addressing social determinants to improve patient care and promote health equity: An American College of Physicians position paper. *Ann Intern Med.* 2018;168(8):577–8.
2. Armstrong FD. Individual and organizational collaborations: A roadmap for effective advocacy. In M. C. Roberts & R. G. Steele (Eds.), *Handbook of pediatric psychology* (pp. 774–784). The Guilford Press.
3. Cushing CC, Friesen CA, Schurman JV. Collaboration with medical professionals in clinical practice: Pediatric abdominal pain as a case example. *Families, Systems, & Health.* 2012;30(4):279.
4. Schurman JV, Friesen CA. Integrative treatment approaches: Family satisfaction with a multidisciplinary paediatric Abdominal Pain Clinic. *Int J Integr Care.* 2010;10:e51.
5. Mikocka-Walus A, Turnbull D, Andrews JM, Moulding N, Wilson I, Holtmann G. Psychogastroenterology: A call for psychological input in Australian gastroenterology clinics. *Intern Med J.* 2009;39(2):127–30.
6. Lamparyk K, Debeljak A, Aylward L, Mahajan L. Impact of integrated care in a pediatric gastroenterology clinic on psychology utilization. *Clinical Practice in Pediatric Psychology.* 2018;6(1):51.
7. Schurman JV, Friesen CA. Leveraging institutional support to build an integrated multidisciplinary care model in pediatric inflammatory bowel disease. *Children.* 2021;8(4):286.
8. Coburn S, Rose M, Sady M, Parker M, Suslovic W, Weisbrod V, et al. Mental health disorders and psychosocial distress in pediatric celiac disease. *J Pediatr Gastroenterol Nutr.* 2020;70(5):608–14.
9. Harris RF, Menard-Katcher C, Atkins D, Furuta GT, Klinnert MD. Psychosocial dysfunction in children and adolescents with eosinophilic esophagitis. *J Pediatr Gastroenterol Nutr.* 2013;57(4):500–5.
10. Lukens CT, Silverman AH. Systematic review of psychological interventions for pediatric feeding problems. *J Pediatr Psychol.* 2014;39(8):903–17.
11. MacKner LM, Greenley RN, Szigethy E, Herzer M, Deer K, Hommel KA. Psychosocial issues in pediatric inflammatory bowel disease: Report of the north american society for pediatric gastroenterology, hepatology, and nutrition. *J Pediatr Gastroenterol Nutr.* 2013;56:449–58.
12. Newton E, Schosheim A, Patel S, Chitkara DK, van Tilburg MA. The role of psychological factors in pediatric functional abdominal pain disorders. *Neurogastroenterology & Motility.* 2019;31(6):e13538.
13. Chu AS, Torres L, Kao G, Gilbert C, Monico EC, Chumpitazi BP. Multidisciplinary care for refractory pediatric functional abdominal pain decreases emergency and inpatient utilization. *J Pediatr Gastroenterol Nutr.* 2022;74(2):248–52.
14. Isaac DM, Wu J, Mager DR, Turner JM. Managing the pediatric patient with celiac disease: A multidisciplinary approach. *J Multidiscip Healthc.* 2016:529–36.
15. Merras-Salmio L, Pakarinen MP. Refined multidisciplinary protocol-based approach to short bowel syndrome improves outcomes. **J** *Pediatr Gastroenterol Nutr.* 2015;61(1):24–9.
16. Sauer BG, West A, McGowan EC. Multidisciplinary eosinophilic esophagitis care: A model for comprehensive patient-centered care through shared decision making between gastroenterology, allergy, and nutrition. *Clin Gastroenterol Hepatol.* 2021;19(11):2226–9.
17. Sharp WG, Volkert VM, Scahill L, McCracken CE, McElhanon B. A systematic review and meta-analysis of intensive multidisciplinary intervention for pediatric feeding disorders: How standard is the standard of care? *J Pediatr.* 2017;181:116–24. e4.
18. Wren AA, Maddux MH. *Integrated multidisciplinary treatment for pediatric inflammatory bowel disease.* MDPI; 2021. p. 169.

Chapter 8

Working with parents and primary caregivers

Kari Freeman Baber and Kelly A. O'Neil Rodriguez

Chapter aims

This chapter explains the essential role of parents and primary caregivers in treating pediatric gastrointestinal (GI) conditions and describes how GI mental health professionals can partner with caregivers to promote youth's adherence, adaptive coping, and daily functioning.

Learning points

- Adjustment to pediatric GI conditions occurs within the family system.
- Social learning, cognitive behavioral theories, and existing research inform caregiving practices that promote health and resilience for youth living with GI conditions.
- Integrating caregivers in GI condition treatment is an essential aspect of pediatric psychogastroenterology care.

Caregivers as essential partners in care

Caregivers are essential partners in pediatric GI condition management. They are typically the first observers of youth's symptoms, guide youth's healthcare utilization, and play a necessary role in condition management until youth capably transition to self-management. Moreover, the biopsychosocial conceptualization (see Chapter 2) recognizes that caregivers shape the social environment in which GI symptoms and management occur. Several decades' worth of research based on ecological systems theory [1] and social learning theory [2] describe the impact of parents' physical and psychological well-being, beliefs, and parenting responses on youth's health, particularly chronic pain [3].

The pediatric chronic pain literature and the emerging evidence base within pediatric GI illness suggest that caregivers' responses are important targets of psychological treatment for pediatric GI conditions [4, 5]. The growing evidence base for pediatric psychogastroenterology practice reflects these considerations. All published, randomized controlled trials of cognitive behavior therapy (CBT) and more than half of the published trials of hypnotherapy for functional abdominal pain (FAP) have included parents in the intervention [6], with at least one intervention trial providing treatment only to parents of affected youth [7]. Similarly, inflammatory bowel disease (IBD)-specific CBT protocols have included sessions uniquely designed for parents and caregivers [8]. Treatment protocols' inclusion of caregivers reflects both the practical reality of pediatric healthcare and the biopsychosocial conceptualization of GI illness. Accordingly, pediatric GI mental health professionals must be prepared to work with caregivers.

DOI: 10.4324/9781003308683-9

Collaborating with caregivers

Caregivers are often most effectively engaged when GI mental health professionals establish a collaborative relationship to which all parties bring distinct and essential expertise. GI mental health professionals must first assess how caregivers understand their children's diagnosis and management. Learning about caregivers' understanding of youth's GI conditions builds rapport and identifies whether families may benefit from additional diagnosis-specific education. In some cases, diagnosis and treatment knowledge may directly impact outcomes of psychological treatment; for example, a recent systematic review indicated that parental knowledge of celiac disease and dietary treatment guidelines is associated with increased dietary adherence [9].

Education may also facilitate shared treatment goals, and this may be especially true for youth living with disorders of gut–brain interaction (DGBI). In a prospective study, parents' chronic pain knowledge and awareness of the biopsychosocial model were positively correlated with expectations for treatment effectiveness in a subspecialty program for FAP [10]. GI mental health professionals must not assume that caregivers have received adequate education prior to referral. A recent systematic review concluded that parents' difficulty in obtaining adequate information about functional constipation and its management is a common source of frustration [11].

While education about GI condition management should be conveyed by medical providers who can answer subsequent questions, GI mental health professionals should expect to serve as the primary educators about psychogastroenterology care, including the purpose and goals of treatment focused on youth's GI symptoms and associated impairment [12]. GI mental health professionals must provide clear, ongoing communication to help caregivers participate effectively in their children's care, beginning with establishing treatment goals and developing a shared biopsychosocial conceptualization. Many families have had limited experience with behavioral healthcare, and even psychologically minded caregivers may be unfamiliar with problem-focused, skill-based treatments typically applied in healthcare settings. While discussing treatment goals within the biopsychosocial framework, GI mental health professionals can begin to highlight how caregivers can help by serving as coaches for youth's GI condition management (see Handout 8.1).

GI mental health professionals are urged to develop culturally responsive conceptualizations so that treatment strategies can be appropriately tailored to caregivers' and families' cultural norms. At the broadest level, caregivers' unique cultural identities and backgrounds may influence their experiences within the healthcare system. Within the family system, cultural identity may shape expectations for caregiving practices and child development (e.g., the age at which caregivers expect children to assume GI condition self-management). Finally, individuals' and family's cultural backgrounds may shape their specific goals for GI condition management and psychogastroenterology care. GI mental health professionals are encouraged to directly assess and incorporate the family's cultural context to inform appropriate intervention strategies. For example, instead of assuming that all caregiving adults in a family will accept and apply a specific behavioral strategy, GI mental health professionals are encouraged to ask about the family's expected roles for caregiving adults; this may be particularly relevant for youth living in multigenerational households including grandparents or other older adults. In order to facilitate culturally responsive psychogastroenterology care, GI mental health professionals are encouraged to inquire directly about the family's caregiving norms and expectations throughout care.

In healthy family systems, caregiver involvement changes over time: while the youngest children are entirely reliant on caregivers to seek and participate in medical evaluation and management, older children typically become increasingly independent in their healthcare. This chapter describes general principles for engaging caregivers as partners in care across three aspects of GI condition management (adherence, coping, daily functioning) based on youth's developmental stage. Throughout, we identify caregiving strategies for infants (<2 years) and toddlers (aged 2–3 years), children (aged 4–9 years), and adolescents (aged 10 and older), while acknowledging that developmental capacity varies even within these general groupings.

Helping caregivers promote adherence

GI condition management varies by diagnosis and disease status and may involve daily or as-needed oral medications, dietary modifications, periodic infusions or injections, routine/monitoring labs, clinic visits, and diagnostic tests and procedures (see Chapters 3 and 4). Engaging in recommended treatments and other healthcare responsibilities can be time-consuming, financially burdensome, and anxiety-provoking for youth and their caregivers. Treatment nonadherence in pediatric GI conditions is highly prevalent, including IBD [13], celiac disease [9], and functional constipation [14]. Chapter 20 describes risk and protective factors related to adherence and disease self-management, which include developmental factors. For example, adolescents with IBD [15] and with celiac disease [16] demonstrate poorer treatment adherence than younger children. However, among adolescents with IBD, greater parental involvement is associated with better medication adherence [17], particularly when family support is balanced with youth involvement [18, 19]. GI mental health professionals can help families identify the appropriate division of healthcare responsibilities based on youth's development and individual mastery [20].

Evidence-based collaboration to promote adherence

There is evidence to support family-based problem-solving skills training [21] and multicomponent adherence intervention in pediatric IBD [22]. Other practical strategies include education (e.g., about the goals of treatment and results of treatment nonadherence), self-monitoring (e.g., tracking medication administration or diet), behavioral strategies (e.g., reminder systems, structured positive reinforcement systems, behavioral contracts), and goal-setting related to specific adherence tasks and promoting adaptive family functioning [21, 23]. Applications vary across development, and examples are described below.

Infants/toddlers

In early childhood, caregivers may be entirely responsible for treatment adherence. GI mental health professionals should facilitate caregivers' appropriate education on the GI condition and treatment and suggest behavioral strategies to support caregiver symptom monitoring and adherence. For example, in cases that involve constipation, GI mental health professionals should provide caregivers of preschool-aged children education about the constipation-withholding cycle (see Chapter 18) and recommend monitoring bowel patterns and medication administration with paper records or mobile apps, setting alarms as reminders to give medication, and positively reinforcing structured toilet sitting adherence.

Children

Beginning in middle childhood, GI mental health professionals should directly assess caregivers' understanding of appropriate healthcare tasks for their children and emphasize that readiness for healthcare responsibilities is based on children's demonstrated skills rather than age [20]. If caregivers express unrealistic expectations (e.g., that a 9-year-old should remember independently all daily medications), GI mental health professionals should normalize caregivers' desire to promote independence, discuss children's current abilities and introduce collaborative problem-solving (see Box 8.1, for example, dialogue supporting a 9-year-old in daily medication adherence).

BOX 8.1 SUPPORTING A 9-YEAR-OLD IN DAILY MEDICATION ADHERENCE

Caregiver: I don't know why she doesn't take her medicine every day – we've talked about it a thousand times!

GI mental health professional: It makes sense you want her to take her medicine on her own; there's so much for you to take care of each day. Most kids of her age aren't ready to remember daily medicines, either. Let's figure out a plan that works for your family, so she'll have some great experience with a consistent routine once she's ready for more independence.

GI mental health professionals may provide education and support for adherence monitoring, positive reinforcement, and problem-solving skills implemented by caregivers. They may also promote adaptive family functioning by enhancing communication skills or family support. For example, GI mental health professionals working with caregivers of school-aged children with celiac disease may offer gluten-free diet education, recommend caregiver adherence monitoring paired with a token economy for children, offer family-based problem-solving skills training focused on social eating situations, or connect caregivers to support groups. See Handout 8.2 for "My coaching plan" to support family-based problem-solving.

Adolescents

Although many adolescents will appropriately take on increasing healthcare responsibilities consistent with growing developmental autonomy, GI mental health professionals should emphasize continued caregiver involvement, as the risk of nonadherence increases during adolescence. GI mental health professionals should encourage ongoing discussions about adolescents' preferences for caregiver involvement. Older adolescents and their families may benefit more than younger adolescents from problem-solving skills training for medication adherence [24], and this may be a primary strategy to introduce. For example, GI mental health professionals may provide problem-solving skills training focused on adolescent and caregiver roles in using a reminder system, goal-setting, and behavioral contracting.

Helping caregivers promote adaptive coping

Families experience a variety of stressors associated with GI symptoms and condition management. Youth with some GI conditions (e.g., IBD or cyclic vomiting syndrome) may experience periods of quiescence, while others experience symptoms relatively constantly, particularly when visceral hypersensitivity is present. Symptoms and medical evaluation may be stressful, and treatments prescribed for GI condition management can be challenging for families to implement. GI symptom-related anxiety, comorbid anxiety disorders or depression, and activity limitations pose additional burdens [5, 25]. Because of these inherent stressors, there have been many attempts to describe and differentiate adaptive coping strategies from maladaptive coping strategies in the context of chronic pain or illness management. Active and accommodative coping strategies (e.g., seeking social support, problem-solving, using relaxation strategies, engaging in distraction, acceptance) are generally associated with improved functioning among youth with chronic pain [26, 27]. In contrast, parental catastrophizing and protective responding are generally associated with maladjustment [4, 5]. Parents often respond protectively to their child's GI symptoms because they want to be empathic/supportive and/or overestimate the potential harm of the GI symptoms. The GI mental health professional should educate caregivers about the long-term benefits of encouraging youth to use active and accommodative coping strategies and shifting their own attention from symptoms and related anxiety to coping and wellness behaviors. It is important to realize this may be difficult for some parents who may associate protectiveness with "being a good parent". These families need additional support to journey from shifting focus away from illness and toward wellness.

Caregiver catastrophizing and protection

Parental catastrophizing may include predictions that the youth's symptoms or conditions will persist, be unmanageable, have catastrophic consequences, or make typical activities impossible. GI-related protection may include expecting less participation in family or other activities when youth are experiencing GI symptoms or engaging in unnecessary accommodations. For example, in celiac disease, protection may include avoiding meals outside the home rather than paying appropriate attention to choosing gluten-free foods across settings. Recent reviews describe consistent evidence that parental catastrophizing about children's pain and protective responding are associated with increased disability [4, 5, 28]. While there are fewer published studies specific to pediatric GI symptoms and findings have been mixed [29], parents' self-reported protectiveness has been associated with increased pain and disability in some samples of children with FAP [30]. Promisingly, decreases in parental catastrophizing following CBT for FAP have been associated with improvement in children's symptoms [31], and results of an experimental study indicated that parental distraction from (vs. attention to) symptoms resulted in decreased discomfort [32]. GI mental health professionals are encouraged to validate and normalize parental inclinations toward protection while also providing guidance about evidence-based, adaptive caregiving responses.

Evidence-based collaboration to promote adaptive coping

Adaptive coping strategies help youth to engage in their daily activities despite their chronic GI illness or symptoms. Evidence-informed treatment protocols for youth with GI conditions have tended to emphasize skills training for relaxation, distraction, and cognitive restructuring focused on pain and GI symptoms [6]. Naturalistic observations align with these protocols. For example, a qualitative analysis by Easterlin and colleagues [33] involving interviews with 18 adolescents with IBD in remission and their caregivers indicated that families derive benefit from a similar set of strategies (positive social support, cognitive strategies for managing emotions, and behavioral strategies for managing pain and anxiety) without undergoing any educational or psychotherapeutic intervention.

Infants and toddlers

GI mental health professionals should encourage caregivers of very young children to model adaptive coping by labeling stressors and their emotional responses and then verbalizing their chosen coping strategies. When caregivers are experiencing significant distress related to children's GI condition, GI mental health professionals may initially ask caregivers to model adaptive coping with stressors that elicit a more manageable emotional response. Ideally, GI mental health professionals can support caregivers to comfortably use this strategy when children are observing GI-related stress, for example "I forgot to give you your medicine before breakfast, so I'm going to set an alarm to remind us to take it before lunch".

Caregivers also can be effective coping coaches by helping their children with the daily practice of relaxation strategies introduced in treatment. Once children demonstrate mastery of a relaxation strategy, caregivers can coach them to use it in response to symptoms or other stressors. This can be especially helpful for caregivers who are inclined toward protection in response to symptoms: rather than reduce demands when children experience discomfort, caregivers can encourage them to use a relaxation strategy or another coping strategy, like distraction. Caregivers should be encouraged to offer praise and immediate positive reinforcement whenever their children exhibit adaptive coping (e.g., "I know you're hurting; you're doing a great job practicing your deep breathing right now"). Young children may be particularly interested in making a "coping kit" – a collection of supports for distraction or soothing – and caregivers can provide practical help and guidance. Some children may also benefit from a sticker chart or simple token economy to provide intermittent, tangible reinforcement for employing adaptive coping strategies.

Children

As children age and become increasingly capable of meta-cognition, they also become more capable of cognitive restructuring focused on GI symptoms and management. GI mental health professionals should encourage caregivers to notice how children describe their symptoms and concerns about condition management between visits. Caregivers can support skill development by helping children notice negative automatic thoughts about symptoms or condition management and then learning skills for cognitive restructuring alongside their children. Caregiver engagement in cognitive restructuring exercises during treatment sessions can also facilitate direct education about catastrophizing as a thinking pattern that tends to increase distress and disability. GI mental health professionals may eventually ask caregivers to support children in applying cognitive restructuring between visits. Children also tend to become more effective partners in collaborative problem-solving during middle childhood.

GI mental health professionals should introduce this skill and facilitate practice in sessions. By providing education and guidance to caregivers during each step of the problem-solving process, GI mental health professionals can support generalization to problems that arise between visits or after treatment ends. Handout 8.2 ("My coaching plan") can support family-based problem-solving and identify specific caregiving behaviors to support adaptive coping.

Adolescents

Adolescents' developmentally appropriate desire for autonomy warrants changes in how caregivers support adaptive coping. Caregivers must be prepared to allow their adolescents to become increasingly independent in coping. Many adolescents describe using smartphone apps for relaxation and distraction. This can create tension with caregivers who perceive their children to be avoiding responsibilities or otherwise "wasting time". GI mental health professionals can support caregivers by guiding a shared functional analysis: if brief use of a smartphone allows the adolescent to cope effectively in ways that facilitate positive adjustment (e.g., distract from pain or nausea or get labs drawn), the GI mental health professional may wish to reinforce how effectively the adolescent is transitioning toward self-management. GI mental health professionals can also suggest apps that include evidence-based strategies for coping with GI symptoms; demonstrating app-based relaxation in treatment sessions may also result in improved acceptability to caregivers.

Caregivers of adolescents may be less aware of the social implications of their children's symptoms or GI condition management as adolescents' socializing is increasingly focused on peer relationships. Caregivers and adolescents may also have different coping goals; for example, caregivers may think it is more essential for adolescents to manage symptoms during the early morning to facilitate timely school arrival, while adolescents may be more concerned with symptom management during the times when peers are socializing.

GI mental health professionals should encourage caregivers to maintain a supportive and validating tone when their children disclose stressors associated with their GI symptoms or management. Caregivers who tend to minimize their adolescents' distress may benefit from education about the importance of a supportive, validating stance. Caregivers should also be encouraged to maintain an open dialogue with adolescents and to provide occasional reminders that they are prepared to support coping strategy use.

Helping caregivers promote daily functioning

Health-related quality of life is negatively affected in pediatric GI conditions (see Chapter 20). Avoidance of daily activities can increase disability and pain severity [34]. Focusing on functional goals and graded engagement in usual daily activities promotes long-term recovery. Additionally, there is evidence that improved daily functioning precedes pain reduction in multidisciplinary treatment for pediatric abdominal pain [35], which offers a compelling rationale for caregivers to prioritize functional goals.

Evidence-based collaboration to promote functioning

There is evidence for cognitive behavioral interventions to promote adaptive functioning with pediatric GI conditions including DGBI [36] and IBD [37] (see Chapters 16 and 20). CBT for chronic GI conditions typically includes psychoeducation, relaxation training, cognitive restructuring, problem-solving skills training, graded engagement/exposure, and caregiver support/training [6, 36, 38]. GI mental health professionals should provide psychoeducation to help caregivers understand the rationale for a focus on daily functioning despite GI symptoms, as well as caregivers' critical roles in supporting children to participate in daily activities and graded engagement/exposure.

Caregivers who demonstrate protective responding appear to be at an increased risk for miscarried helping [39]. "Miscarried helping" is a maladaptive, dynamic process that can occur in pediatric chronic health conditions, whereby a caregiver's early responsibility to help with managing the condition or its symptoms can inadvertently contribute to negative caregiver–child interactions and poor adjustment as caregiver demands child involvement increase and children resist to assert autonomy [40]. Hypervigilance to their children's symptoms and excessive inquiries about – or monitoring of – GI symptoms can also reflect overly protective caregiving.

There is evidence that internet-delivered CBT for adolescents with chronic pain and their parents can reduce parental miscarried helping and protective behaviors [41]. GI mental health professionals may find it helpful to normalize and validate caregivers' protective responses before asking them to partner on taking a different approach (see Box 8.2).

BOX 8.2 ADDRESSING PARENTAL OVERPROTECTION

Caregiver: It's so hard to tell him he needs to get out of bed and go to school when he always feels so terrible in the morning.

GI mental health professional: Of course, that's hard. When he's sick with flu, staying home in bed might be exactly the right thing – he has a contagious illness and his body needs rest to recover, and that feeling of nausea may be an accurate sign that he's going to vomit. However, the approach that's right for an acute illness doesn't work as well for chronic illness. Resting doesn't make his nausea any better and has so many downsides. Staying in bed prevents him from getting to school and being eligible for extracurricular activities. His care team also believes that getting moving in the mornings would help him feel better. Would you be willing to consider another approach?

Early childhood

Although preschool-aged children likely have fewer out-of-home activities that may be missed due to their chronic GI condition, there are still critically important aspects of physical, emotional, and social development that can be negatively affected by symptoms and treatment. Additionally, caregivers of young children are likely more influential than caregivers of older children or adolescents in modeling responses to illness [3]. GI mental health professionals should educate caregivers about the importance of encouraging children's participation in daily activities that support healthy early childhood development (e.g., independent play, peer interactions, and growing independence in routines of sleep, eating, and toileting). GI mental health professionals should offer psychoeducation and training regarding caregivers' roles in encouraging daily activities and graded engagement/exposure. For example, in collaborating with a caregiver of a preschool-aged child with very early onset IBD who slept independently from caregivers until an extended hospitalization, the GI mental health professional may first normalize a post-discharge regression in sleep routines in the context of an acute medical situation, then assess the family's interest and values around returning to independent sleep, and finally collaborate with the family to develop an acceptable plan for graded engagement including gradual exposure with positive reinforcement for brave behavior.

Middle childhood

GI mental health professionals working with caregivers of slightly older children should provide psychoeducation about normal developmental changes that impact caregivers' roles in supporting children's daily activities. Extracurricular and other social activities outside the home become increasingly rewarding during middle childhood. At the same time, caregivers

– especially those who catastrophize – may have difficulty supporting youth to engage in these activities. For example, in working with caregivers of school-aged children with irritable bowel syndrome who have limited social activities due to symptoms, GI mental health professionals may educate caregivers about the rationale for focusing on functioning and rehearse adaptive responses to symptoms in ways that support de-catastrophizing (e.g., "I know your belly is bothering you, and I know you'll be able to use your coping plan to stay at the party").

Adolescence

Adolescents are moving toward greater autonomy and less parental input, but parental responses and behaviors continue to influence symptoms and daily functioning well into adolescence [41]. Thus, caregivers continue to have an important role in promoting adaptive functioning, although perhaps primarily through modeling of adaptive coping and support for graded engagement. For example, in working with caregivers of adolescents with eosinophilic esophagitis who avoid eating outside of the home due to dietary restrictions and related anxiety, GI mental health professionals may educate caregivers about how to model coping with illness-specific anxiety and how to support teenagers with graded engagement (e.g., first facilitate eating at extended family members' homes, next in a restaurant with family, then at peers' homes or with peers at a restaurant).

Supporting effective family-provider communication

GI mental health professionals should empower and support caregivers to communicate with their children's medical teams about barriers to treatment adherence, adaptive coping, and age-appropriate daily functioning. GI mental health professionals may support caregivers in problem-solving, defining specific barrier(s) to communicate with the care team, and behavioral rehearsal of effective communication strategies. It may be helpful for GI mental health professionals to facilitate coordination between the healthcare team and schools or community agencies to address barriers. When language or cultural differences are present, GI mental health professionals should also support families' access to medical interpreters for all communication with the medical team (e.g., office visits, telephone calls) and support medical colleagues in culturally responsive care.

When caregivers need more care

Caregivers may have difficulty effectively engaging in their children's care because of their own healthcare or other needs. When these needs are unmet, resulting caregiver stress may mutually exacerbate youth stress and illness, negatively impacting adherence, coping, and functioning. Parents of youth with GI conditions are more likely than parents of healthy children to have their own chronic illnesses and to experience anxiety, depression, somatic symptoms [5, 25], and parenting stress [42]. They also may be balancing multiple caregiving demands, including the needs of healthy siblings who are also at risk for emotional and behavioral challenges [43]. Caring for children with chronic illnesses, including GI conditions, can also create strains on employment with associated impacts on financial stability [44]. When caregivers' competing demands interfere with effective treatment for the target GI symptoms and associated impairment, GI mental health professionals should offer empathy, normalize the need for additional support, and provide referrals or other resources when possible.

Caregivers who lack social support related to youth's chronic illness management may benefit from referral to support groups or group interventions, some of which are accessible online [45, 46]. Caregivers who are experiencing significant mental health concerns should be referred for appropriate treatment. Caregivers who describe significant family conflict or who are unable to provide developmentally appropriate support or autonomy for their children with GI conditions may need family therapy, which is distinct from engaging caregivers as coping coaches in psychogastroenterology care. Finally, GI mental health professionals may need to work with colleagues or community partners to help caregivers access practical resources (e.g., financial assistance). GI mental health professionals are encouraged to clearly communicate to caregivers that pursuing such additional resources may make them even more effective in supporting their children with GI conditions.

Pearls of wisdom

- Caregivers need to be involved in their child's psychogastroenterology care – this aligns with the pediatric healthcare model and is supported by the growing evidence base. Invite caregivers to be active partners in psychogastroenterology care and be direct in communicating their role in treatment.
- Establishing effective collaboration often begins with validating caregivers' experience related to their child's GI condition. Keep in mind how difficult it may be for caregivers to witness their children experiencing physical and/or emotional discomfort.
- Be curious about caregivers. Consider how their upbringing and their own experiences with the healthcare system may impact their experience of their children's care and their responses and expectations for their children. Consider these factors in your biopsychosocial conceptualization and tailor evidence-based strategies accordingly.
- Just as youth with GI conditions benefit from developmentally appropriate education (including simpler terms or analogies), caregivers are likely to appreciate language that recognizes their expertise and knowledge, including about their child's GI condition.
- Using medical terms appropriately and matching the caregivers' language reinforces the GI mental health professional's role as a knowledgeable member of the healthcare team and may lead to increased buy-in for psychogastroenterology care.

Summary

Caregivers are essential members of the healthcare team for youth with GI conditions. Caregivers' responses to youth's GI conditions impact youth adjustment and GI condition management. Therefore, caregiver cognitions and behaviors are appropriate targets for education and intervention. Collaborative partnership empowers caregivers to supplement their existing expertise and caregiving practices with evidence-based strategies for GI condition management. Caregivers may benefit from education and support to apply developmentally appropriate strategies to promote adherence, adaptive coping, and age-appropriate daily functioning.

Recommended readings

For youth and caregivers:

- Coakley, R. (2016). *When your child hurts: effective strategies to increase comfort, reduce stress, and break the cycle of chronic pain.* Yale University Press.

- Oliva-Hemker, M., Ziring, D., Saeed, S.A., Bousvaros, A. (2017). *Your child with inflammatory bowel disease: A family guide for caregiving*. JHU Press.
- Palermo, T.M., Law, E.F. (2015). *Managing your child's chronic pain.* Oxford University Press.
- Sileo, F.J., Potter, C.S. (2021). *When Your Child Has a Chronic Medical Illness: A Guide for the Parenting Journey*. American Psychological Association.

For mental health professionals:

- Palermo, T.M. (2012). *Cognitive-behavioral therapy for chronic pain in children and adolescents*. Oxford University Press.

References

1. Bronfenbrenner U. *The ecology of human development: Experiments by nature and design*. Harvard University Press; 1979.
2. Bandura A, Walters RH. *Social learning theory*. Prentice Hall; 1977.
3. Palermo TM, Valrie CR, Karlson CW. Family and parent influences on pediatric chronic pain: A developmental perspective. *American Psychologist*. 2014;69(2):142.
4. Donnelly TJ, Palermo TM, Newton-John TR. Parent cognitive, behavioural, and affective factors and their relation to child pain and functioning in pediatric chronic pain: A systematic review and meta-analysis. *Pain*. 2020;161(7):1401–19.
5. Newton E, Schosheim A, Patel S, Chitkara DK, van Tilburg MA. The role of psychological factors in pediatric functional abdominal pain disorders. *Neurogastroenterology & Motility*. 2019;31(6):e13538.
6. Abbott RA, Martin AE, Newlove-Delgado TV, Bethel A, Thompson-Coon J, Whear R, et al. Psychosocial interventions for recurrent abdominal pain in childhood. *Cochrane Database Syst Rev*. 2017(1).
7. Levy RL, Langer SL, Van Tilburg MA, Romano JM, Murphy TB, Walker LS, et al. Brief telephone-delivered cognitive-behavioral therapy targeted to parents of children with functional abdominal pain: A randomized controlled trial. *Pain*. 2017;158(4):618.
8. Stapersma L, van den Brink G, van der Ende J, Szigethy EM, Groeneweg M, de Bruijne FH, et al. Psychological outcomes of a cognitive behavioral therapy for youth with inflammatory bowel disease: Results of the HAPPY-IBD randomized controlled trial at 6-and 12-month follow-up. *J Clin Psychol Med Settings*. 2020;27:490–506.
9. Myléus A, Reilly NR, Green PH. Rate, risk factors, and outcomes of nonadherence in pediatric patients with celiac disease: A systematic review. *Clin Gastroenterol Hepatol*. 2020;18(3):562–73.
10. Hale AE, Smith AM, Christiana JS, Burch E, Schechter NL, Beinvogl BC, et al. Perceptions of pain treatment in pediatric patients with functional gastrointestinal disorders. *Clin J Pain*. 2020;36(7):550–7.
11. Thompson AP, Wine E, MacDonald SE, Campbell A, Scott SD. Parents' experiences and information needs while caring for a child with functional constipation: A systematic review. *Clin Pediatr*. 2021;60(3):154–69.
12. van Tilburg MA. Psychogastroenterology: A Cure, Band-Aid, or Prevention? *Children*. 2020;7(9):121.
13. Spekhorst LM, Hummel TZ, Benninga MA, van Rheenen PF, Kindermann A. Adherence to oral maintenance treatment in adolescents with inflammatory bowel disease. *J Pediatr Gastroenterol Nutr*. 2016;62(2):264–70.
14. Koppen IJN, van Wassenaer EA, Barendsen RW, Brand PL, Benninga MA. Adherence to polyethylene glycol treatment in children with functional constipation is associated with parental

illness perceptions, satisfaction with treatment, and perceived treatment convenience. *J Pediatr.* 2018;199:132–9. e1.
15. LeLeiko NS, Lobato D, Hagin S, McQuaid E, Seifer R, Kopel SJ, et al. Rates and predictors of oral medication adherence in pediatric patients with IBD. *Inflamm Bowel Dis.* 2013;19(4):832–9.
16. Mager DR, Marcon M, Brill H, Liu A, Radmanovich K, Mileski H, et al. Adherence to the gluten-free diet and health-related quality of life in an ethnically diverse pediatric population with celiac disease. *J Pediatr Gastroenterol Nutr.* 2018;66(6):941–8.
17. Reed-Knight B, Lewis JD, Blount RL. Association of disease, adolescent, and family factors with medication adherence in pediatric inflammatory bowel disease. *J Pediatr Psychol.* 2011;36(3):308–17.
18. Feldman EC, Durkin LK, Greenley RN. Family support is associated with fewer adherence barriers and greater intent to adhere to oral medications in pediatric ibd. *J Pediatr Nurs.* 2021;60:58–64.
19. Greenley RN, Kunz JH, Biank V, Martinez A, Miranda A, Noe J, et al. Identifying youth nonadherence in clinical settings: Data-based recommendations for children and adolescents with inflammatory bowel disease. *Inflamm Bowel Dis.* 2012;18(7):1254–9.
20. Reed-Knight B, Blount RL, Gilleland J. The transition of health care responsibility from parents to youth diagnosed with chronic illness: A developmental systems perspective. *Families, Systems, & Health.* 2014;32(2):219.
21. Greenley RN, Kunz JH, Walter J, Hommel KA. Practical strategies for enhancing adherence to treatment regimen in inflammatory bowel disease. *Inflamm Bowel Dis.* 2013;19:1534–45.
22. Maddux M, Ricks S, Delurgio S, Hommel K. A pilot study evaluating the impact of an adherence-promoting intervention among nonadherent youth with inflammatory bowel disease. *J Pediatr Nurs.* 2017;35:72–7.
23. Holbein CE, Carmody JK, Hommel KA. Topical Review: Adherence Interventions for Youth on Gluten-Free Diets. *J Pediatr Psychol.* 2018:392–401.
24. Greenley RN, Gumidyala AP, Nguyen E, Plevinsky JM, Poulopoulos N, Thomason MM, et al. Can You Teach a Teen New Tricks? Problem Solving Skills Training Improves Oral Medication Adherence in Pediatric Patients with Inflammatory Bowel Disease Participating in a Randomized Trial. *Inflamm Bowel Dis.* 2015;21(11):2649–57.
25. Cushman G, Shih S, Reed B. Parent and family functioning in pediatric inflammatory bowel disease. *Children*:2020;7(10) :188.
26. Claar RL, Baber KF, Simons LE, Logan DE, Walker LS. Pain coping profiles in adolescents with chronic pain. *Pain.* 2008;140(2):368–75.
27. Walker LS, Baber KF, Garber J, Smith CA. A typology of pain coping strategies in pediatric patients with chronic abdominal pain. *Pain.* 2008;137(2):266–75.
28. Harrison LE, Timmers I, Heathcote LC, Fisher E, Tanna V, Duarte Silva Bans T, et al. Parent responses to their child's pain: Systematic review and meta-analysis of measures. *J Pediatr Psychol.* 2020;45(3):281–98.
29. Van Der Veek SM, Derkx H, De Haan E, Benninga MA, Plak RD, Boer F. Do parents maintain or exacerbate pediatric functional abdominal pain? A systematic review and meta-analysis. *J Health Psychol.* 2012;17(2):258–72.
30. DuPen MM, Van Tilburg MA, Langer SL, Murphy TB, Romano JM, Levy RL. Parental protectiveness mediates the association between parent-perceived child self-efficacy and health outcomes in pediatric functional abdominal pain disorder. *Children.* 2016;3(3):15.
31. Levy RL, Langer SL, Romano JM, Labus J, Walker LS, Murphy TB, et al. Cognitive mediators of treatment outcomes in pediatric functional abdominal pain. *Clin J Pain.* 2014;30(12):1033.
32. Walker LS, Williams SE, Smith CA, Garber J, Van Slyke DA, Lipani TA. Parent attention versus distraction: Impact on symptom complaints by children with and without chronic functional abdominal pain. *Pain.* 2006;122(1–2):43–52.

33. Easterlin MC, Berdahl CT, Rabizadeh S, Spiegel B, Agoratus L, Hoover C, et al. Child and family perspectives on adjustment to and coping with pediatric inflammatory bowel disease. *J Pediatr Gastroenterol Nutr*. 2020;71(1):e16–e27.
34. Simons LE, Kaczynski KJ. The fear avoidance model of chronic pain: Examination for pediatric application. *J Pain*. 2012;13(9):827–35.
35. Beinvogl BC, Burch E, Snyder J, Schechter NL, Hale AE, Riley B, et al. Tu1779 Improved functioning precedes improvement of abdominal pain in pediatric patients with functional gastrointestinal disorders. *Gastroenterology*. 2020;158(6):S-1157.
36. Baber K, Rodriguez KAON. Cognitive behavioral therapy for functional abdominal pain disorders. *Handbook of cognitive behavioral therapy for pediatric medical conditions*. 2019:201–17.
37. Levy RL, Van Tilburg MAL, Langer SL, Romano JM, Walker LS, Mancl LA, et al. Effects of a cognitive behavioral therapy intervention trial to improve disease outcomes in children with inflammatory bowel disease. *Inflammatory Bowel Diseases*. 2016;22(9):2134–48.
38. Szigethy E, Weisz JR, Findling RL. *Cognitive-behavior therapy for children and adolescents*. American Psychiatric Pub;2012.
39. Fales JL, Essner BS, Harris MA, Palermo TM. When helping hurts: Miscarried helping in families of youth with chronic pain. *Journal of pediatric psychology*. 2014;39(4):427–37.
40. Anderson BJ, Coyne JC, editors. "Miscarried helping" in the families of children and adolescents with chronic diseases. An adaptation of this paper was presented at the National Institute of Child Health and Human Development Conference on Compliance to Health-Promoting Behavior in Children, Washington, DC, July 1989; 1991: University of Florida Press.
41. Palermo TM, Law EF, Fales J, Bromberg MH, Jessen-Fiddick T, Tai G. Internet-delivered cognitive-behavioral treatment for adolescents with chronic pain and their parents: A randomized controlled multicenter trial. *Pain*. 2016;157(1):174.
42. Judd-Glossy L, Ariefdjohan M, Ketzer J, Curry S, Schletker J, Edmonds T, et al. Analysis of patients' and caregivers' psychosocial functioning in colorectal conditions: Comparison of diagnosis, gender, and developmental functioning. *Pediatr Surg Int*. 2021;37:437–44.
43. Pinquart M. Behavior problems, self-esteem, and prosocial behavior in siblings of children with chronic physical health conditions: An updated meta-analysis. *J Pediatr Psychol*. 2023;48(1):77–90.
44. Stawowczyk E, Kawalec P, Kowalska-Duplaga K, Mossakowska M. Productivity loss among parents of children with inflammatory bowel diseases in relation to disease activity and patient's quality of life. *J Pediatr Gastroenterol Nutr*. 2020;71(3):340–5.
45. Coakley R, Wihak T, Kossowsky J, Iversen C, Donado C. The comfort ability pain management workshop: A preliminary, nonrandomized investigation of a brief, cognitive, biobehavioral, and parent training intervention for pediatric chronic pain. *J Pediatr Psychol*. 2018;43(3):252–65.
46. Douma M, Maurice-Stam H, Gorter B, Krol Y, Verkleij M, Wiltink L, et al. Online psychosocial group intervention for parents: Positive effects on anxiety and depression. *J Pediatr Psychol*. 2021;46(2):123–34.

Chapter 9

Caring for youth and families with complex medical and psychosocial concerns

Bradley Jerson and Amy E. Hale

Chapter aims

This chapter will review approaches for treating youth living with gastrointestinal (GI) conditions who present with complex medical and/or psychosocial variables that require adaptation of standard pediatric psychogastroenterology strategies. Identification of "complex" issues will be discussed, followed by recommendations for modifying treatment conceptualization and planning.

Learning points

- Adapt typical psychogastroenterology interventions for commonly encountered complexities, including medical and psychiatric comorbidities, which can attenuate treatment effectiveness.
- Navigate treatment resistance from youth, families, or other medical or community-based providers.
- Strengthen partnerships with youth living with GI conditions and their families through relationship building, improved communication, and collaborative problem-solving.

Common characteristics of complex cases

The work of a GI mental health professional is often rewarding, but treatment does not always proceed smoothly. In this chapter, common challenges faced when working with complexities in pediatric psychogastroenterology treatment, along with recommendations for navigating them, will be reviewed. The information that follows is designed to supplement and bolster the other chapters within this handbook, offering guidance for when the plan falls apart and/or the mental health professional simply feels stuck. First, common medical, psychological, and social comorbidities which can complicate treatment planning are reviewed. Next, common questions and misconceptions about treatment are highlighted. Finally, detailed recommendations are provided for navigating points of resistance or confusion when working with youth and their families, medical teams, and schools.

Diagnostic comorbidity

There are commonly seen diagnostic comorbidities which can complicate standard psychogastroenterology interventions when not sufficiently considered. The list that follows is not exhaustive

DOI: 10.4324/9781003308683-10

and only represents a small sampling of the possible comorbidities. It is strongly recommended to seek consultation with other medical team members or mental health professionals to learn more about specific comorbidities that may affect conceptualization and treatment planning. Additionally, the best approach is to always ask the youth and family directly how these may be influencing daily functioning and participation in treatment. Handout 9.1 outlines ways to recognize and respond when comorbidities impact treatment engagement.

GI-related comorbidities

Bowel urgency, pain, nausea, vomiting

For youth with underlying GI conditions (e.g., inflammatory bowel disease, celiac disease, eosinophilic esophagitis), gastroenterologists strive to address active GI symptomatology and also mucosal healing and histologic inflammation. What, then, is someone living with a GI condition to do when endoscopy and laboratory values come back "looking great", but they continue to experience bowel urgency, dysphagia, fatigue, or pain? Because those living with chronic GI disorders frequently also experience symptoms of disorders of gut–brain interaction (DGBI) [1], this frustrates families and providers alike. For irritable bowel syndrome (IBS), for example, there are numerous proposed mechanisms that may influence symptoms co-occurring with quiescent inflammatory bowel disease (IBD; e.g., visceral hypersensitivity, central sensitization, previous mucosal disruption and immune dysfunction, psychological distress, and autonomic nervous system (ANS) activation).

GI mental health professionals can support youth living with IBD by acknowledging gratitude for mucosal healing and histologic remission while simultaneously honoring frustration associated with functional impairments related to concurrent DGBI. Many families may also benefit from psychoeducation that comorbid IBD and DGBI are not only possible but common. This will additionally lead to increased motivation for youth participation in psychogastroenterology treatment to address ongoing GI symptoms. See Box 9.1 for a sample dialogue discussing refractory symptoms amid reassuring test results.

BOX 9.1 DISCUSSING REFRACTORY SYMPTOMS AMID REASSURING TEST RESULTS

"We are so glad to see that your endoscopy and colonoscopy is looking great – however, we also understand that your symptoms are still so frustrating and exhausting. It must be really annoying that you're still feeling this way even when we tell you that treatment is working. I promise we believe you. Sometimes even after inflammation heals, the GI system continues to be reactive; it can be confusing because similar symptoms might be because of inflammation, or they might be because the nervous system and GI tract has been on high alert for a long time. It's frustrating either way, but we will take a slightly different approach than only medication that we would normally use to address the inflammation".

Communication and reassurance needs regarding comorbid disorders and any potential overlap with DGBI symptoms vary greatly depending on developmental stage and learning style.

For children or older adolescents with developmental delays, often the reassurance that their symptoms are hurtful but not harmful is enough. Older adolescents may require more detailed answers and should be asked directly about diagnostic questions or concerns they have. For example, sometimes older adolescents worry that their caregivers and medical teams may be withholding information regarding their illness and unless addressed directly may continue to worry.

Dysautonomia and other disruptions in the ANS

Orthostatic intolerance and dysautonomia are becoming increasingly recognized as commonly co-occurring in individuals with chronic GI symptomatology [2]. Symptoms include dizziness, lightheadedness, nausea, motion sensitivities, and worsened symptoms in the morning [3]. GI mental health professionals can inquire about particular patterns or other sensations showing up at particular times of day or with activity demands. When youth are working on increasing physical activity and improving sleep hygiene as part of their GI treatment plan, these symptoms may be of concern because they can interfere with youth school schedules requiring early wake-up. In addition, students are expected to maintain prolonged concentration during the school day and may have physical demands walking across school campuses. Thankfully, behavioral interventions for dysautonomia are often complementary to those for GI symptoms including increased fluids, regular snacks, and increasing physical activity. Clarifying recommendations with the medical team is essential to reducing family hesitancy for treatment engagement.

Food-related concerns

Sometimes eating specific foods puts a youth in physical danger, complicating the treatment approach to disordered feeding. For example, the ingestion of gluten by youth diagnosed with celiac disease leads to damage to the small intestine. Whenever there are feeding-related changes, GI mental health providers should compare behavioral changes regarding food to the actual recommendations given by GI providers and dietitians. Quality of life should also be considered as there can be times that youth will make dietary changes that are more restrictive than those recommended. Providers should help families distinguish from food *sensitivities* observed to be triggers of symptoms for GI discomfort but which are *not* fundamentally dangerous or unsafe. For the latter, treatment may include purposeful exposure to foods that cause discomfort for the sake of challenging and ultimately limiting situational avoidance and anxiety about the food. Someone with celiac disease, however, should never be asked to consume gluten as a way of reducing food hypervigilance. In general, the treatment goal should be to implement the least restrictive diet possible so that youth living with GI conditions are able to eat and enjoy a wide variety of foods across social situations. Once medical clearance is obtained, encouraging youth of all ages to experiment in systematic ways with different foods and quantities of specific foods may serve to both help expand their diets and increase their sense of confidence in their ability to predict and manage reactions to foods. Assessment of youth and caregiver anxiety related to eating fears is important at this stage of treatment as well as the goal is not to eradicate fear but to create a sense of adaptive anxiety essential to maintaining health.

Autism spectrum disorder (ASD), attention deficit hyperactivity disorder (ADHD), and other sensory processing concerns

Within this diverse group of comorbidities, an individual's learning and/or sensory experience can complicate GI treatment. This is particularly relevant because of the high rates of youth with ASD and comorbid GI distress [4]. Many children with ASD present with sensory processing difficulties causing sensitivity to smells, tastes, textures, temperature, and appearance of food. Mealtimes thus may be a source of distress and frustration, and restrictive eating patterns and preferences toward processed food high in carbohydrates can influence constipation and other GI symptoms. Behavioral rigidity can make learning new behaviors challenging for youth with ASD, so the scaffolding steps and pacing of a typical exposure and skill-building plan may need to change.

Treatment modifications for neurodiverse youth may need to consider issues of proprioception (i.e., difficulty recognizing their own bodily signals and making sense of themselves within their own bodies and physical space) and attentional challenges, which can make focusing on learning and/or practicing "boring" relaxation skills especially difficult. Adopting a flexible treatment approach and partnering with the youth's other providers (e.g., occupational therapists, speech and language pathologists, ABA specialists, and/or developmental behavioral pediatricians) to construct personalized treatment plans are essential.

Clinical recommendations

- Develop a clear interdisciplinary conceptualization considering how all diagnoses and symptoms interconnect. Put the conceptualization and treatment plan in writing in order to help unify specific language choices and recommendations across treating providers.
- Identify what is driving impairment or avoidance to prioritize treatment targets. GI symptoms may be the referral reason, but not necessarily the place to start.

Anxiety disorders and obsessive-compulsive disorders (OCD)

Youth living with chronic GI symptoms often have normative levels of anxiety about their physical sensations, and families often shift routines to minimize physical discomfort for their children. Research indicates that anxiety disorders are highly comorbid with GI symptoms, and that the link between anxiety and GI symptoms is bidirectional. As with any form of initially normative worry (e.g., concern about having a bowel accident in school), concern about symptoms can easily shift from adaptive to impairing, and reasonable accommodation can rapidly spiral into ever-increasing avoidance (e.g., total school refusal because of fear of having a bowel accident). It is imperative to spend adequate time identifying the anxiety theme at the core of behavioral avoidance. For example, a student may have school-specific anxiety surrounding classroom presentations, and this may result in sensations of abdominal pain or nausea. Distinguishing the anxiety theme is essential to inform exposure-based intervention planning. Avoiding a classroom presentation due to worry of needing to urgently use the bathroom is different from avoiding due to perceived social judgment and experiencing associated somatic symptoms. GI-symptom-specific anxiety itself is important to distinguish and respect if identified. This may feel like a "chicken or the egg" situation and is expanded upon in Box 9.2.

BOX 9.2 THE CHICKEN OR THE EGG? GI SYMPTOMS AND ANXIETY DISORDERS

Many health professionals are familiar with the idea that GI symptoms accompany anxiety, but the relationship between these is actually much more complex. Take the case of a child with a history of reflux and abdominal pain: slightly anxious about "getting sick", over time they become increasingly hypervigilant to digestive sensations. They avoid breakfast and lunch to manage their experience of symptoms at school, worrying about vomiting in class. Their hypervigilance eventually generalizes to refusal of long car rides or sleepovers at friends' houses and requests for frequent reassurance. Although the child may have had subclinical anxiety previously, it was the onset of GI discomfort and avoidance behaviors that led to the development of a clinically significant specific phobia of vomiting (i.e., emetophobia).

There are almost limitless examples of how GI and mental health symptoms can become intertwined. Secondary to increased avoidance, rigidity, and withdrawal associated with untreated GI symptoms, social anxiety, generalized anxiety, OCD, depression, and other disorders are all common developments.

As noted in Chapter 16, behavioral and exposure-based treatments all tend to work well for GI symptoms. Identifying specific mechanisms driving behavioral avoidance is essential for personalized treatment plans. Of note, even though GI symptoms might be the referral reason, they may not be the appropriate initial target; it could be more useful to target the co-occurring mental health disorder. For example, youth living with significant IBS often report frequent and prolonged bathroom visits, and thus there is natural anxiety about bowel urgency. However, if a child establishes rules and routines and cannot leave the bathroom for 2 hours until they fully evacuate with a "just right" feeling and follow a specific cleaning ritual involving the use of 25 wet wipes, this might be best conceptualized through a treatment lens of OCD. This differentiation between GI symptoms and mental health disorders is particularly essential when youth present with disordered eating routines (see Chapters 10–13). Handout 9.2 highlights a variety of evidence-based treatment recommendations when GI symptoms are not determined to be the primary driving mechanism.

Given the pervasive way that both anxiety and GI symptoms can impact daily functioning, caregivers often feel a strong sense of helplessness and may wish to outsource responsibility for change to the mental health professional. Education regarding the role of caregivers as coaches and between-session supports for youth learning to face their fears is critical, since continued caregiver reassurance and accommodation can stymie progress. Utilization of developmentally appropriate books, videos, and other resources explaining anxiety across the lifespan and various evidence-based approaches can be valuable in these situations. A full discussion of these resources is outside the scope of this handbook, but several are listed in Handout 9.2.

Clinical recommendations

- Identify what is driving impairment or avoidance to prioritize treatment targets. GI symptoms may be the referral reason, but not necessarily the place to start.
- Emphasize exposure therapy and reduced situational avoidance, combined with reduced parental accommodation and increased support, for all anxiety symptoms – both GI related and generalized.

The role of trauma

Stress, trauma, and physical symptoms

Many mental health professionals attribute GI symptoms and other childhood somatic symptoms to acute stress or trauma. In reality, many youths with chronic GI conditions have indeed experienced overlapping trauma and adverse childhood experiences (ACEs) [5], and conceptualizing physical expressions of trauma responses is indeed foundational in pediatric evidence-based trauma-informed therapies (e.g., TF-CBT). Also, living with a GI condition can itself have the potential to be traumatizing (e.g., embarrassing symptoms, invasive evaluations). It is essential to assess and validate the lived experiences of youth and how they have navigated their GI journeys (see Chapter 2 for further discussion). Navigating trauma disclosures later in treatment is discussed in Box 9.3 and Handout 9.3.

With this acknowledged, many youths with GI symptoms will *not* report a trauma history and the assumption that GI symptoms necessarily reflect trauma exposure or acute stress is not supported by the existing literature. Given this, mental health professionals should not "go digging" for a trauma history; to do so risks communicating a distrust of the stated personal experience and jeopardize the therapeutic relationship. As an example, many medical and mental health professionals are instructed to view encopresis (fecal incontinence or soiling) as a red flag for abuse or trauma and may unintentionally carry a bias of overreaching for signs of trauma.

BOX 9.3 NAVIGATING TRAUMA DISCLOSURES

As a trusting therapeutic alliance grows, sometimes youth choose to disclose a previous trauma. When this happens, the mental health professional can use this opportunity to validate the developing therapeutic alliance and explore whether this disclosure should change the focus of their work or if continuing with GI-focused treatment continues to be the identified therapeutic goal. For young children, this may involve parental insights on trauma-related behaviors, but for adolescents and young adults, respect for autonomy in therapy should be prioritized.

Clinical recommendations

- Assess for trauma history but do not assume its presence.
- Acknowledge that chronic medical symptoms and associated healthcare experiences may be developmentally disruptive and potentially traumatizing themselves.

Social determinants of health (SDOH)

The cumulative burdens of systemic racism, discrimination, poverty, barriers to accessing equal and equitable adequate medical care, limited school resources, and food insecurity can also significantly influence etiology, morbidity, and treatment of youth living with GI symptoms. When conceptualizing complex cases, GI mental health professionals must incorporate these factors into an understanding of youth experiences (see Chapter 6 for more details) and also recognize the role of cumulative trauma that interconnects these pieces. Unfortunately, these factors are still rarely assessed within the course of standard gastroenterology practice. Thus, the astute GI mental health professional will enhance and build family trust and deepen the therapeutic relationship by identifying and making space for discussion of SDOH (see Chapters 6 and 7) as they relate to symptom presentation and treatment implementation.

Clinical recommendation

- Prioritize discussion of SDOH, bias, and discrimination in medical care to promote inclusive healthcare experiences. For example, modeling and explaining the importance of consistently using preferred gender pronouns in documentation and clinical discussions is a simple step toward reducing perceived medical stigma and discrimination in LGBTQIA+ youth.

Addressing difficulties in the therapeutic alliance and misconceptions about treatments

One of the most common challenges for GI mental health professionals is the formation of a strong therapeutic alliance. Families navigating GI uncertainty frequently perceive mental health referrals as a dismissal of their symptoms. As such, it is essential to work toward forming a warm, supportive relationship with families who enter treatment feeling unheard, frustrated, and skeptical. Addressing the misconceptions about psychogastroenterology is critical to the success of treatment. See Box 9.4 for some common statements indicating potential barriers, underlying issues, and potential responses to address the misconception about treatment.

BOX 9.4 RESPONDING TO COMMONLY EXPRESSED TREATMENT CONCERNS

Statement 1: "This isn't psychological, it's a medical problem".

Barriers: Perceived dismissal of symptom legitimacy, lack of understanding about biopsychosocial model.

Response: *I totally agree that this isn't just psychological! You aren't seeing me because your doctor thinks this is "all in your head" or anything silly like that. You're been referred to me because the human brain is in charge of processing all physical sensations, and we're learning from science that the most effective treatments address both what's happening in the gut and also teach the brain what to do with the info it's getting. Working with a GI mental health professional isn't a replacement for also working with your medical doctor, it's just another part of the treatment that we know works well.*

Statements 2 and 3: "I'm already seeing a therapist" or "The last therapist said I'm fine!"

Barriers: Lack of provider understanding about psychogastroenterology, misdiagnosis.

Response: *I can see why you're not sure about this meeting! Let's see how this goes. GI therapy is different from "regular therapy" because we use active strategies to directly target your symptoms, and research shows some of these skills and strategies work even better than medication. If you have GI symptoms that are interfering with your quality of life, we usually recommend a one-time consult or a short course of treatment to make sure you're getting the best treatment. My job is to get a full picture of who you are and how symptoms are showing up, identify what science-backed strategies we can add to your treatment plan, and make sure you know what treatment options exist. Sound okay?*

Statement 4: "I'm referring them to you because they have so much anxiety".

Barriers: Provider misunderstanding about the anxiety–symptom relationship, belief that anxiety is always the mental health professional's treatment target.

Response: *Thanks for the referral! I'll make sure to talk with them about the biopsychosocial model. I'll go over how anxiety and other psychological processes can sometimes trigger or exacerbate GI symptoms but don't necessarily cause them, and reassure them that they'll keep following up with you so they don't feel like seeing a GI mental health professional is dismissing them or saying this is "just anxiety". Looking forward to meeting them!*

Statement 5: "He never talks to anyone about these things, so we shouldn't bother".

Barriers: Shy youth, caregiver ambivalence about mental health, perception that GI therapy requires significant emotional vulnerability, familial discomfort with acknowledging GI symptoms.

Response: *That's a normal concern for some teens! As long as he's willing to answer some questions about his experience it will be okay. Therapy can be easier if kids are super chatty, but psychogastroenterology is skills-focused so it's more about willingness to experiment with skills and strategies than it is talking about someone's deepest darkest feelings with a total stranger. That would be hard for anyone.*

Statement 6: "My child is just doing this for attention. They could poop in the toilet if they wanted to".

Barriers: Caregiver frustration, misunderstanding about encopresis, insecurity about parenting skill or relationship with their child.

Response: *This is such a stressful problem for every family! It can sure seem like accidents are purposeful, but actually kids usually feel really bad about them – they just don't know how to handle them. Usually, it is really just that they have some pooping skill deficits and we need to re-teach some of those basic skills. Let's see how it goes!*

Statement 7: "How long is this therapy supposed to take?"

Barriers: Uncertainty about treatment, concern about waste of time, effort, or money.

Response: *Great question – you've had these symptoms a long time and I bet you are DONE with them! The gut and the brain have a complicated relationship so I can't give you an exact number of sessions, but one thing that can make a difference is when you are willing to experiment with different skills and strategies. If the only time you practice them is during our appointments, I don't think you'll see much change ... but if you are doing a bunch of practice and coming back to session noticing what's working and where you are getting stuck, what's falling apart, etc. that can help speed up progress.*

Each suggested response includes two elements: (1) joining with the speaker and identification/acknowledgment of the underlying issue and (2) clarification of the misunderstanding. Regardless of whether this or other language is used, it is essential that both these aspects are included. If only the barrier is named without clarification, then the listener will not experience a therapeutic shift. If the GI mental health professional proceeds straight to the clarification without identifying and validating the concern, the listener will not be receptive to new information. Of note, barriers in the therapeutic alliance may appear for both youth and their caregivers. With younger children, addressing any barriers with caregivers should be prioritized as much as alliance with the child to maximize treatment success.

Handling refractory symptoms within refractory systems

When symptoms are refractory, GI mental health professionals must consider whether the ideal treatment plan needs to be adjusted to fit a youth's real-life context. Underlying issues that may contribute to refractory symptoms, as well as key collaborations gaining traction, are outlined below.

Underlying issue: Misaligned treatment goals

Sometimes the reason why a treatment plan is ineffective is because there has been a miscommunication regarding either the symptoms being experienced or expectations regarding specific treatment demands. An example of the former is that "vomiting" can look different across multiple individuals and an accurate understanding of what *type* of vomiting is taking place (e.g., functional vomiting, rumination, cyclic vomiting syndrome) can enhance treatment planning. To identify if treatment is failing because of misaligned goals, the GI mental health professional may trial a time-limited, detailed, symptom-tracking log and use photos/videos to clarify the youth's experience. Symptom logging on a routine basis is not recommended, as in the case of DGBI, this can amplify symptoms of pain or nausea, but a few days of symptom-tracking can be invaluable.

An equally important consideration is miscommunication regarding the required youth and family level of involvement in treatment. Successful treatment invariably involves the practice of relaxation strategies, exposure hierarchies, sleep hygiene modifications, active coping strategies, and/or consistent implementation of behavioral plans. All of these require active youth engagement and caregiver collaboration. When refractory symptoms are reported, an assessment of treatment adherence potentially followed by motivational interviewing surrounding behavioral change may be indicated. It is perfectly reasonable for an adolescent to conclude that their GI symptoms bother them less than the effort involved in changing sleep hygiene, but that is not the same thing as "Nothing is working!" Especially for adolescents who are functioning well, their preferences regarding treatment engagement should be prioritized.

At times, a caregiver may become fixated on making their child entirely symptom-free before stopping treatment, but mental health professionals should be ready to validate that the adolescent – the individual who actually has to do the treatment activities – should be able to make their decisions about cost/benefit analysis of treatment engagement. Additionally, new caregivers of infants or toddlers understandably have expectations for their children's "perfect health". Social media portrayals of ideal feeding, toilet training, and sleep success stories can lead caregivers to have unhelpful judgments of themselves when their experiences are misaligned. This can lead to increased distress regarding normative childhood GI presentations (e.g., constipation, delayed toileting, food intolerances) and must be assessed.

Underlying issue: Stigma

Individuals living with GI conditions have reported significant stigmatization secondary to their chronic health and GI concerns, with a substantial proportion perceiving discriminatory attitudes or behaviors from others because of their illness [6, 7]. The presence of stigma can influence one's attitudes toward accessing and engaging in appropriate care and also negatively impact mental health functioning. Stigma permeates medical systems when individual healthcare providers unconsciously make diagnostic and treatment decisions influenced by their own biases [8, 9]. Unfortunately, the invisibility of GI symptoms also poses a barrier to school personnel believing in student distress and thus delaying treatment collaboration [10]. Additionally, general stigma and disgust surrounding digestive issues remain pervasive in many cultures. Patient and family-run social media groups pertaining to chronic health conditions can provide opportunities for felt acceptance and belonging in oft-misunderstood medical conditions. A note of caution – these groups can also inadvertently promote misinformation and an unhelpful fixation on illness (vs. recovery) behaviors. Open treatment discussion about the use of social media to access information and peer support is essential.

Underlying issue: Systemic barriers to optimal treatment implementation

Sometimes treatment is hampered by inadequate resources at familial and/or systemic levels. Resistance to engagement in a treatment plan may be overt (e.g., a school refusing to allow a student to do a gradual reentry process), or covert (e.g., a caregiver that agrees to participate in a behavioral plan but does not follow it). Caregivers of infants and toddlers particularly, who are caught between competing needs and systemic barriers, may struggle to provide idealized care. Open acknowledgment of their particular challenges and problem-solving regarding their hierarchy of needs may be important for treatment success. Regardless of how it presents, the GI mental health professional should approach any nonadherence with curiosity rather than judgment, since a lack of treatment engagement often reflects a resource deficit rather than a compassion or motivational deficit (see Box 9.5 for example).

BOX 9.5 SYSTEMIC BARRIERS IN ACTION

A well-meaning provider recommends that a 5-year-old with encopresis do four structured, supervised, 5-minute toilet sits per day with accompanying rewards and consequences. Unfortunately for a single caregiver working two jobs, with multiple children at home, implementing it may be out of reach because resources of time, consistency, attention, and energy are simply not available. The difficulty in this case is not lack of willingness, but the level of demands already present on the caregiver. To facilitate more appropriate treatment planning, a nonjudgmental and proactive consideration of contextual factors is critical. To do this, one might say: "Before we finalize this week's plan, let's be super realistic: how might this fit between work and kids' schedules? What parts of the day are especially challenging? I care more about creating a plan that'll feel doable rather than one that's nice on paper but not really going to work for you and your family".

Treatment difficulties may not arise from limited caregiver motivation or development of a poor treatment plan. Rather, the sheer demand already present in a family's ecosystem can make implementation untenable. This can be true for behavioral plans, buying special foods for a specific diet, enrolling a child in weekly physical therapy, or arranging transportation for partial school days within a gradual school reentry plan. Resource deficits can also be seen in broader school and community systems as well. Some school districts may be overwhelmed by the mismatch between existing student needs and available resources. In the community, there may be few available mental health providers, and/or providers may be out of reach because of scheduling and financial constraints. See Handout 9.4 for an outline of levels of care that can support various types of treatment needs.

Key collaborations for troubleshooting treatment nonadherence

When a GI mental health professional sees that treatment is stymied and/or recommendations are not being followed, a thoughtful discussion with the youth and caregiver to assess barriers and to adjust the treatment plan to fit their real-world experience and resources is indicated. Below are three potential collaborations that can help effectively navigate refractory symptoms and work to ensure realistic treatment plans.

Key collaboration: (1) School and/or coach

Why this matters: When a youth is struggling to implement a school or sport reentry plan, forming a collaborative relationship with the school or coach is essential. Sometimes having a conversation with a provider (e.g., GI mental health professional) can reinforce the legitimacy of the child's experiences, and knowing that there is a clear treatment plan can relieve a school administrator or coach's anxiety about whether or not a child will be successful. Sometimes schools also have resources or flexibility of which students and families may be unaware, and coaches can become much more flexible about attendance and game-day policies than they might have previously communicated.

How to do it: For further discussion of working with multidisciplinary team members including school personnel, please see Chapter 7. Even when reaching out to schools or coaches that the family has reported has been hostile, it is strongly recommended to start from the assumption that they want to help the student be successful and that they also have limited resources. Obtaining a release of information from the caregiver, discussing with the youth what the most stressful parts of school or sports have been, and setting the expectation that you'll be reaching out to try and enlist help (not calling to yell at them) are all important. See Box 9.6 for more strategies on optimizing this partnership with a school and/or coach.

BOX 9.6 TIPS FOR ENHANCING TREATMENT COLLABORATION WITH A SCHOOL AND/OR COACH

- Identify your role specifically related to GI symptoms.
- Acknowledge the reality of student functioning at school (good or bad!) and the school's current efforts.
- Provide the framework that your goal is to be a resource for the student's success at school versus telling them how to care for this student.
- For example, "Thanks so much for taking the time to connect! I've been working with Sam as part of multidisciplinary care for their GI symptoms. I was hoping to hear more about what you are observing and see how we can collaborate on Sam's reentry process. I know you're juggling a lot so I'm grateful for your time. Can you tell me what you're seeing and what the current challenges are from your perspective?"

Key collaboration: (2) Multidisciplinary team (e.g., pediatrician, dietitian, GI medical team)

Why this matters: Sometimes a GI mental health professional becomes aware that there are divergent approaches within the treatment team, making it challenging for the youth to make progress. This can take many forms, ranging from stigmatizing language and conceptualization to conflicting treatment approaches. A medical provider may write a letter excusing youth from school despite active school reentry planning. Someone might prescribe an unrealistic food intake goal for someone in avoidant/restrictive food intake disorder (ARFID) treatment, and another might recommend talk therapy instead of a medical/behavioral plan.

How to do it: See Chapter 7 for a discussion of working on multidisciplinary teams. When the GI mental health professional determines that there are conflicting approaches, they can serve as a "quarterback" to organize a discussion regarding treatment goals and recommendations.

Key collaboration: (3) Partner with caregivers

Collaborative goals: Youth living with GI conditions often require a significant level of caregiver support. This may be developmentally appropriate or a result of developmental regressions secondary to illness experiences. When individual caregiver variables may be impeding progress in treatment (e.g., because of caregiver anxiety, distress tolerance, lack of scaffolding experience), referral to caregiver-specific treatment may be indicated.

How to do it: Chapter 8 provides a robust discussion of working with caregivers. Some evidence-based programs for specific needs are detailed in Handouts 9.2 and 9.4.

Clinical recommendations

- Regularly assess, in a warm and nonjudgmental manner, for invisible barriers to treatment engagement: misalignment between family experience and intended treatment plan, impact of stigma, and/or resource deficits.
- Explore treatment focus and level of engagement with the youth and caregiver when encountering roadblocks. If the latter is a potential problem, access motivational interviewing and consider adjusting treatment, including changing the frequency and focus.
- Proactively seek out important collaborations with treatment team stakeholders and normalize expectations. Assume that the youth, caregiver, school, and others involved are doing the best they can with the resources they have.

Pearls of wisdom

- Take time to establish rapport with youth and validate the awkwardness of talking about embarrassing digestive sensations and the frustrations of ongoing medical evaluations interfering with childhood. This immediately sets you apart from others who have likely been viewed as judgmental and dismissive.
- Counteract fragmentation in care with direct, concise, and consolidated information and conceptualization and next steps toward functional improvement. This is a tremendous gift to a family to be able to hold all the moving pieces together with intentional treatment planning.
- Remain curious, not defensive, about treatment ambivalence and openly evaluate for roadblocks.

Summary

When dealing with complex clinical presentations in youth and families, consider the diagnoses, the treatment focus and dose, and potential barriers to engagement. It is essential to examine the developmental and family ecosystems of youth and provide psychoeducation to families and medical providers accordingly. Consider the need for multidisciplinary care including the gastroenterology provider as well as dieticians, physical therapists, speech and language pathologists, and occupational therapists. Digestive functioning is closely interconnected with other internal and external systems, and the relationships can be complicated and messy. When this complexity presents, thoughtful collaboration from a place of honesty, kindness, and respect is recommended. In doing this, you also honor the reality of the youth's experience of suffering, of a potentially invalidating medical community, and even the hopelessness they have felt along their journeys.

Recommended readings

For youth and caregivers

- Zoffness, R. (2019). *The Chronic Pain and Illness Workbook for Teens: CBT and Mindfulness-Based Practices to Turn the Volume Down on Pain.* New Harbinger Publications.

For mental health professionals

- van Tilburg. M.A.L. (2020). Psychogastroenterology: A Cure, Band-Aid, or Prevention? *Children* (Basel), 2020 Sep 3;7(9):121.

References

1. Damianos JA, Charabaty A, Dunleavy KA. Recognizing and managing irritable bowel syndrome in quiescent inflammatory bowel disease. *Practical Gastroenterology*. 2022;9:32–49.
2. Saurman V, Yue L, Feinstein L. Health related quality of life survey in pediatric patients with autonomic dysfunction and gastrointestinal symptoms. *J Pediatr Gastroenterol Nutr*. 2021:S437–S8.
3. Boris JR, Moak JP. Pediatric postural orthostatic tachycardia syndrome: Where we stand. *Pediatrics*. 2022;150(1):e2021054945.
4. McElhanon BO, McCracken C, Karpen S, Sharp WG. Gastrointestinal symptoms in autism spectrum disorder: A meta-analysis. *Pediatrics*. 2014;133(5):872–83.
5. Park SH, Videlock EJ, Shih W, Presson AP, Mayer EA, Chang L. Adverse childhood experiences are associated with irritable bowel syndrome and gastrointestinal symptom severity. *Neurogastroenterol Motil*. 2016;28(8):1252–60.
6. Laird KT, Smith CA, Hollon SD, Walker LS. Validation of the health-related felt stigma and concealment questionnaire. *J Pediatr Psychol*. 2020;45(5):509–20.
7. Wakefield EO, Belamkar V, Litt MD, Puhl RM, Zempsky WT. "There's Nothing Wrong With You": Pain-related stigma in adolescents with chronic pain. *J Pediatr Psychol*. 2021;47(4):456–68.
8. Feingold JH, Drossman DA. Deconstructing stigma as a barrier to treating DGBI: Lessons for clinicians. *Neurogastroenterol Motil*. 2021;33(2):e14080.
9. Sasegbon A, Vasant DH. Understanding racial disparities in the care of patients with irritable bowel syndrome: The need for a unified approach. *Neurogastroenterol Motil*. 2021;33(5):e14152.
10. Logan DE, Coakley RM, Scharff L. Teachers' perceptions of and responses to adolescents with chronic pain syndromes. *J Pediatr Psychology*. 2006;32(2):139–49.

Part 2

Psychological approaches in pediatric psychogastroenterology

Chapter 10

Feeding difficulties

Introduction

Hayley H. Estrem, Jaclyn Pederson, and Kaitlin B. Proctor

Learning points

- Provide an overview of the relevant feeding difficulty problems and diagnoses, including pediatric feeding disorder (PFD) and avoidant restrictive food intake disorder (ARFID).
- Review the best practices to address feeding difficulties for youth living with gastrointestinal (GI) disorders.

Chapter aims

This chapter will provide an overview of pediatric feeding problems including commonly used terms and diagnoses used to describe pediatric feeding problems. This chapter will work to synthesize currently available literature and terminology to facilitate pediatric psychogastroenterology practice.

Feeding difficulty introduction

Feeding infants and children is something that is often assumed to be easy, even instinctual. It can be distressing when parents find themselves struggling with a youth who does not feed well. Infants and toddlers evidence a wide range of responses to the introduction of food, including a developmentally normative food neophobic or "picky eating" stage from about 18 to 36 months of age. However, the wide spectrum of developmentally normative feeding behaviors observed over the course of development may make diagnosis and access to treatment for clinically significant feeding difficulty more challenging for many families. Clinically significant feeding difficulty for youth is generally agreed to occur at increasingly higher rates, and the chances of experiencing a feeding difficulty increase if a youth has a co-occurring medical or developmental condition such as being born prematurely, having a developmental delay or disability, or having a congenital abnormality [1, 2].

Feeding is an integral part of development; nutrition during the first 1,000 days of a child's life is critical for development and long-term health [3]. Not only are youth with developmental delay or medical conditions at a greater risk for feeding problems, but they are also more vulnerable to insults from malnutrition. Pressure to deliver nutrition for these youth is heightened, and parents of youth with feeding problems will often try a variety of ultimately ineffective techniques to feed, including coaxing, distraction, bargaining, and feeding only preferred foods. Youth with feeding disorders may present for care evidencing malnutrition, suboptimal or faltering growth, reliance on feeding tubes or oral nutritional supplements, and severe

DOI: 10.4324/9781003308683-12

psychosocial impairment resulting from the feeding concerns. Youth's medical, gross, and oral motor skills and developmental strengths and difficulties significantly influence the degree and progression of their feeding concerns.

Feeding difficulties become significant when a youth cannot or will not eat sufficient volume or variety of foods in an age-normative way to the point that it affects their growth and development and/or there is marked psychosocial impairment from the compensations or adaptations caregivers have had to make to accomplish feeding. Developmentally normative "picky eating" occurs along a spectrum but can be differentiated from a feeding disorder by the persistence, severity of dietary restriction, and intensity of the emotional or behavioral response to food presentation. "Picky eating" generally improves over time, does not impact growth, development, or health, and does not consistently evoke a strong, negative youth response to the presentation of new or non-preferred foods. Conversely, feeding disorders typically remain stable or worsen over time and do compromise the health or progression of age-typical food intake. Many parents of youth with feeding disorders report needing to expend extraordinary amounts of time and energy to get their youth to eat. Others find they are only successful if they offer their youth certain foods that they will accept (such as processed snack foods), or in a certain container or temperature [4]. This makes life difficult when social events often involve food, like holidays, birthday parties, or attending a school lunchtime environment that cannot be completely controlled. Even finding babysitters or family members willing and able to successfully feed a child can be hard when a youth has feeding difficulty.

Over time, pediatric feeding difficulties have been called by different names depending on the discipline or the professional describing the problem, and so it has been described in the literature as pediatric feeding difficulty, disorder, problems, failure to thrive (organic and non-organic), infantile anorexia, dysphagia, and avoidant/restrictive food intake disorder (ARFID) among others [5]. Two of the most recent and commonly used diagnoses are ARFID and pediatric feeding disorder (PFD) [6], both of which will be discussed in more detail. It is also relevant to note that this is a chapter about *feeding* difficulties. The term "feeding" reflects the interactional and relational component of providing nourishment to infants and children wherein a caregiver assists, leads, or facilitates providing food and directing mealtimes. "Eating" is an action and process that is self-led by an individual.

Multidisciplinary assessment is important in the diagnosis and management of feeding disorders. Referral networks and collaboration with medical, nutrition, and feeding skill providers (such as speech-language pathologists) are important for clients with suspected feeding disorders. It is important whenever feeding disorder is suspected for youth to have medical assessment to rule out underlying causes for discomfort that may make eating uncomfortable or unsafe. A nutritional assessment is indicated for severely restricted or age-atypical intake, as the limited dietary variety that can come with restrictive or selective diets can cause nutritional deficiencies (or excesses) with or without the context of underweight. Finally, a feeding skill assessment should be considered for youth who present with neurological or motor conditions that may impact swallowing safety or the ability to consume age-appropriate textured foods.

Relevant feeding difficulty diagnoses for mental healthcare professionals

This chapter will discuss primarily PFD and ARFID. In 2013, the *DSM-5* revised the diagnosis of "pediatric feeding difficulties of infancy and early childhood", recategorizing feeding disorders alongside eating disorders and developing the new diagnostic label of ARFID. This diagnosis and change in organization reflects ARFID as a lifespan disorder characterized by avoidant or restrictive eating absent weight or body image concerns [7, 8]. In 2022, the ICD-10 added pediatric feeding disorder (PFD) with acute and chronic classifications based on a multidisciplinary consensus definition [6]. There are some differences between PFD and ARFID, including the typical age and medical/feeding skill profile of affected youth. PFD may be more frequently applied to infants and toddlers, whereas ARFID may be more commonly applied to children and adolescents [9]. Another is that the use of each diagnosis may be discipline-specific; for example, ARFID is a psychiatric diagnosis. The shared space between the two diagnoses and how mental healthcare providers might collaborate for multidisciplinary care if needed is highlighted in Handout 10.1 (also see Figures 10.1 and 10.2).

Pediatric feeding disorder (PFD)

PFD is defined as the impaired oral intake that is not age-appropriate and has medical, nutritional, feeding skill, and psychosocial domains [6]. This multidomain approach leverages the International Classification of Function, Disability, and Health versus a disease-specific lens to ensure all facets of feeding experience are being considered during assessment and management.

PFD is a disturbance in oral intake of nutrients, inappropriate for a child's chronological age (vs. developmental age), lasting at least two weeks and associated with one or more of the following:

Medical dysfunction, as evidenced by any of the following:

(1) Cardiorespiratory compromise during oral feeding.
(2) Aspiration or recurrent aspiration pneumonitis.

Nutritional dysfunction, as evidenced by any of the following:

(1) Malnutrition.
(2) Specific nutrient deficiency or significantly restricted intake of one or more nutrients. resulting from decreased dietary diversity.
(3) Reliance on enteral feeds or oral supplements to sustain nutrition and/or hydration.

Feeding skill dysfunction, as evidenced by any of the following:

(1) Need for texture modification of liquid or food.
(2) Use of modified feeding position or equipment.
(3) Use of modified feeding strategies.

Psychosocial dysfunction, as evidenced by any of the following:

(1) Active or passive avoidance behaviors by the child when feeding or being fed.
(2) Inappropriate caregiver management of child's feeding and/or nutrition needs.
(3) Disruption of social functioning within a feeding context.
(4) Disruption of caregiver–child relationship associated with feeding.

Symptoms can be further classified into acute PFD (<3 months' duration) and chronic PFD (≥3 months' duration). The impaired oral intake occurs in the absence of the cognitive processes

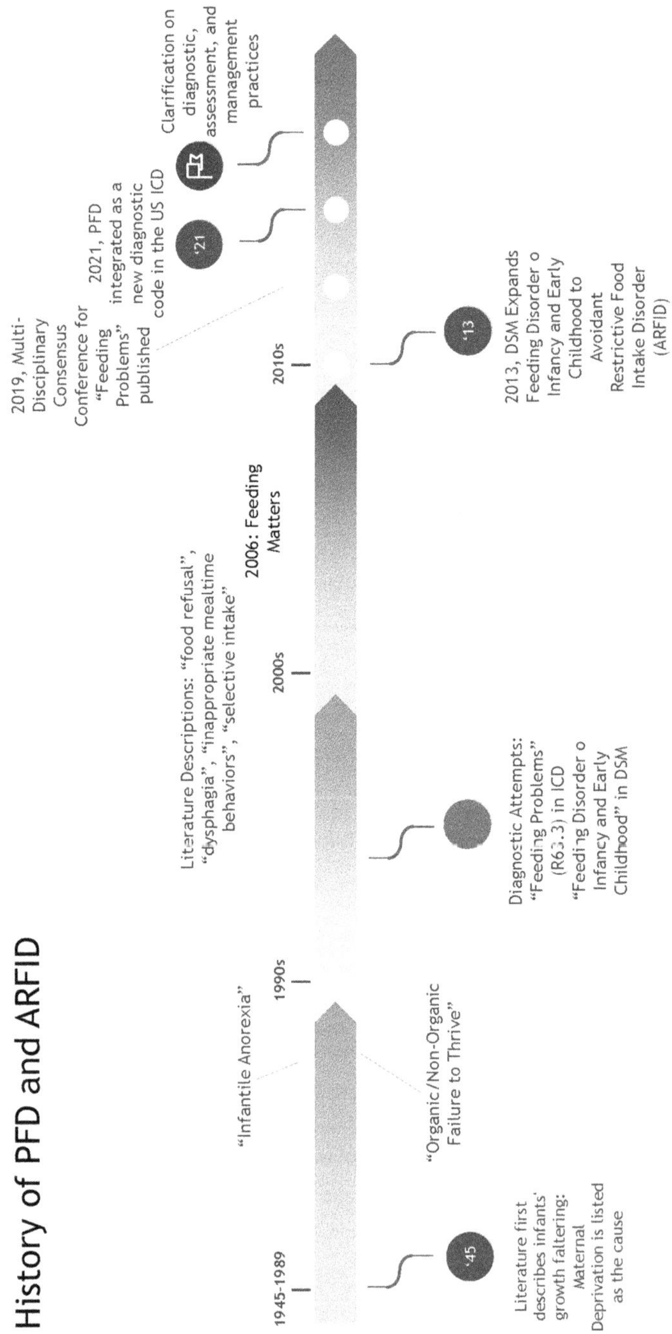

Figure 10.1 **History of PFD and ARFID (Source: Pederson and adapted from [5, 6]).**

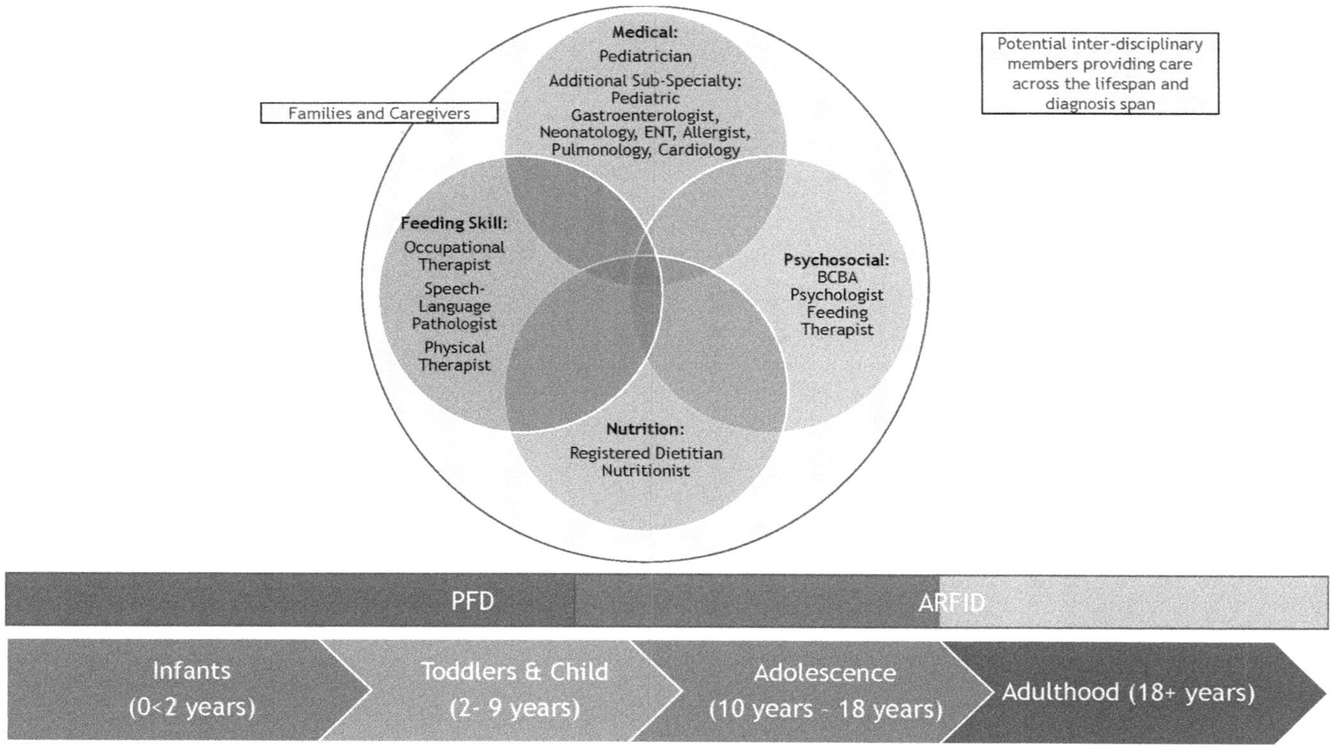

Figure 10.2 Patient ages per diagnostic code use (Source: Pederson and adapted from [6, 9]).

consistent with eating disorders. The pattern of oral intake is not due to a lack of food or congruent with cultural norms. These two codes for PFD were added to the US-ICD-10 in 2021. The codes help to improve health outcomes for patients with PFD by standardizing and clarifying coding, advancing quality improvement efforts, and advancing research inclusive of inter- or multidisciplinary treatment approaches. A recent prevalence study analyzed a series of diagnostic and treatment codes that would qualify for the new definition of PFD [1]. Results demonstrated that PFD is more prevalent than many common childhood conditions.

Avoidant/restrictive food intake disorder (ARFID)

Introduced to the *DSM-5*, ARFID is a lifespan diagnosis that subsumed the previous pediatric feeding disorder diagnosis [10, 11]. For the purposes of this book chapter, we are considering only pediatric cases of ARFID. A recent scoping review of ARFID studies found that the ARFID diagnosis is typically used with older children compared to the average PFD case [12]. Those with ARFID are also more independent eaters on the feeding-to-eating developmental spectrum.

The diagnostic criteria for ARFID [11] are an eating or feeding disturbance as manifested by failure to meet nutritional and/or energy needs associated with one (or more) of the following:

(1) Significant weight loss (or failure to gain weight or faltering growth).
(2) Significant nutrient deficiency.
(3) Dependent on enteral feeding or oral nutritional supplements.
(4) Marked interference with psychosocial functioning.

This eating disturbance also cannot be better explained by:

(1) Lack of available food or a cultural food practice.
(2) Anorexia nervosa, bulimia nervosa, or any other disorder of body image related to weight.
(3) A concurrent medical or mental disorder.

Thomas et al. [13] proposed a three-dimensional model for the neurobiology of ARFID, which we will adopt in this text to organize the next chapters on feeding difficulty. This model posits that there are neurobiological underpinnings, which drive and maintain ARFID symptoms resulting in three primary behavioral manifestations [14]:

(1) Lack of interest in eating or food (e.g., skips meals, eats little, food refusal).
(2) Selective eating or limited variety, oftentimes associated with sensory sensitivity (e.g., avoids fruits or vegetables or mushy foods).
(3) Fear of aversive consequences (e.g., choking phobia, avoidance of bloating).

Often youth will have a combined presentation of the three maintaining mechanisms proposed in the model, to varying degrees of severity. At times, a youth with a medical diagnosis such as dysphagia, reflux, or failure to thrive may not yet have received a diagnosis of PFD and/or ARFID but may still display symptoms consistent with feeding difficulties. Please note in Figure 10.2 that the diagnoses of PFD and ARFID may be applied to the same case because ARFID is a mental health diagnosis and PFD can be used by a multidisciplinary team.

Notably, this chapter will not include a discussion of eating disorder diagnoses such as anorexia nervosa and bulimia nervosa that involve patient body image distortion. Instead, the chapter will focus on the severe, persistent, restrictive feeding presentation observed in youth that may be maintained by several factors but is not related to attempts to control body size or weight. A clinically important distinction observed in practice is that a verbal, school-aged child with a feeding disorder may endorse being comfortable or even motivated to gain weight if they can do it with a preferred food, vehicle, or reduced aversive eating experiences like nausea or early satiety.

State of practice

A recent descriptive survey of community feeding treatment providers was conducted to assess the landscape of practice in community settings [15]. Speech-language pathologists (SLPs) followed by occupational therapists (OTs) were the most represented treatment professionals in the community setting providing feeding intervention. These disciplines represent the feeding skill domain. This work emphasizes the multidomain nature and complexity of atypical pediatric feeding. Of the few mental health professionals who did participate in the survey, the majority were employed in multidisciplinary feeding clinics, which typically treated severe cases. There are a small number of multidisciplinary treatment programs in the United States, so it is likely that youth without geographical proximity or access to these services as well as youth with lower severity, but clinically relevant feeding problems, may present to community providers. The following provides broad foundational clinical recommendations for the assessment and treatment of feeding disorders. Chapters 11–13 will also provide specific and applied recommendations.

Generalized best practices to address feeding difficulties

A critical first piece of the clinical assessment of feeding concerns is to differentiate between "picky eating" and ARFID/PFD symptoms. Several measures have been validated to support accurate assessment and intervention planning [16, 17] (also see recommended readings and Handouts 10.2 and 10.3). Differentiating features include the chronicity, severity/persistence, and level of emotional and behavioral response that occur when new or non-preferred foods are presented. Without intervention, feeding disorders typically do not improve and may actually worsen over time; may result in poor growth, the omission of entire food groups, or the acceptance of a very small number of foods; and may be associated with intense refusal behaviors or emotional responses (e.g., tantrums, aggression) in food-related situations. Assessment should also include a review of parent and primary caregiver strategies previously employed to address feeding concerns, prior therapies or medical conditions and response to intervention, psychosocial impairment due to the feeding problems, and the impact on the parent–youth relationship related to feeding and mealtimes as one or multiple of these may be appropriate targets for intervention. Feeding intervention does not have a gold standard, "one-size-fits-all approach", and requires tailoring for each youth depending on the factors driving and maintaining feeding problems. The following core practices are foundational in feeding interventions.

Engage appropriate consultation

Before beginning behavioral feeding intervention, it is important for mental health professionals to have a comprehensive picture of areas that may potentially underlie or exacerbate a youth's feeding problems [6]. For example, a youth with a history of reflux or family history of food allergies may benefit from medical evaluation to ensure there are no ongoing medical conditions that may cause pain or discomfort with eating. Ongoing medical symptoms may inadvertently reinforce or perpetuate feeding aversion if the youth continues to experience discomfort while eating. Youth with developmental or motor skill differences may benefit from being evaluated by a feeding skill provider (such as a speech-language pathologist or occupational therapist) to assess the youth's feeding skills, including swallowing safety and ability to consume higher textured foods if these are not already in the child's diet. Finally, a youth who exhibits significant dietary restriction by omitting entire or multiple food groups, who is evidencing growth stunting or weight loss, or who relies heavily on the formula for nutrition, likely will benefit from working with a dietitian to develop a plan to ensure nutrition needs are being met.

Establish a predictable, consistent mealtime structure

Often, parents and caregivers facing feeding difficulties will try many different strategies to address these problems and may frequently alternate their approaches. To support optimal learning, mealtimes should follow a consistent and predictable structure [18]. For infants/toddlers, this may mean ensuring that the child sits in their highchair for about 5 minutes while food is presented or is present at the table while family members are eating; for school-aged children, this may mean having clear mealtime expectations for behavior (e.g., sitting with the family, having a consistently implemented reward system for target behaviors like new food practices) with clear start and end times for meals.

Offer meals and snacks on a predictable schedule matched to the youth's developmental level and abilities

Generally, having eating time spaced throughout the day and scheduled at consistent times helps support hunger and appetite regulation. Special consideration may be required for youth who are tube/formula-fed, have volume tolerance limitations, and/or have medical conditions requiring deviation from this guideline. Collaborating with treating medical and nutrition providers can help to optimize a youth's schedule to allow regular opportunities to eat by mouth. Children who can sit safely unsupported should be offered meals in structured seating/at the table [18].

Leverage behavioral strategies to maximize the effectiveness of parental attention

Parents and caregivers should be coached to provide specific, labeled praise for all appropriate mealtime behaviors or approximations toward desired mealtime behaviors (e.g., praising a youth's willingness to interact with a food) as well as high-quality, positive social attention during meals [19]. Relatedly, minimizing coaxing, negotiating, arguing, or nagging during meals and coaching parents in the use of differential attention (ignoring inappropriate behaviors and attending to appropriate mealtime behaviors) are encouraged to maintain positive mealtime interactions.

Use antecedent-based strategies to increase a child's willingness to engage with new foods

For neurotypical preschool-aged children and older, several antecedent-based strategies (e.g., changes to the way the feeding demand is presented) may help enhance the child's willingness to interact with, try, and consume new or non-preferred foods. Two such antecedent-based strategies are (1) altering the amount of food presented and (2) incorporating closed-ended choices [20]. See Box 10.1 for a description of visualizing antecedent-based challenges.

BOX 10.1 VISUALIZING ANTECEDENT-BASED CHALLENGES

- Picture the visual difference between a full bowl of peas and one pea being offered on the plate – even if the task is to only eat one pea from the bowl, visually this will appear like a much more difficult challenge to a child who is reluctant to try that food.
- Another antecedent-based strategy is to incorporate developmentally appropriate, closed-ended choices. Following the previous example, a child might be given the choice to select to try a small bite (half pea), medium-sized bite (one pea), or big bite (two peas).

Pearls of wisdom

- "Picky eating" is normative; highly restrictive/selective food intake that persists, interferes with growth or adequate nutrition, and/or interferes with youth/family functioning warrants an additional assessment.
- Infants/toddlers may not be able to verbalize gut or other problems. They simply notice eating makes them uncomfortable and then decide to stop eating. This makes a lot of sense to them but veils the real reason for eating problems.

Summary

Feeding disorders commonly co-occur with medical and developmental conditions. Youth experiencing clinically significant feeding problems represent a heterogeneous group with different clinical manifestations and hypothesized mechanisms driving or maintaining feeding concerns. It takes a network or team of professionals from the medical, skill, nutrition, and psychosocial domains to address all the possible needs of youth and family with feeding difficulties. The following chapters will provide information about three common maintaining mechanisms of feeding difficulty with recommendations for assessment and treatment intervention. Feeding disorders occur in a heterogeneous population, and best practice recommendations support the integration of multidisciplinary intervention to comprehensively address feeding concerns.

Recommended readings

For youth and caregivers

- Feeding Matters, Power of Two: Parent-to-parent support program: https://www.feedingmatters.org/resources-support/.

- Feeding Matters Family Guide: https://www.feedingmatters.org/wp-content/uploads/2020/09/FeedingMattersFamilyGuide.pdf.
- Thomas, J. J., Becker, K. R., and Eddy, K. T. (2021). *The Picky Eater's Recovery Book: Overcoming Avoidant/Restrictive Food Intake Disorder*. Cambridge University Press.

For mental health professionals

- Open Access manuscript PFD Case Report Forms for each domain in the supplemental material: https://pubmed.ncbi.nlm.nih.gov/35687655/.
- Thomas, J. J. and Eddy, K. T. (2018). *Cognitive-behavioral therapy for avoidant/restrictive food intake disorder: children, adolescents, and adults*. Cambridge University Press.

References

1. Kovacic K, Rein LE, Szabo A, Kommareddy S, Bhagavatula P, Goday PS. Pediatric feeding disorder: A nationwide prevalence study. *J Pediatr*. 2021;228:126–31. e3.
2. Lefton-Greif MA, Arvedson JC. Pediatric feeding and swallowing disorders: State of health, population trends, and application of the international classification of functioning, disability, and health. *Semin Speech Lang*. 2007;28(03):161–5.
3. Schwarzenberg SJ, Georgieff MK. Advocacy for improving nutrition in the first 1000 days to support childhood development and adult health. *Pediatrics*. 2018;141(2):e20173716.
4. Estrem H, Thoyre S, Knafl K, Pados B, Van Riper M. "It's a long-term process": Description of daily family life when a child has a feeding disorder. *J Pediatr Health Care*. 2018;32(4):340–7.
5. Estrem HH, Pados BF, Park J, Knafl KA, Thoyre SM. Feeding problems in infancy and early childhood: Evolutionary concept analysis. *J Adv Nurs*. 2017;73(1):56–70.
6. Goday PS, Huh SY, Silverman A, Lukens CT, Dodrill P, Cohen SS, et al. Pediatric feeding disorder: consensus definition and conceptual framework. *J Pediatr Gastroenterol Nutr*. 2019;68(1):124–9.
7. Attia E, Becker AE, Bryant-Waugh R, Hoek HW, Kreipe RE, Marcus MD, et al. Feeding and eating disorders in DSM-5. *Am J Psychiatry*. 2013;170(11):1237–9.
8. Sharp WG, Stubbs KH. Avoidant/restrictive food intake disorder: A diagnosis at the intersection of feeding and eating disorders necessitating subtype differentiation. *Int J Eat Disord*. 2019;52(4):398–401.
9. Estrem HH, Park J, Thoyre S, McComish C, McGlothen-Bell K. Mapping the gaps: A scoping review of research on pediatric feeding disorder. *Clin Nutr ESPEN*. 2022.
10. American Psychiatric Association. *Diagnostic and statistical manual of mental disorders* (5th ed., text rev.). Washington, DC: American Psychiatric Association; 2022.
11. American Psychiatric Association. *Diagnostic and statistical manual of mental disorders* (5th ed.). Arlington, VA: American Psychiatric Association; 2013.
12. Bourne L, Bryant-Waugh R, Cook J, Mandy W. Avoidant/restrictive food intake disorder: A systematic scoping review of the current literature. *Psychiatry Res*. 2020;288:112961.
13. Thomas JJ, Lawson EA, Micali N, Misra M, Deckersbach T, Eddy KT. Avoidant/restrictive food intake disorder: A three-dimensional model of neurobiology with implications for etiology and treatment. *Curr Psychiatry Rep*. 2017;19:1–9.
14. Thoyre SM, Pados BF, Park J, Estrem H, McComish C, Hodges EA. The pediatric eating assessment tool: Factor structure and psychometric properties. *J Pediatr Gastroenterol Nutr*. 2018;66(2):299–305.
15. Sharp W, Estrem, H., Romeo, C., Pederson, J., Proctor, K., Gillespie, S., & Marshall, J. Assessing the treatment landscape for children with pediatric feeding disorder: A survey of multidisciplinary providers. Child: Care, Health, & Development (Accepted for publication with revisions).
16. Lane-Loney SE, Zickgraf HF, Ornstein RM, Mahr F, Essayli JH. A cognitive-behavioral family-based protocol for the primary presentations of avoidant/restrictive food intake disorder (ARFID): Case examples and clinical research findings. *Cogn Behav Pract*. 2022;29(2):318–34.

17. Silverman AH, Berlin KS, Linn C, Pederson J, Schiedermayer B, Barkmeier-Kraemer J. Psychometric properties of the infant and child feeding questionnaire. *J Pediatr.* 2020;223:81–6. e2.
18. Sharp WG, Volkert VM, Scahill L, McCracken CE, McElhanon B. A systematic review and meta-analysis of intensive multidisciplinary intervention for pediatric feeding disorders: How standard is the standard of care? *J Pediatr.* 2017;181:116–24. e4.
19. Thomas JJ, Eddy KT. *Cognitive-behavioral therapy for avoidant/restrictive food intake disorder: Children, adolescents, and adults.* Cambridge: Cambridge University Press; 2018.
20. Thomas JJ, Becker KR, Eddy KT. *The Picky eater's recovery book: Overcoming avoidant/restrictive food intake disorder.* Cambridge: Cambridge University Press; 2021.
21. Sharp WG, Silverman A, Arvedson JC, Bandstra NF, Clawson E, Berry RC, et al. Toward better understanding of pediatric feeding disorder: A proposed framework for patient characterization. *J Pediatr Gastroenterol Nutr.* 2022;75(3):351.

Chapter 11

Feeding difficulties

Food refusal

Meghan A. Wall, Andrea Begotka, and Cindy Kim

Chapter aims

This chapter provides a practical guide to address food refusal and difficulty with weight gain for youth using behavioral strategies within a multidisciplinary care model.

Learning points

- Understand various underlying conditions or reasons for food refusal from infancy through childhood.
- Introduction to behavioral strategies to address food refusal and improve weight gain.
- Practical application of behavioral strategies with an emphasis on caregiver support and participation.

Youth presenting with an apparent lack of interest in eating or food can be perplexing for parents and gastrointestinal (GI) mental health professionals. The drive to eat is basic and life-sustaining, so why do some youth present with food refusal? The origins of food refusal vary based on the developmental stage when symptoms first present. Across the developmental spectrum, GI mental health professionals can apply behavioral and cognitive interventions to address food refusal and promote weight gain. Infants and toddlers with a history of invasive medical interventions such as surgery, intubation, and prolonged feeding tube dependence may present with subsequent food refusals associated with aversive or negative feeding experiences. Prolonged hospitalization, illness, or neurodevelopmental delays may all inhibit the development of oral motor skills during critical periods of feeding development. These may include neurodevelopmental disorders such as autism, cerebral palsy, oral motor dysfunction, sensory disorganization, negative mealtime behavior, and psychosocial challenges. Infants and toddlers with food refusal may present with delayed feeding milestones, nutritional risk, or preference for feeding while sleeping.

In youth who present with food refusal, it is important to assess whether symptoms are new onset or have been present since infancy or toddlerhood and how symptoms have changed over time. Behaviorally, children oftentimes present with food rules and rigidities, limited interest in food or eating, and negative behaviors when prompted to eat or when presented with non-preferred foods. These children may experience difficulties with motor strength and/or coordination, texture progression, sensory processing, or inadequate feeding skills. Children may also

DOI: 10.4324/9781003308683-13

develop these symptoms after a traumatic feeding event such as choking. See Chapter 13 for details on the fear of aversive consequences of eating.

Young children will display food refusal if eating is uncomfortable due to pain or fear. Thus, psychosocial issues around eating such as anxiety, avoidance, and oppositional behaviors may be stemming from an early history of painful and/or unpleasant feeding experiences. This behavioral avoidance of food can then continue into later childhood or even adolescence. When adolescents experience food refusal, symptoms frequently have been present for some time and oftentimes accommodated. For new-onset food refusal in adolescence, the differential diagnosis may include esophageal or abdominal pain, dysphagia, nausea, or avoidance of eating after a traumatic feeding event.

Food refusal in youth has detrimental consequences not only for the target child who may fail to gain weight or suffer malnutrition but also for parents and the entire family system. Food refusal is associated with parental stress, decreased self-esteem, and feelings of rejection. With early disruptions in the feeding relationship, there are also associated disruptions in bonding. Caregivers of infants and toddlers with food refusal tend to display less physical contact or forceful touch, are less affectionate, and have decreased play interactions. Poor parental coping can often result in the parent experiencing anxiety, depression, anger, frustration, or resentment. Parents may have difficulty reading or responding appropriately to their child's cues for hunger and satiety. It is not uncommon to find a parent is either overcontrolling or undercontrolling in their parenting approach. See Table 11.1 for a summary of contributing factors associated with food refusal.

Once food refusal is well established, youth may appear healthy, but parents may be making extreme accommodations to maintain their child's nutritional health. The child may be either drinking all of his/her calories through supplemental beverages or only eating one type of food and therefore malnourished. Usually, some occurrences of forced feeding, grazing, or distracted feeding are common. Parents may resort to allowing their child to only eat preferred foods, making excessive accommodations to get their child to eat, or feeding a child who is able to self-feed. Parents are already so stressed with feeding their child and usually believe they are "doing what they have to do to get nourishment into their child". As a result of these feeding challenges, parents may in turn resort to not offering new foods, giving into their child's demands, and becoming socially isolated for fear of judgment from family or friends.

Community-based treatment of food refusal

Diagnostically, youth with symptoms of food refusal may fit the criteria for both pediatric feeding disorder (PFD) and avoidant restrictive food intake disorder (ARFID). See Chapter 10 for a more detailed discussion of these two diagnoses and their use to classify symptoms of feeding difficulties. Given that feeding is multifactorial, a multidisciplinary team approach is the best intervention to ensure the integration of a variety of domains/disciplines and to address the feeding problem holistically. This chapter includes strategies and handouts for use with less medically complex youth when treated in a community-based setting where a multidisciplinary team may not be feasible/available. This chapter is not intended to promote community-based treatment for youth who are severely underweight. All youth presenting with food refusal should be under the care of a pediatrician throughout behavioral intervention, and it is the responsibility of the GI mental health professional to engage in regular coordinated care.

Table 11.1 Summary of contributing factors associated with food refusal

Medical factors *Prematurity* • Complex medical course, prolonged neonatal intensive care unit (NICU) stay, intubation • Neurological impairment (e.g., cerebral palsy, autism) *Allergies* • Food-related allergies • Eosinophilic esophagitis	*Structural anomalies* • Orofacial – cleft lip and palate, dental issues • Cardiorespiratory – chronic lung and/or heart disease, vocal fold paralysis, bronchopulmonary dysplasia, laryngeal cleft • GI (e.g., esophageal atresia, malrotation, omphalocele) *Invasive medical interventions* • Surgery • Intubation • Prolonged nasogastric (NG) tube	*GI concerns* • Reflux • Constipation • Motility
Nutritional factors *Weight* • Difficulty maintaining or gaining weight	*Macro/micro nutritional deficiencies* • Diet-related deficiencies due to restriction or refusal.	*Inadequate diet diversity* • Missing entire food groups
Feeding skill *Oral motor* • Oral motor skills for managing food bolus or solid foods • Problems with motor strength or coordination, texture progression • Age-appropriate feeding skills	*Oral sensory* • Hyper- or hypo-sensory arousal • Oral aversion	*Pharyngeal* • Inefficient swallow • Airway protection
Psychosocial/behavioral *Developmental* • Delay in cognition • Behavior rigidities • Learned aversion • Brand or food selectivity ***Caregiver*** • Environmental – meal schedule and structure • Unresponsive vs. overresponsive • Caregiver depression and/or anxiety impacting relationship	*Emotional* • Anxiety • Trauma • Aversive or negative feeding experiences	*Social* • Disordered parent–child relationship • Culture-specific norms

Strategies to address food refusal

Setting up meals for success

Environmental control

Environmental control is intended to minimize distraction during meals/snacks and help the child focus on eating and drinking for improved intake. It is necessary to have a controlled feeding environment before focusing on specific refusal behaviors. Caregivers should provide appropriate food/beverages based on a child's development rather than age [1]. For example, many children with food refusal will have difficulties with transitioning from liquid feedings to table foods. In addition, textures and tastes vary across foods, and generally certain foods are more easily introduced (easily dissolvable snack foods) than others (tougher-to-chew foods). Presenting food that is more advanced than the child's developmental level will likely result in refusal behaviors and possible safety risks for the child. Consult with a speech and language pathologist as needed to determine appropriate textures for a child. Children should eat all meals and snacks at a designated table with developmentally appropriate seating [2]. The feeding environment at home should have little to no distractions, so the child and caregiver can focus on eating and drinking. However, this can be challenging outside of the home (e.g., school, day-care), but accommodations in these settings to minimize distractions are recommended.

Meal schedule and structure

Setting up and being consistent with a mealtime schedule will promote appetite and improve oral intake and behaviors [2, 3]. Grazing or continuous access to food or caloric beverages will decrease the child's appetite and result in reduced intake. The optimal schedule would allow for 2–3 hours between scheduled meals/snacks so the child can get fully hungry before the next feeding. Meals should not exceed 30 minutes to ensure sufficient time to get hungry for the next meal/snack and prevent increased refusal behavior when the child loses focus and interest in eating.

It is important to maximize the calories children consume within meals (see Handouts 11.1 and 11.2 for a practical guide to address food refusal in youth aged 0–4 and ages 5 and older, respectively). Offering high-calorie foods and beverages will increase the calories consumed in meals without increasing the overall volume. Consult with a registered dietitian for guidance. To ensure the child doesn't fill up on a nutritious beverage, it is best to offer a few sips periodically throughout the meal. For children who prefer to drink rather than eat, a nutritious beverage can be given once the target volume goal of food has been met. Limit food offerings to three to four foods on the plate per meal to prevent overwhelming the child. When these strategies have been consistently followed and a child still demonstrates low appetite or lack of expected weight gain, consult with the child's physician regarding the use of an appetite stimulant [4].

Increasing positive feeding behaviors

Positive reinforcement

The goal of behavioral feeding therapy is to increase desirable feeding behaviors. Positive reinforcement is defined as adding something reinforcing to the environment when the targeted behavior occurs, thus increasing the likelihood of the behavior happening again [5]. For example, when a child accepts a bite of food, the caregiver provides specific praise, clapping, or preferred food to reinforce taking the bite. It is important to not accidentally reinforce food refusal by providing attention to refusal behavior. Therefore, it is best to attend to positive behaviors and actively ignore or refrain from reinforcing negative behaviors, which is called differential reinforcement [6]. If the child refuses and the caregiver provides attention through coaxing, prompting, or negotiating, the refusal behavior likely will increase in the future. Over time, the child learns that the desirable behaviors get attention. For older children and adolescents, caregivers may find a daily or weekly reward chart helpful to reinforce good eating at mealtimes.

Desensitization

Desensitization is a strategy used to help youth, generally older than 5 years, to increase their acceptance of food over time with gradual repeated exposures [7]. Desensitization improves willingness to try a food using gradual steps (e.g., touch, smell, taste/lick, chew, and swallow) [8]. Handout 11.2 includes a worksheet on how to create a food exposure hierarchy for gradual exposure to foods that are challenging for the child, allowing for gradual desensitization. Additional examples along with a therapist's session guide are also available in Handout 11.2.

Fading

Fading can be used to achieve larger volumes of accepted food or drink by gradually increasing each bite or drink size. This would involve starting with a crumb-sized bite of food, then a rice-sized bite, etc., up to a full-sized bite of food with reinforcement for completing each step (see Figure 11.1).

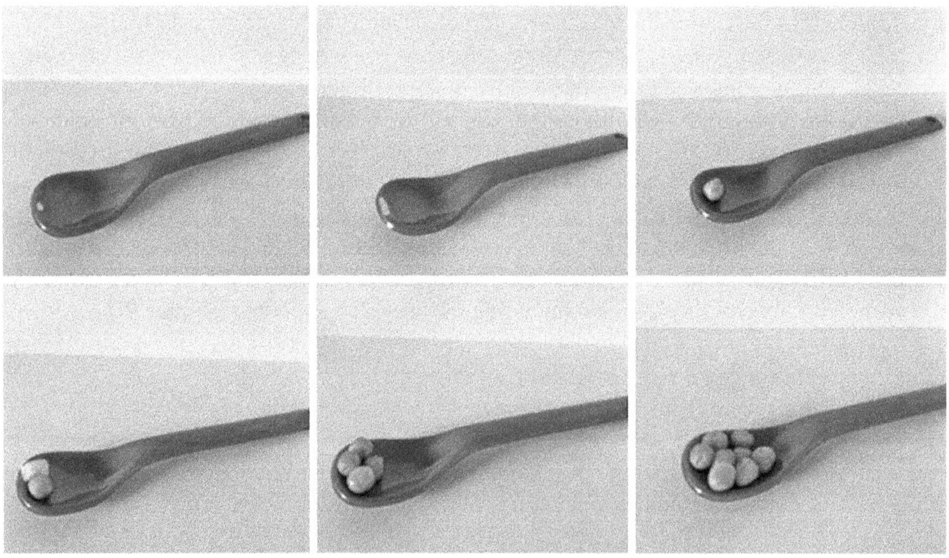

Figure 11.1 Bite-size fading (Source: Authors).

Decreasing undesirable feeding behavior

Escape extinction

Studies have shown that the function of most children's refusal behavior during mealtimes is to escape/avoid taking a bite [9, 10]. Escape extinction is the most widely known strategy to address food refusal and is typically achieved by keeping the spoon at a child's lips until the child takes the bite, while ignoring the refusal behaviors. A common strategy for youth aged 5 and older is to keep a plate with a bite of new food present until the child takes the bite. Research suggests that combining escape extinction with positive reinforcement improves outcomes [11, 12]. This strategy can be difficult to implement in youth with high hates of refusal behaviors (e.g., pushing the spoon away, hitting the feeder) and is best conducted in the context of a multidisciplinary feeding program with behaviorally trained therapists.

Caregiver training

Caregiver education and training is a critical component of behavioral feeding therapy to master the techniques and skills that help feeding success generalize to the home. Typically, caregiver training includes a variety of teaching methods including psychoeducation, written material, modeling, live coaching, and family meals in a similar setting to the home. The next section (see also Handouts 11.1 and 11.2) will provide examples of when caregiver education and training are needed throughout the treatment of food refusal for youth.

Practical guide to address food refusal

Improving feeding for youth of all ages is a process that requires ongoing collaboration between the therapist and a youth's caregivers. The path to improving food refusal is a process that involves the active participation of a youth and their caregivers during each therapy session and implementation of recommendations at home between sessions. The specific strategies used vary based on the developmental level of the youth, the goals identified by the caregivers (and youth if 10 years and older), and which behaviors need to be addressed. This section reviews the strategies that are commonly used across age groups.

Feeding strategies across the life span

0–2 years

Feeding therapy for children under 2 years old is focused primarily on caregiver-directed strategies to address food refusal. Therapy focuses on education, modeling, and training of caregivers in the areas of setting up mealtime, increasing positive feeding behaviors, and decreasing refusal behaviors.

2–4 years

When a child is developmentally a toddler to school age, the approach is akin to that used with children two and under, but now caregivers are also encouraged to incorporate strategies demonstrated in outpatient feeding therapy. Children in this age range are often motivated by preferred food and/or items so contingency management strategies can be highly effective in increasing volume. Using appetite stimulants and decreasing tube feedings when appropriate can also increase appetite and oral intake.

5–9 years

Cognitive behavior therapy (CBT) can be used in addition to the aforementioned strategies when the child's cognition is adequately advanced. For some children, this can be as young as 5 years, but sometimes not until a few years older than that. If the child is able to engage, cognitive therapy helps with identifying and then changing negative thoughts about foods and/or eating so that the child is no longer afraid of the food or something bad happening when he/she eats more volume or variety. For example, a mental health professional will teach a child to identify the worry or negative thought regarding trying new foods.

Once identified, the child will learn to challenge these thoughts by generating neutral to positive alternative thoughts (e.g., "maybe I will like this food", "this food will help give me strong muscles", "I like foods similar to this food"). Another strategy is to explore the sensory experience of the food by stating what the food looks like, smells like, feels like, and tastes like. These should also be kept as neutral observations ("the food is brown and crunchy") versus negative comments ("its smells bad and looks like mud"). An additional cognitive strategy is to help the child identify what is the worst thing that will happen if they don't like the food and how to handle that. For example, if the youth states "it will taste bad", help them come up with what they can do if it tastes bad (e.g., take a drink of water or bite of preferred food).

Behavioral strategies can complement cognitive therapy if the child is still anxious when taking bites and/or gagging with bites. Mental health professionals may use distraction such as conversations about a preferred topic while the child eats the challenge foods. Distraction can be weaned as anxiety levels decrease with repeated exposure. Youth can be reminded to chew on their side or back teeth so it does not get on the middle of their tongue which can result in a gag reflex. Appetite stimulant medication and tube weaning when appropriate are also useful for this age range to increase appetite and oral intake.

10+ years (including adolescence)

For older youth, the mental health provider should complete a thorough assessment of the feeding difficulties and rule out an eating disorder (e.g., anorexia nervosa, bulimia) as these treatments are very different from food refusal on its own. Once ruling out other feeding/eating disorders, a psychologist or therapist should work directly with the adolescent using CBT to identify and change negative thoughts regarding eating to be positive and adaptive thoughts which can lead to more oral intake. The adolescent should help with goal setting and treatment planning, then the mental health professional coaches the adolescent through the implementation of treatment strategies. Caregivers are taught how to support their adolescent's progress using positive reinforcement and reminders to follow the plan. General mental health is also essential to address if there are any concerns outside of feeding (e.g., generalized anxiety, depression, attention deficit hyperactivity disorder) to eliminate this possible barrier.

Summary

Children and adolescents can struggle with food refusal for a variety of reasons including medical, developmental, and/or behavioral. Multidisciplinary care is recommended when working with children and adolescents with more significant food refusal and/or complex medical conditions to increase acceptance of food and weight gain. Increasing oral volumes to promote weight gain and/or reduction in supplemental feedings is a process that changes and evolves with a youth's growth and developmental needs. Emphasizing patience, flexibility, and a strong commitment to change is essential when establishing treatment goals and expectations with families. A child's diet may require modifications to the type, texture, and volumes they are able to consume and requires collaboration with other disciplines to ensure the best and safest care. Caregivers are an important part of the treatment process. Caregiver collaboration, training, and support are essential for success in feeding therapy (Table 11.2).

Table 11.2 Summary of common psychological and behavioral issues and suggested assessment questions/comments and interventions

Psychological and behavioral issues

Common issue: Lack of appetite, low volumes at mealtimes.

Suggested assessment questions/comments: Assess the current feeding schedule with a 3-day food record listing times and amounts of food and liquids the child eats and drinks throughout the day. This will help the provider identify ways to potentially improve the mealtime schedule/structure to maximize appetite, increase food and/or beverage calories to help with weight gain, and give suggestions for other foods to possibly try if diet expansion is a goal. Assess for constipation, distractibility, and caregiver expectations for food textures and self-feeding.

Suggested intervention: Parent education and implementation of scheduled meals and snacks with developmentally appropriate textures and utensils using Feeding Plan Worksheet. Positively reinforce taking bites and drinks. Address other barriers to volume (e.g., manage constipation, limit distractions, and avoid attending to undesirable mealtime behavior).

Common issue: Dependence on milk or formula.

Suggested assessment questions/comments: Parents may report that their child drinks most of their nutrition rather than eating solid foods, even when they have the appropriate oral skills to chew and swallow solids.

Suggested intervention: Parent education on mealtime structure, escape extinction, positive reinforcement, and bite-size fading strategies for solid foods. Present sips of liquid spaced throughout the meal so the child does not fill up on liquid early in the meal and then refuse solids.

Common issue: Child cries when placed in the highchair.

Suggested assessment questions/comments: Assess for prior negative experiences with introduction and use of highchair. Assess for possible underlying triggers or antecedents resulting in negative transitions to the chair and how caregivers respond when child cries in the highchair.

Suggested intervention: Consult with an occupational therapist to determine developmentally appropriate seating. Improve transitions to mealtimes (e.g., avoid transitioning from a highly preferred activity to the highchair). Provide positive reinforcement when placed in highchair. If child cries while in highchair, wait until calm before removing from highchair.

Common issue: Inability to achieve expected weight gain.

Suggested assessment questions/comments: Assess child's appetite and if child consumes higher volumes for a certain meal in the day. Assess barriers to appetite (e.g., medication side effects, filling up on water in a meal, grazing). Compare child's average daily caloric intake to dietitian's estimation of daily caloric needs for weight gain. Consider the child may have a gut issue that makes them uncomfortable with eating.

Suggested intervention: Consult with physician about potential gut issues (e.g., constipation/reflux) associated with feeding refusal, as well as introduction of appetite stimulant. Incorporate meal schedule and structure, reduce behaviors that may lead to early satiety (e.g., limit excessive water consumption before or during meal). Offer high-calorie food and/or beverage at all meals to meet daily caloric needs set by dietitian. Maximize volume during meals when child demonstrates the greatest appetite.

Pearls of wisdom

- Long after contributing medical factors resolve, learned aversions and negative feeding behaviors may remain, resulting in food refusal. Behavioral interventions are key in promoting positive mealtimes and increased oral intake. CBT can be used in older children and adolescents to address unhelpful beliefs impeding adequate oral intake.
- Feeding is a process. It is essential for families to have patience, flexibility, and a strong commitment to change.
- Oral volume should be the primary goal for underweight youth while dietary variety and feeding skill advancement should be a secondary goal.

Recommended readings

For youth and caregivers:

- Rowell, K., McGlothlin, J., Morris, S.E. *(2015). Helping Your Child with Extreme Picky Eating: A Step-by-Step Guide for Overcoming Selective Eating, Food Aversion, and Feeding Disorders.* New Harbinger Publications.
- Williams, K.E., & Seiverling, L.J. (2018). *Broccoli Boot Camp: Basic Training for Parents of Selective Eaters.* Woodbine House.

For mental health professionals:

- Thomas, J.J., Eddy, K.T. (2019). *Cognitive-Behavioral Therapy for Avoidant/Restrictive Food Intake Disorder.* Cambridge University Press.
- Arvedson, J.C., Brodsky, L., & Lefton-Greif, M.A. (2020). *Pediatric Swallowing and Feeding: Assessment and Management.* Plural Publishing.

References

1. Arvedson JCB, Brodsky L, Lefton-Greif, MA. *Pediatric swallowing and feeding: Assessment and management 3ed: Plural Publishing*; 2019 July 26, 2019. p. 562.
2. Silverman AH. Behavioral management of feeding disorders of childhood. *Ann Nutr Metab.* 2015;66(Suppl 5):33–42.
3. Linscheid TR. Behavioral treatments for pediatric feeding disorders. *Behav Modif.* 2006;30(1):6–23.
4. Sant'Anna AM, Hammes PS, Porporino M, Martel C, Zygmuntowicz C, Ramsay M. Use of cyproheptadine in young children with feeding difficulties and poor growth in a pediatric feeding program. *J Pediatr Gastroenterol Nutr.* 2014;59(5):674–8.
5. Skinner BF. *Science and human behavior.* Cambridge, Massachusetts: Simon and Schuster; 1965.
6. Patel MR, Piazza CC, Martinez CJ, Volkert VM, Christine MS. An evaluation of two differential reinforcement procedures with escape extinction to treat food refusal. *J Appl Behav Anal.* 2002;35(4):363–74.
7. Thomas JJ, Becker KR, Kuhnle MC, Jo JH, Harshman SG, Wons OB, et al. Cognitive-behavioral therapy for avoidant/restrictive food intake disorder: Feasibility, acceptability, and proof-of-concept for children and adolescents. *Int J Eat Disord.* 2020;53(10):1636–46.
8. Thomas JJ, Eddy KT. *Cognitive-behavioral therapy for avoidant/restrictive food intake disorder.* New York: Cambridge University Press; 2019. p. 181.

9. Bachmeyer MH, Piazza CC, Fredrick LD, Reed GK, Rivas KD, Kadey HJ. Functional analysis and treatment of multiply controlled inappropriate mealtime behavior. *J Appl Behav Anal.* 2009;42(3):641–58.
10. Piazza CC, Fisher WW, Brown KA, Shore BA, Patel MR, Katz RM, et al. Functional analysis of inappropriate mealtime behaviors. *J Appl Behav Anal.* 2003;36(2):187–204.
11. Piazza CC, Patel MR, Gulotta CS, Sevin BM, Layer SA. On the relative contributions of positive reinforcement and escape extinction in the treatment of food refusal. *J Appl Behav Anal.* 2003;36(3):309–24.
12. Reed GK, Piazza CC, Patel MR, Layer SA, Bachmeyer MH, Bethke SD, et al. On the relative contributions of noncontingent reinforcement and escape extinction in the treatment of food refusal. *J Appl Behav Anal.* 2004;37(1):27–42.

Chapter 12

Feeding difficulties

Food selectivity

Kaitlyn Mosher, Robert Dempster, Valentina Postorino, and T. Lindsey Burrell

Chapter aims

This chapter aims to define food selectivity and its impact on health and psychosocial functioning, provide actionable recommendations to reduce food selectivity in practice, and offer special considerations for vulnerable populations.

Learning points

- Food selectivity is a common childhood concern, ranging from mild to severe.
- Behavioral intervention, including antecedent manipulation, reinforcement, and persistence, is the most well-supported intervention to address these concerns.
- Youth with autism spectrum disorder (ASD) have an increased risk of having a feeding problem, most often food selectivity.

Brief overview of food selectivity

Food selectivity, or eating a narrow variety of foods, is one of the most common feeding problems observed in childhood [1, 2]. Among the feeding and eating disorders described in the *Diagnostic and Statistical Manual of Mental Disorders, 5th Edition* (*DSM-5*), the diagnosis of avoidant/restrictive food intake disorder (ARFID) most aligns with food selectivity [3]. Food selectivity may range from mild to severe, with moderate or greater severity increasing the risk for nutritional and medical complications [4–7]. Therefore, youth with moderate or severe food selectivity often require intervention to avoid negative health outcomes [8, 9]. Food selectivity and picky eating share similar features, however, they are distinct in terms of duration and intensity. For further clarification regarding differences in picky eating and food selectivity, see Figure 12.1.

Evidence-based interventions overview

Due to the severity and chronicity of food selectivity, intervention is required to preclude the impact on health and psychosocial functioning. Studies have reported that behavioral interventions are the most well-supported interventions for severe feeding disorders [10, 11]. Behavioral interventions that target feeding issues often combine a formalized meal structure

DOI: 10.4324/9781003308683-14

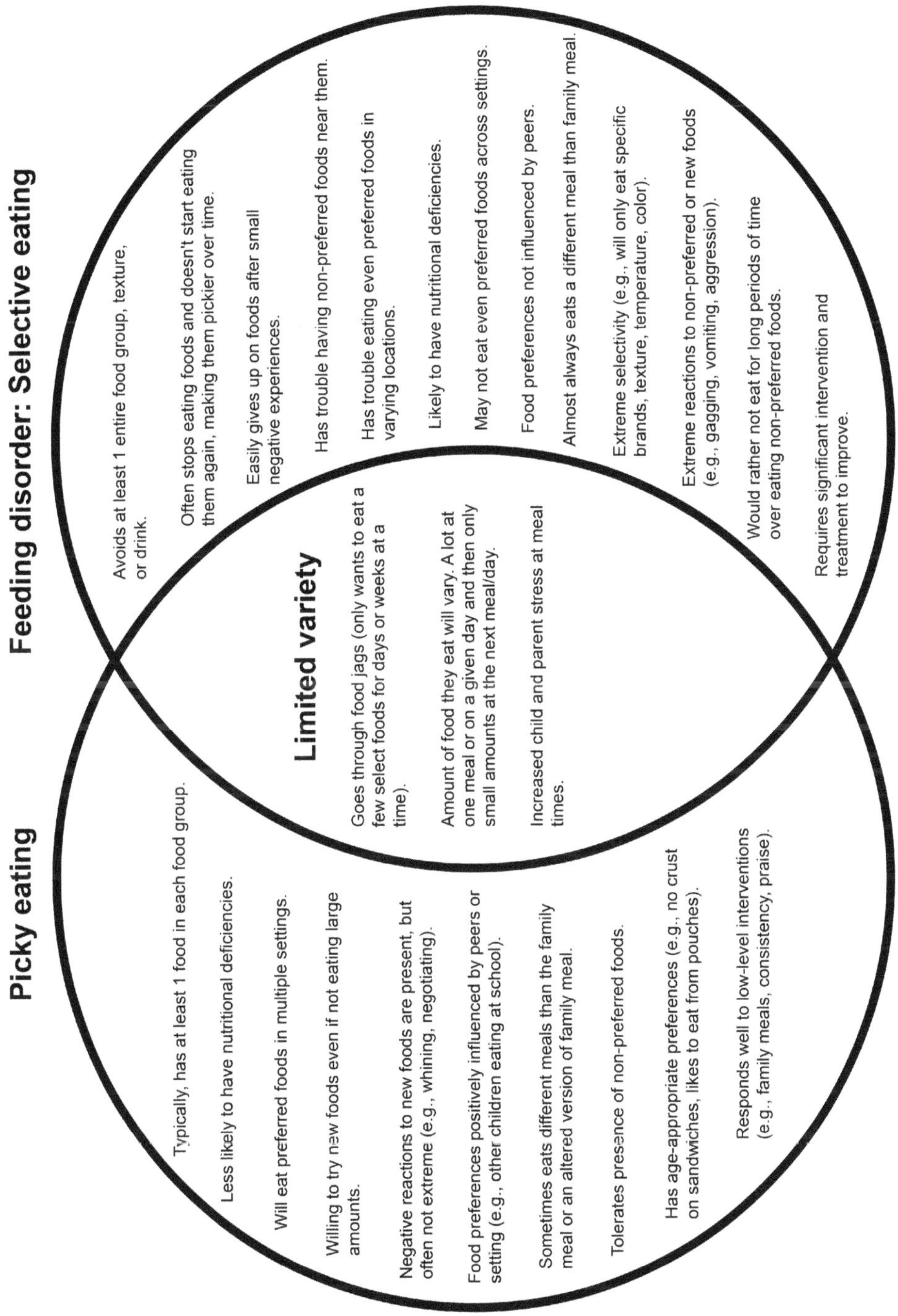

Figure 12.1 Picky eating and selective eating (Source: Authors).

with consequence-based procedures (e.g., escape extinction, differential reinforcement of alternative behaviors) and antecedent manipulations (e.g., reduced bite volume or modified food texture) to promote consumption.

Parent and family factors

Disruptive mealtime behavior and food selectivity can become a significant stressor and negatively impact families' overall quality of life. Research indicates parents of youth with food selectivity are significantly more likely to experience high levels of parental stress compared with parents of youth without food selectivity [12, 13]. See Figure 12.2 for explanation of a common parent–child interaction related to food selectivity.

Parent training

Parent training (PT) is generally recognized as an evidence-based treatment for youth with disruptive behavior [14]. PT is a type of parent-mediated intervention in which parents are the agents of change in using techniques to modify youth's behavior [15]. PT is especially fitting for treating feeding problems because disruptive mealtime behavior is one of the most reported concerns for parents of youth with feeding problems [16, 17]. Therefore, PT is imperative in both teaching prosocial feeding behavior and generalizing skills and strategies across contexts and environments [18]. Given the value of parents in youth's treatment, they should be considered primary interventionists (parent teaches youth directly) or complementary to intervention (GI mental health professional works with youth directly and then generalizes skills to parents).

Treatment planning

Before working on expanding dietary variety, it is important to solidify foundational feeding behaviors to add structure and develop good meal hygiene practices: (1) have 2–3-hour gaps between meals and snacks, (2) sit at a table or other defined space (e.g., counter, TV stand) for up to 10 minutes, and (3) tolerate being in the presence of non-preferred foods (e.g., sitting at the table when others are eating). See Figure 12.3 for further conceptualization of short- and long-term goals related to improving variety.

Behavioral strategies to increase appropriate mealtime behaviors

The first step in addressing selective eating includes altering the environment to increase the likelihood of expanding dietary variety and improving mealtime behavior. See Handout 12.1 for rationale and behavioral strategies to decrease food selectivity.

Reinforcement and selective attention

Reinforcement can be used as an effective tool to increase variety and decrease inappropriate feeding behaviors when combined with escape extinction [19, 20]. However, reinforcement is only successful when a child is not receiving attention (e.g., scolding, negotiating) for disruptive mealtime behaviors such as making negative statements about the food (e.g., "it's gross"), gagging, spitting out the food, whining or crying, or pushing the plate away.

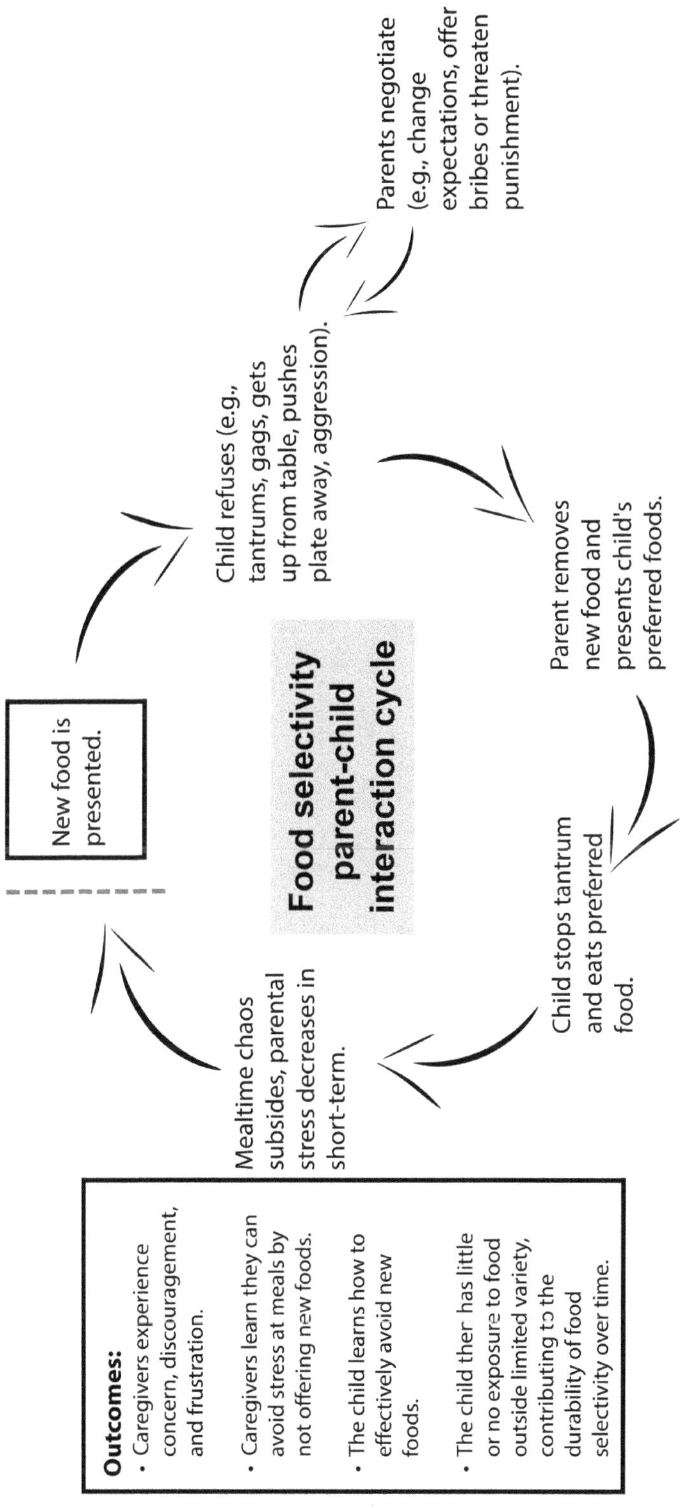

Figure 12.2 Parent–child feeding interaction (Source: Authors).

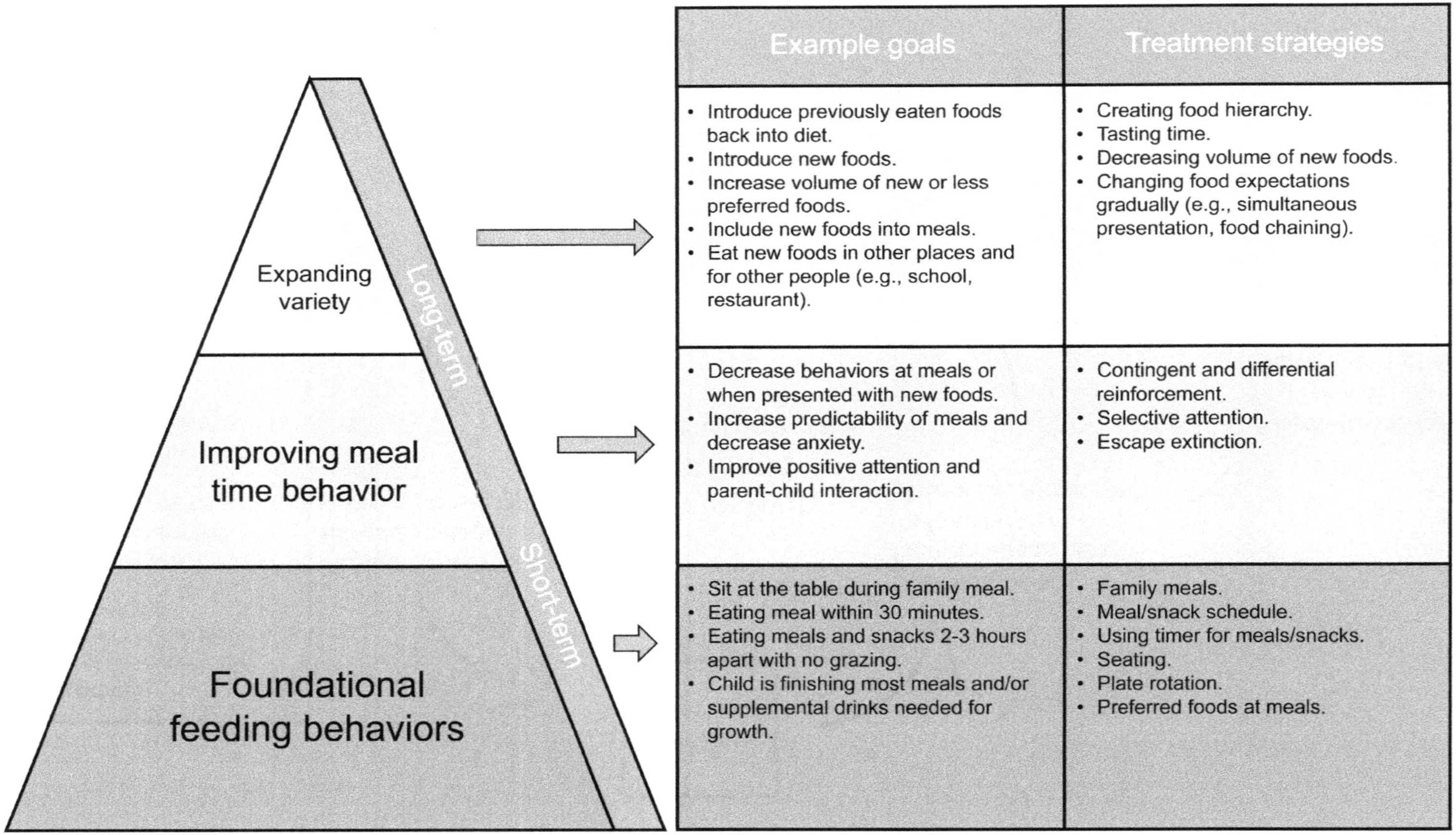

Figure 12.3 Treatment goals for food selectivity (Source: Authors).

It is important to note that youth engage in disruptive mealtime behavior because they are effective in avoiding the demand and elicit reactions from parents. As these behaviors often become more intense when they are *initially* ignored, it is imperative to prepare parents through modeling and coaching so that they are effectively able to persist in ignoring these behaviors at home. By removing attention for disruptive mealtime behaviors, reinforcement of desired behaviors becomes more powerful and differentiated to the child. For example, parents of a child who typically gags and spits out new foods should be encouraged to specifically praise their child for swallowing the new food quickly and to ignore any gagging that occurs. Handout 12.2 outlines the different types of reinforcement commonly used to increase dietary variety.

Reinforcement considerations

Set clear expectations ahead of time

Parents should establish a reward system and clearly explain this to the child before meals or food tasting begins. If rewards are offered once refusal has occurred, the refusal behavior may be inadvertently reinforced.

Limit rewards at other times of the day

Rewards for positive food behaviors are more motivating if they are not accessible at other times of the day. Any tangible reinforcers (e.g., toys or electronics) should be designated only for, or withheld before, meals.

Be thoughtful when using food rewards

Though some youth are especially motivated by certain foods and supplemental drinks, it is important to ensure nutritional foods (e.g., formula/supplements) are not withheld when there are growth concerns. This is another reason to encourage families to work on new foods at a separate snack time to not impact intake if the child is refusing the new food. Many youth lose appetite when presented with a novel food, which can limit the reinforcing properties of food rewards. In addition, research related to utilizing food as reinforcement is mixed [21, 22], and several organizations (e.g., American Academy of Pediatrics, American Psychological Association) have spoken out against using food to reinforce behaviors.

Creating food hierarchies

One of the most fundamental interventions targeting expanding dietary variety is the process of selecting target foods. A food hierarchy allows a provider and family to have a list of foods, ranked easiest to hardest, which bolsters motivation and a reasonable starting point for the child. This activity is often an engaging way to encourage youth to interact with food in a non-threatening way early in therapy and can be utilized in most developmental stages.

The following steps can be adjusted for different ages and situations:

Step 1: Establish goals, provide rationale, and prepare for creating the hierarchy. Discuss short- (e.g., eating a dropped or inconsistently consumed food) and long-term goals (e.g., eating vegetables) with parents to establish expectations. It is also very helpful to have pictures of food, play food, or real food available to provide a visual for food selection in Step 2.

Step 2: Have parents select foods they would like their child to eat. Then provide the youth with a chance to add any other foods they are interested in trying.
Step 3: Explain how to rank the foods that have been selected. This can be done by rank-ordering foods, giving foods a rating of 1–10 difficulty, or designating foods into categories such as red, yellow, or green. Other children may benefit from reducing the number of foods to rank and asking specific questions (e.g., "would crackers or bananas be easier?").

Once the hierarchy is established, treatment can begin targeting the easiest foods and then gradually moving up the hierarchy once success is achieved. The food hierarchy can also be utilized as a working document that is modified by the parent or child once exposure has begun and progress with foods can be re-evaluated.

Tasting time

Once the treatment foods have been established, tasting practices can begin. Researchers have found that daily taste exposures lead to a significant increase in the targeted food group [23]. For youth who have mild selectivity, this may be able to take place within the meal. However, for many youth and families, this can add to the overall stress of meal times and further negatively impact the parent–child relationship [8]. Conducting frequent tasting exposures, separate from mealtimes, can be one of the most effective ways to introduce new foods. The steps to a snack "Tasting time" are outlined below. This intervention is most successful if it can be modeled and practiced within session before being implemented at home.

Tasting time protocol

The parent will implement tasting time with a designated new food or choice between two foods at a pre-determined time of day when the child is likely to be hungry. The amount expected to eat should be very small initially. Parents will establish the reward for completing the bite and set a 5-minute timer. Tasting time ends when youth complete the feeding demand or the 5 minutes has elapsed. Parents should be coached to only provide brief reminders of the expectation and use differential attention to attend to appropriate and ignore inappropriate mealtime behaviors. See Handouts 12.3 and 12.4 for tasting time instructions and reward plan.

The amount of food the child is expected to eat increases slowly every 2–3 successful days (e.g., child completing demand before timer goes off). The demand should be gradually increased over time (e.g., from 1 to 2 small bites, 3 to 5 bites, 5 to 10 bites). A food can be considered "graduated" or "preferred" once a child eats the established volume goals for the child (e.g., half serving size).

Selecting tasting time foods

Sometimes even the first food on the hierarchy may be too great of a demand, or the child cannot engage in creating a food hierarchy due to developmental age or engagement. Initial tasting time goals can be very small (e.g., a different flavor or brand of preferred food, a food the child previously liked). Some youth who need a more gradual approach benefit from simultaneous presentation and stimulus fading which includes the presentation of a preferred food and new food at the same time. For example, a child who enjoys yogurt could have a bite of yogurt with a small piece of fruit and gradually the yogurt would be reduced and the bite of fruit would be larger. One way to use a similar strategy includes adding elements of the food as the child becomes more successful (e.g., first pizza crust, then pizza crust with sauce).

Another gradual method includes food chaining, which aims to expand food repertoire by emphasizing similar features (e.g., flavor, texture) between accepted food items and new food items (e.g., moving from fries to roasted potatoes [24]). For youth whose selectivity relates to texture, it may be beneficial to introduce foods in their preferred texture first. For a child who has an easier time with softer foods, introducing applesauce before apples may be helpful, whereas a child who primarily eats crackers and crunchy foods may do better with banana chips and veggie straws before soft fruits and vegetables.

These strategies benefit youth of all ages. However, adolescents require more thoughtful consideration about choice, autonomy, and personal motivation. For considerations when working with adolescents on food selectivity, see Handout 12.5.

Generalization and maintenance

Once a food is graduated from tasting time, it should be included as one of the child's meal foods. As foods higher in nutritional value are graduated and included in meals, parents should be encouraged to gradually replace some of the less nutritious foods from the meal. Generally, transitioning tasting time foods into meals is successful as the child has had extensive practice with that food. However, sometimes meal structure and reinforcement for finishing meals need to be revisited. It is often helpful for parents to have a running updated list of the graduated foods to avoid falling back into old routines of eating the most preferred foods.

Eating the family meal

Parents often desire for their child to be able to eat any food the family is having for dinner. One way to achieve this goal is targeting frequently prepared foods during tasting time. It can also be encouraged for family to have a "bonus bowl" of a small amount of the family meal that the child is encouraged, but not required, to try. Eating the family meal may be a long-term goal that can be established by targeting the foods from family meals in tasting time and then generalizing them back into family meals.

Eating away from home

It is often important to youth and their families that they are able to eat in other places aside from their home (e.g., school, restaurant). This can be challenging for many youth with selective eating. For tips on generalizing feeding improvement to various settings, see Handout 12.6.

Special considerations for ASD

Children with ASD, a neurological developmental disability characterized by social communication deficits, restricted interests, and repetitive behaviors [3], are more likely than their peers to have co-occurring feeding concerns [1, 25]. Food selectivity by type, texture, and presentation are the most common feeding problems observed in youth with ASD [9, 26, 27]. Sensory challenges, internalizing and externalizing behaviors, and rigid mealtime rituals are some of the underlying factors that contribute to food selectivity in this population [12, 28–30].

Gastrointestinal (GI) concerns

Children with ASD are more likely than their peers to be hospitalized due to GI concerns and exhibit specific GI symptoms such as abdominal pain, constipation, and diarrhea [31]. The presentation of GI and related concerns may differ from standard presentations or may not be reported given communication impairment in this population [32]. Parents often rely on nonverbal behavior and bodily signs to determine if a child with ASD is experiencing GI discomfort [33]. This can result in youth with ASD having GI discomfort for longer before it is recognized or diagnosed. Thus, youth with ASD may be especially at-risk for food refusal and selectivity related to or originating from GI discomfort. Given the elevated risk for GI concerns and nutrient deficiencies in this population, these concerns should be evaluated prior to clinical intervention to ensure that underlying medical issues are addressed prior to treatment and to inform prioritization of goals.

Nutritional deficiencies and nutrition-related medical diseases

Research suggests that youth with ASD are not different from their non-ASD peers in height, weight, and body mass index (BMI); however, they are 5 times more likely to exhibit feeding problems and consume less calcium and protein compared to typically developing peers [5, 6]. The increased risk for nutrient deficiencies and related medical diseases indicates a need for a lower threshold for dietary analysis and blood work to identify underlying deficiencies. Results should guide priorities for feeding interventions that may include focusing on increasing animal proteins, fortified dairy, fruits, and vegetables, depending on the individualized needs of the child.

Impact of disruptive behavior in youth with ASD and food selectivity

Youth with ASD often have co-occurring behavior problems [34, 35]. These behaviors also often occur during mealtimes of youth with ASD [16, 28, 36]. Other reports have also found that greater repetitive and ritualistic behaviors and sensory sensitivity also influence mealtime problem behavior and feeding problems [28]. This may explain some of the increased rigidity around specific food brands, presentation, and preparation often observed in this population. Due to these factors, there are a number of factors to consider when treating youth with ASD and food selectivity, see Handout 12.7 for a summary.

Pearls of wisdom

- Behavioral and anxiety management strategies are helpful in increasing exposure to new foods but cannot make youth *like* the food.
- It is much better to start slow and build momentum than to start with a food that is too challenging and stall treatment progress.
- Make sure the family has a road map of how your individual treatment step (e.g., licking a potato chip) will lead to their desired outcome (e.g., eating fruits and vegetables at meals).

Summary

Food selectivity involves eating a narrow variety of foods that can have short and long-term impacts on the child's health and the child and family's psychosocial functioning. Due to the impact of food selectivity, treatment is necessary to expand dietary variety. Behavioral intervention with a GI mental health professional and via PT has the most support to expand dietary variety. Gradual demand progression through antecedent manipulation, reinforcement, and persistence with the demand is critical to treatment success. The gradual treatment progression involves establishing foundational feeding behaviors, reducing disruptive mealtime behavior, and expanding dietary variety. These treatment strategies are necessary for all youth with food selectivity, but youth with ASD may require an even more gradual approach and other special considerations.

Recommended readings

For youth and caregivers:

- Williams, K. E., & Seiverling, L. J. (2018). *Broccoli boot camp: Basic training for parents of selective eaters*. Woodbine House.

For mental health professionals:

- Thomas, J. J., & Eddy, K. T. (2018). *Cognitive-behavioral therapy for avoidant/restrictive food intake disorder: children, adolescents, and adults*. Cambridge University Press.

References

1. Bandini LG, Anderson SE, Curtin C, Cermak S, Evans EW, Scampini R, et al. Food selectivity in children with autism spectrum disorders and typically developing children. *J Pediatr*. 2010;157(2):259–64.
2. Esteban-Figuerola P, Canals J, Fernández-Cao JC, Arija Val V. Differences in food consumption and nutritional intake between children with autism spectrum disorders and typically developing children: A meta-analysis. *Autism*. 2019;23(5):1079–95.
3. American Psychiatric Association. *Diagnostic and statistical manual of mental disorders* (5th ed., text rev.). Washington, DC: American Psychiatric Association; 2022.
4. Ma NS, Thompson C, Weston S. Brief report: Scurvy as a manifestation of food selectivity in children with autism. *J Autism Dev Disord*. 2016;46(4):1464–70.
5. Neumeyer AM, O'Rourke JA, Massa A, Lee H, Lawson EA, McDougle CJ, et al. Brief report: Bone fractures in children and adults with autism spectrum disorders. *J Autism Dev Disord*. 2015;45(3):881–7.
6. Sharp WG, Berry RC, McCracken C, Nuhu NN, Marvel E, Saulnier CA, et al. Feeding problems and nutrient intake in children with autism spectrum disorders: A meta-analysis and comprehensive review of the literature. *J Autism Dev Disord*. 2013;43(9):2159–73.
7. Sharp WG, Postorino V. Food selectivity in autism spectrum disorder. *Clinical handbook of complex and atypical eating disorders*. New York: Oxford University Press; 2017:126–48.
8. Greer AJ, Gulotta CS, Masler EA, Laud RB. Caregiver stress and outcomes of children with pediatric feeding disorders treated in an intensive interdisciplinary program. *J Pediatr Psychol*. 2008;33(6):612–20.
9. Sharp WG, Jaquess DL, Morton JF, Miles AG. A retrospective chart review of dietary diversity and feeding behavior of children with autism spectrum disorder before and after admission to a day-treatment program. *Focus Autism Other Dev Disabl*. 2011;26(1):37–48.
10. Lukens CT, Silverman AH. Systematic review of psychological interventions for pediatric feeding problems. *J Pediatr Psychol*. 2014;39(8):903–17.
11. Sharp WG, Jaquess DL, Morton JF, Herzinger CV. Pediatric feeding disorders: A quantitative synthesis of treatment outcomes. *Clin Child Fam Psychol Rev*. 2010;13(4):348–65.

12. Postorino V, Sanges V, Giovagnoli G, Fatta LM, De Peppo L, Armando M, et al. Clinical differences in children with autism spectrum disorder with and without food selectivity. *Appetite*. 2015;92:126–32.
13. Silverman AH, Erato G, Goday P. The relationship between chronic paediatric feeding disorders and caregiver stress. *J Child Health Care*. 2021;25(1):69–80.
14. Michelson D, Davenport C, Dretzke J, Barlow J, Day C. Do evidence-based interventions work when tested in the "real world?" A systematic review and meta-analysis of parent management training for the treatment of child disruptive behavior. *Clin Child Fam Psychol Rev*. 2013;16:18–34.
15. Bearss K, Burrell TL, Stewart L, Scahill L. Parent training in autism spectrum disorder: What's in a name? *Clin Child Fam Psychol Rev*. 2015;18:170–82.
16. Burrell TL, Scahill L, Nuhu N, Gillespie S, Sharp W. Exploration of treatment response in parent training for children with autism spectrum disorder and moderate food selectivity. *J Autism Dev Disord*. 2023;53(1):229–35.
17. Vaz PC, Volkert VM, Piazza CC. Using negative reinforcement to increase self-feeding in a child with food selectivity. *Journal of Applied Behavior Analysis*. 2011;44(4):915–20.
18. Aponte CA, Brown KA, Turner K, Smith T, Johnson C. Parent training for feeding problems in children with autism spectrum disorder: A review of the literature. *Children's Health Care*. 2019;48(2):191–214.
19. Reed GK, Piazza CC, Patel MR, Layer SA, Bachmeyer MH, Bethke SD, et al. On the relative contributions of noncontingent reinforcement and escape extinction in the treatment of food refusal. *J Appl Behav Anal*. 2004;37(1):27–42.
20. Vollmer TR, Bacotti JK, Lloveras LA. Extinction and differential reinforcement. *Handbook of applied behavior analysis interventions for autism*. Cham: Springer International Publishing; 2022. p. 539–54.
21. Fedewa AL, Davis MC. How food as a reward is detrimental to children's health, learning, and behavior. *J Sch Health*. 2015;85(9):648–58.
22. Roberts L, Marx JM, Musher-Eizenman DR. Using food as a reward: An examination of parental reward practices. *Appetite*. 2018;120:318–26.
23. Touyz LM, Wakefield CE, Grech AM, Quinn VF, Costa DS, Zhang FF, et al. Parent-targeted home-based interventions for increasing fruit and vegetable intake in children: A systematic review and meta-analysis. *Nutr Rev*. 2018;76(3):154–73.
24. Fishbein M, Cox S, Swenny C, Mogren C, Walbert L, Fraker C. Food chaining: A systematic approach for the treatment of children with feeding aversion. *Nutr Clin Pract*. 2006;21(2):182–4.
25. Curtin C, Hubbard K, Anderson SE, Mick E, Must A, Bandini LG. Food selectivity, mealtime behavior problems, spousal stress, and family food choices in children with and without autism spectrum disorder. *J Autism Dev Disord*. 2015;45:3308–15.
26. Cermak SA, Curtin C, Bandini LG. Food selectivity and sensory sensitivity in children with autism spectrum disorders. *J Am Diet Assoc*. 2010;110(2):238–46.
27. Williams KE, Field DG, Seiverling L. Food refusal in children: A review of the literature. *Res Dev Disabil*. 2010;31(3):625–33.
28. Johnson CR, Turner K, Stewart PA, Schmidt B, Shui A, Macklin E, et al. Relationships between feeding problems, behavioral characteristics and nutritional quality in children with ASD. *J Autism Dev Disord*. 2014;44(9):2175–84.
29. Mazurek MO, Petroski GF. Sleep problems in children with autism spectrum disorder: Examining the contributions of sensory over-responsivity and anxiety. *Sleep Med*. 2015;16(2):270–9.
30. Suarez MA, Nelson NW, Curtis AB. Longitudinal follow-up of factors associated with food selectivity in children with autism spectrum disorders. *Autism*. 2014;18(8):924–32.
31. McElhanon BO, McCracken C, Karpen S, Sharp WG. Gastrointestinal symptoms in autism spectrum disorder: A meta-analysis. *Pediatrics*. 2014;133(5):872–83.
32. Buie T, Campbell DB, Fuchs III GJ, Furuta GT, Levy J, VandeWater J, et al. Evaluation, diagnosis, and treatment of gastrointestinal disorders in individuals with ASDs: A consensus report. *Pediatrics*. 2010;125 Supplement 1(Supplement_1):S1–S18.

33. Holingue C, Poku O, Pfeiffer D, Murray S, Fallin MD. Gastrointestinal concerns in children with autism spectrum disorder: A qualitative study of family experiences. *Autism*. 2022;26(7):1698–711.
34. Mazurek MO, Kanne SM, Wodka EL. Physical aggression in children and adolescents with autism spectrum disorders. *Res Autism Spectr Disord*. 2013;7(3):455–65.
35. Postorino V, Sharp WG, McCracken CE, Bearss K, Burrell TL, Evans AN, et al. A systematic review and meta-analysis of parent training for disruptive behavior in children with autism spectrum disorder. *Clin Child Fam Psychol Rev*. 2017;20:391–402.
36. Sharp WG, Burrell TL, Berry RC, Stubbs KH, McCracken CE, Gillespie SE, et al. The autism managing eating aversions and limited variety plan vs parent education: A randomized clinical trial. *J Pediatr*. 2019;211:185–92. e1.

Chapter 13

Feeding difficulties

Difficulty swallowing and the fear of aversive consequences

Nancy L. Zucker, Ilana B. Pilato, and Sarah LeMay-Russell

Chapter aims

This chapter will provide a detailed understanding of the emergence of fears of aversive consequences broadly and more specifically in youth with avoidant/restrictive food intake disorder (ARFID), practice guidance on differentially assessing ARFID from other related psychiatric disorders, and guidance on tools to address these fears in youth.

Learning points

- Describe the phenomenology of fears of aversive consequences and the emergence of the maladaptive fear network.
- Understand the differential diagnosis and diagnostic challenges when fears of aversive consequences manifest in ARFID relative to other psychiatric disorders such as specific phobia of vomiting or anorexia nervosa (AN) as well as when further medical diagnostic tests are warranted.
- Describe how a fear of aversive consequences presents in youth and how to assess these fears in youth.
- Practical recommendations will be given, including tools to address a fear of aversive consequences in youth.

The phenomenology of fears of aversive consequences: A cycle of somatic avoidance

Fear may play a crucial role in the initiation, exacerbation, and/or maintenance of many forms of pediatric gastrointestinal (GI) disorders. Fear is adaptive when individuals fear sensations or situations that pose a legitimate threat. Fear can become maladaptive when individuals learn to fear situations and stimuli that have an extremely low probability of causing harm. This can occur through learning processes of association. Not only will individuals learn to fear threatening stimuli, but they may also learn to fear situations and stimuli perceived to be linked with these threatening stimuli but which are, in fact, harmless. This can result in an elaborate fear network that encompasses a vast and nuanced array of harmless stimuli. People then act to avoid stimuli or circumstances with the potential to evoke fear. Thus, this elaborate fear network is coupled with a profoundly inhibited behavioral repertoire in which activities that are life-sustaining, life-promoting, and rewarding are avoided due to the potential threat of harm.

DOI: 10.4324/9781003308683-15

The purpose of this chapter is to explore the role of maladaptive fear-learning in the context of eating challenges in pediatric GI disorders. The chapter will (1) examine how this fear-learning network may function when the initial feared stimulus is a somatic sensation, such as the tightening of the throat, swallowing, or sensations of nausea or vomiting, (2) describe a model in which the factors that may increase vulnerability to the emergence of a GI disorder may also increase vulnerability to the emergence of an elaborate fear network, and (3) use a model to guide the choice of different intervention techniques that may be useful for the management of fear in youth. The chapter will also elucidate pragmatic challenges for differential diagnosis and assessment. Finally, the chapter describes some specific intervention approaches using the fear of swallowing as an example of maladaptive somatic fear. The term fear of aversive consequences (FOAC) will be used to encapsulate somatic sensations related to eating and digesting food that may be feared.

The emergence of a maladaptive fear network

Fear spreads. It is quite adaptive for a fear of something that poses a legitimate threat (i.e., has a high probability of causing harm) to generalize to similar objects or circumstances. For example, if an individual burns themselves on a hot stove-top, they don't need to replicate the experience to discern whether or not other hot stove-tops are harmful. It is also advantageous for that individual to generalize learning beyond the category of stoves to the broader category of hot surfaces. They do not need to directly experience contact with every hot surface to learn that such surfaces are probably best avoided. It is highly efficient and adaptive to create categories of things that have a high likelihood of harm and learn to avoid that category, even without having directly experienced harm from the majority of objects in that category, as a system for the preservation of life. However, the system is even more sophisticated than that. Individuals can also learn to distinguish sensations, stimuli, or situations that may predict future harm. In this example, thereby avoiding touching a stove-top that is starting to warm up. One challenge in harnessing fear as an adaptive protection device is the establishment of an optimal fear gradient – defining the boundaries around which fear would be adaptive versus impairing.

As shown in Figure 13.1, an individual experiences a real threat – they nearly choke. The proximal rings around this event represent reasonable reactions to threat: it would be safer for the individual in the future if they took smaller bites and ate more slowly, if, in fact, these were problems prior to the choking incident – of course, even this "adaptive" response could be taken to an extreme if the individual started taking such small bites that eating a sufficient quantity was challenging and/or if the length of mealtime started causing impairment in other areas. As the individual moves further and further out from the actual fear, the response to the threat becomes increasingly maladaptive. Avoiding all solid foods and then liquids represents an overgeneralized fear response to a threatening event.

It is important to consider how a maladaptive fear gradient may occur. To begin (for a sensation to become feared), it must first be perceived. For that reason, youth at risk for the emergence of pediatric GI disorders may be at a disadvantage given the burgeoning evidence documenting increased visceral hypersensitivity in individuals with various forms of GI disorders [1–3]. Visceral hypersensitivity is defined as the increased perception of sensations from the viscera (see [4] for some thoughts on the origins of visceral hypersensitivity). This sensitivity has been associated with increased pain and with more intense GI symptoms [1, 2], a feature that persists over time. Quite simply, youth with visceral hypersensitivity may notice and experience more intense sensations from their bodies (see Steps 1 and 2 of Figure 13.2).

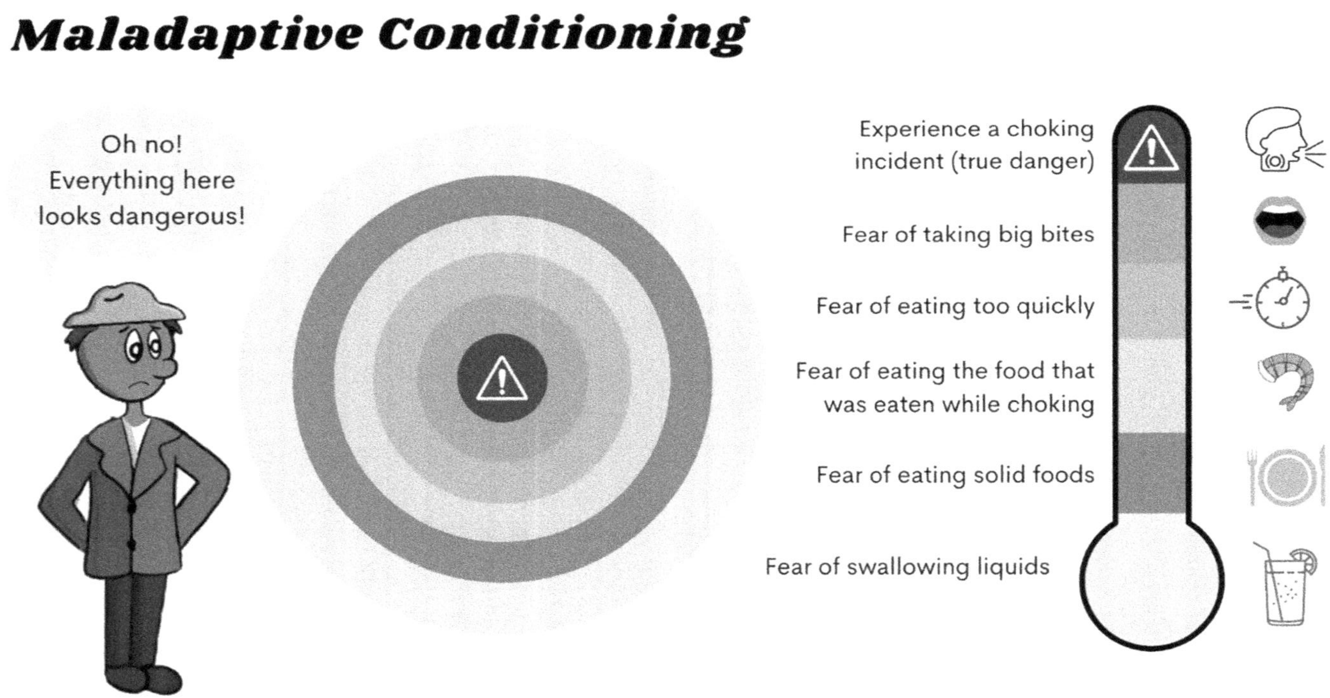

Figure 13.1 An example of a maladaptive fear gradient following a choking incident (Source: Julia Gianneschi).

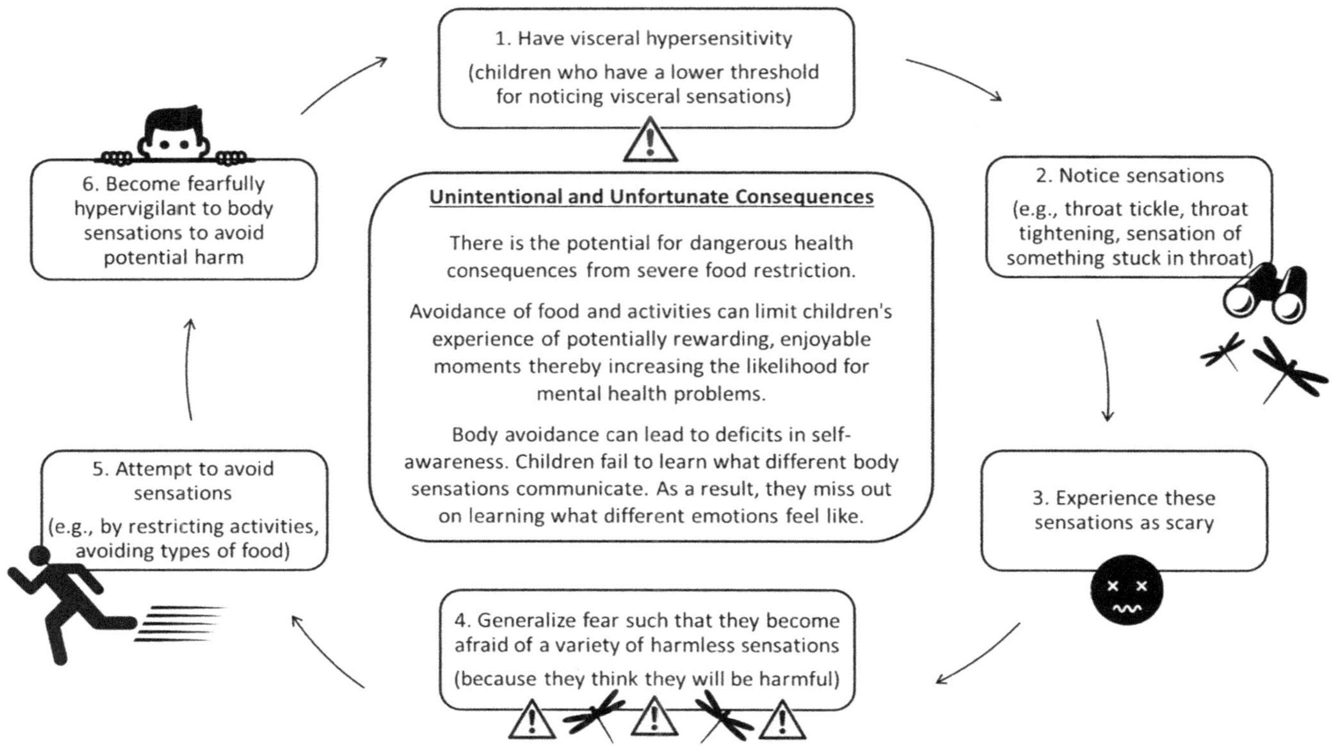

Figure 13.2 Cycle of somatic avoidance resulting from fear generalization (Note: A hypothetical model of fear generalization that may result in maladaptive avoidance; Source: Julia Gianneschi).

Certain bodily sensations signal threat or potential threat such as pain, choking, burning, vomiting, or gagging (see Chapter 15 for more information about the assessment of and psychophysiology of pain). Given the potential for harm, one's perceptual system prioritizes these threatening sensations or stimuli. In his model of fear-learning, Joseph LeDoux describes a "high road" and a "low road" that communicates to neural circuits responsible for detecting threats such as the limbic circuit [5]. The low road to the central node of the limbic circuit, the amygdala, is a rapid superhighway that detects and signals potential threats based on gross, perceptual features (e.g., sudden movement, an encroaching dark shadow) before the more integrated higher-order "high road" information has had time to figure out what the stimuli actually is – aka whether it is indeed threatening. This rapid low road to the limbic circuit facilitates an initial "knee-jerk" response to potential threats that helps us to be prepared to protect ourselves in the case of true danger (see Step 3 of Figure 13.2). However, it is also responsible for a startle response, such as when the vacuum robot quickly enters the room and is mistaken for a rodent. In regard to maladaptive fear conditioning, one can imagine that one could have overgeneralized "knee-jerk" responses to a variety of sensations with a low probability for threat (see Step 4 of Figure 13.2). Given that youth with visceral hypersensitivity notice more sensations and feel sensations more intensely, it is a reasonable hypothesis that they might also have a more potent "knee-jerk" response when they experience an intense sensation. However, it is important to note that this same cycle of fear avoidance can develop in any child that has experienced a fearful event, such as a choking incident.

Next, avoidance can occur. If one had a "knee-jerk" fear response to the typical sensations that constitute chewing and swallowing food, it would be very distressing and challenging to eat. Let's walk through an example. Imagine a child who has had a choking incident, a scary event for anyone. The child could learn to fear a variety of oral and throat sensations because they fear that these sensations may predict a future choking incident. Because eating and drinking are two behaviors that elicit sensations of chewing and swallowing food, the child may start to avoid activities such as eating certain types of food that elicit similar sensations. If this avoidance becomes severe, it may result in the aversive consequences listed in Figure 13.1 – the severe health consequences of food avoidance. Notwithstanding, there are social and emotional consequences to extreme avoidance. Avoiding food often means avoiding people, as eating is a very social activity (e.g., team sports, dinners, class parties, birthday parties). Food avoidance can quite rapidly contribute to the diminishment of activities that bring joy and thus set the stage for mental health problems (see Step 5 of Figure 13.2). Finally, the paradoxical combination of hypervigilance toward body sensations and yet attempts to avoid the experience of somatic sensations can interfere with the emergence of self-awareness and, more profoundly, one's sense of self (see Step 6, Figure 13.2). Individuals learn by reactions to experiences – what feels pleasurable, scary, etc.

Finally, paradoxical events can occur. Fear can exacerbate the very sensations that one is trying to avoid (see Step 6, Figure 13.2). The muscles of the throat can tighten when one is anxious, causing sensations that may exacerbate one's perceived threat of choking. Respiratory symptoms of anxiety, such as shortness of breath, can add to fears of choking. One can become more nauseous and vomit when one is anxious. These somatic sensations, if perceived as threatening, add to the cycle of fear and increase hypervigilance and potentially amplify attention to innocuous visceral sensations. The end result is that the individual may have increased awareness of their body, an awareness that is perceived via the lens of threat.

Now that there is an understanding of the experience of somatic fears and the learning framework that may exacerbate these fears, it is important to explore treatment planning and intervention. Of course, as GI mental health professionals, it is also important to determine whether a child (and caregivers') fears are adaptive or maladaptive. Therefore, it is necessary to understand the assessment of fear with particular focus on differential diagnosis as GI mental health professionals need to ensure that the child's fears are not exacerbated by an untreated medical condition that is contributing to harm.

Differential diagnosis of fears of aversive consequences

In order to treat a fear of an aversive consequence, one needs to define and differentiate this from other challenges that overlap in presentation. In this section, we will discuss ARFID, dysphagia, AN, and specific phobias, and how one might differentiate these conditions which all have some variation of fears of somatic sensations.

ARFID, a diagnosis codified in the *Diagnostic and Statistical Manual of Mental Disorders*, 5th edition (*DSM-5*) [6] is characterized by a pattern of restrictive or avoidant eating resulting in malnourishment, a low body weight, dependence on enteral feeding or supplements, and/or a significant impact on their psychosocial functioning [7]. Data support that youth with ARFID are significantly younger than those diagnosed with AN, with one study finding the age of onset to be 8 years old, compared to 16 years old in those with AN [8]. Though prevalence and incidence rates of ARFID have yet to be established, a recent study identified 23% of youth presenting to a pediatric neurogastroenterology clinic had symptoms of ARFID. Those with ARFID may restrict or avoid food for several reasons including a poor appetite or general disinterest in eating, sensory sensitivity, and/or a fear of aversive consequences such as vomiting or choking. Importantly, the eating restriction or avoidance cannot be attributed or better explained by what would be expected of a concurrent medical condition.

Dysphagia, or a physiological difficulty swallowing [9], may exist in isolation or in the context of other conditions. In youth, this may arise as youth achieve developmental milestones (e.g., sensory differentiation and integration or fine motor coordination) [10] or can be associated with factors such as premature birth [11], neurological difficulties [12], reflux [13], and congenital physiological malformations [14]. Dysphagia may have all of the same negative health and psychological consequences as FOAC, but the major distinction is that dysphagia is a skill-based deficiency [15]. Dysphagia is a physiological inability to swallow, and an eating disorder (such as ARFID) is the difficulty of swallowing that cannot solely be relegated to a physiological cause.

Assessment tools for dysphagia in pediatric populations include self-report screening tools (e.g., the Schedule for Oral-Motor Assessment [16] and the Dysphagia Disorder Survey [17]), radiographic assessments that illustrate throat function (e.g., videofluoroscopic swallow study [18], and fiberoptic endoscopic evaluation of swallow [19]). If these test results are negative, then difficulties with swallowing cannot be attributed to a sensorimotor or related deficit. This can be reassuring to both caregivers and GI mental health professionals as it allows for treatment planning that can include the inclusion of a variety of food textures when appropriate without fears that such foodstuffs have the potential to cause harm.

AN is an eating disorder characterized by significant food restriction driven by the pursuit of weight or body shape change, leading to subsequent weight loss, medical consequences of starvation and malnourishment, and impairment in functioning [7]. In the context of food restriction in AN, individuals frequently describe fears around food and eating. Furthermore, those with severe malnourishment and starvation symptoms may experience significant GI distress when eating [20]. This GI distress can, in turn, lead to a fear of GI sensations, further reinforcing beliefs that food is threatening and associated with food restriction, ultimately perpetuating the cycle [21]. Those with AN have been found to have heightened visceral sensitivity which can increase a fear of these physiological sensations [22]. This sensitivity can perpetuate the belief that food is unsafe and should be avoided, further worsening their behavior. Though AN and ARFID have similar presentations, ARFID is distinct in that those with ARFID do not experience disturbance in their experience of their shape and weight; therefore, food restriction is not used as a means of weight loss or to impact their shape [23].

In sum, those with AN may experience a FOAC; however, it is also important to assess other motivations for food restriction. If there is a concern that eating will contribute to weight gain, fear that they will become fat, or will change their body shape in a negative way, this may be a sign that AN is a more appropriate diagnosis. See the assessment section below for diagnostic tools to help differentiate AN from ARFID and FOAC more broadly.

Specific phobias are characterized as persistent, identifiable, and excessive fear(s) of a specific object or experience that typically elicit extreme anxiety leading to avoidance of the object of fear. Common phobias in youth include the dark, insects, clowns, injections, and others. Specific phobias of choking (pseudodysphagia), vomiting (emetophobia), and swallowing (phagophobia) are less common and are scarce in the literature [24–26], yet cause significant distress and can impact eating to similar levels of severity as ARFID or AN, which can also result in the same physiological consequences. It is common for these three phobias to develop following a traumatic event such as experiencing or witnessing a choking or vomiting episode; however, sometimes these fears appear idiopathically [25]. Individuals with ARFID typically have numerous motivations driving their food avoidance that may include FOAC but often includes sensory aversions and diminished experiences of reward from food. Research on the overlap and distinctiveness of FOAC in ARFID and specific phobias is sparse. Fear generalization is documented in both disorders. For example, in emetophobia, individuals may avoid eating to prevent vomiting, but also would likely avoid others who might vomit or any other experience that may induce vomiting such as riding a roller coaster or, in adult women, getting pregnant [26]. In ARFID cases where FOAC is present, individuals may generalize food-related anxieties from just one food (e.g., chicken) to entire food groups (e.g., all poultry or all meats), leading to broad food avoidance and restriction [27]. Evidence of fear generalization in ARFID beyond food is an area in need of further study.

Assessment of fears in youth

Assessment of fears in children ideally should integrate data from multiple reporters including youth and parents (see Handout 13.1 for an overview of existing screening instruments for fear of choking, vomiting, and eating). Additionally, given the limited screening measures available, it is important for providers to conduct a thorough medical evaluation in which youth and parents are queried about fears related to eating so that untreated medical contributions to difficulties with chewing and swallowing food can be delineated and treated [27].

Integrating treatment approaches into the fear-learning model

Treatment of somatic fears typically aims to create new learning experiences that demonstrate the safety of a previously feared stimulus. Inhibitory learning is one theoretical model proposed to explain how treatments for anxiety work [28]. New memories of safety compete for accessibility with older memories of fear. For example, imagine that an individual always ate scrambled eggs with bacon every morning without exception. If the person thought of scrambled eggs, they would think: bacon. But then they started having new experiences. Scrambled eggs with sausage, with toast, with hash browns, with sliced tomatoes, with cheese. Now, the thought of scrambled eggs conjures up innumerable possibilities. So it is with treatments for somatic fear; innumerable new experiences that occur with manageable uncertainty and without danger allow for different experiences of body sensations. Handout 13.2 lists the elements of the fear model (see Figure 13.2) and some possible treatment approaches.

A toolbox of strategies to address fears of aversive consequences

Given that many children with maladaptive fear-learning have trait-level heightened sensitivity to interceptive sensations [29, 30], it is recommended that providers encourage children to explore their body sensations with curiosity. This can be done in the context of interoceptive exposures, using an acceptance-based approach with the goal of building pleasurable memories that compete with previously established fearful ones. For example, rather than attempting to terminate or extinguish uncomfortable sensations, children can be taught to explore them and recognize interoceptive sensations as a source of information communicating needs such as hunger, fatigue, or an emotional experience. Children can then be provided with the tools to decipher these sensations' meanings and link them to adaptive actions that will allow them to meet particular needs. Practitioners teach families to use a playful approach and conduct exposures in a nonjudgmental and inquisitive manner so that children can meet uncertainty with lightness rather than anxiety.

Honoring children with the title of feeling and body investigators ("FBI" agents), specialists who gather clues about their bodies, provides the framework for these acceptance-based interoceptive exposures [30, 31]. The initial perception of a sensation should then be altered by linking sensations to different playful characters. Figure 13.3 depicts examples of characters associated with different throat sensations. Rather than experiencing fear when they notice an uncertain sensation in their throat, children link these experiences with characters: "Oh, that's Sizzling Sylvia, Tight-Wad Ty, or Stuck Sasha". Next, children design body investigations that manipulate these sensations and are intended to demonstrate how "wicked smart" and strong the body is. For example, each session begins by having youth listen to and manipulate their heart rate. In the spirit of keeping exposures playful, this bodily sensation is named Henry Heartbeat, with curiosity children explore raising and lowering it using in-session experiments (e.g., running around the room or taking deep breaths). Children are then encouraged to consider what they have learned about the wisdom of their bodies during this investigation (e.g., "my heart is smart and can adapt!").

To help children encode this new memory, children add a drawing of what they have learned to a life-sized outline of their body. Similar explorations can be conducted with other bodily sensations (e.g., noticing Gaggy Greg or Victor Vomit). Through these investigations, children not only learn to approach the exploration of bodily sensations with curiosity rather than fear, but also link the information gathered to important information about their experiences and needs. While the strategies described were developed for young children, older children and adolescents may also appreciate and enjoy this approach. For these age groups, it is best to let the children/adolescents decide or develop their own characters. However, the investigative framework, scientific data collection of body symptoms, and design of investigations that probe body symptoms work well. The investigations are simply more sophisticated!

Youth are also taught to have a playful and curious approach to satiety cues as they eat new foods, which are called food adventures. For example, parents are encouraged to facilitate

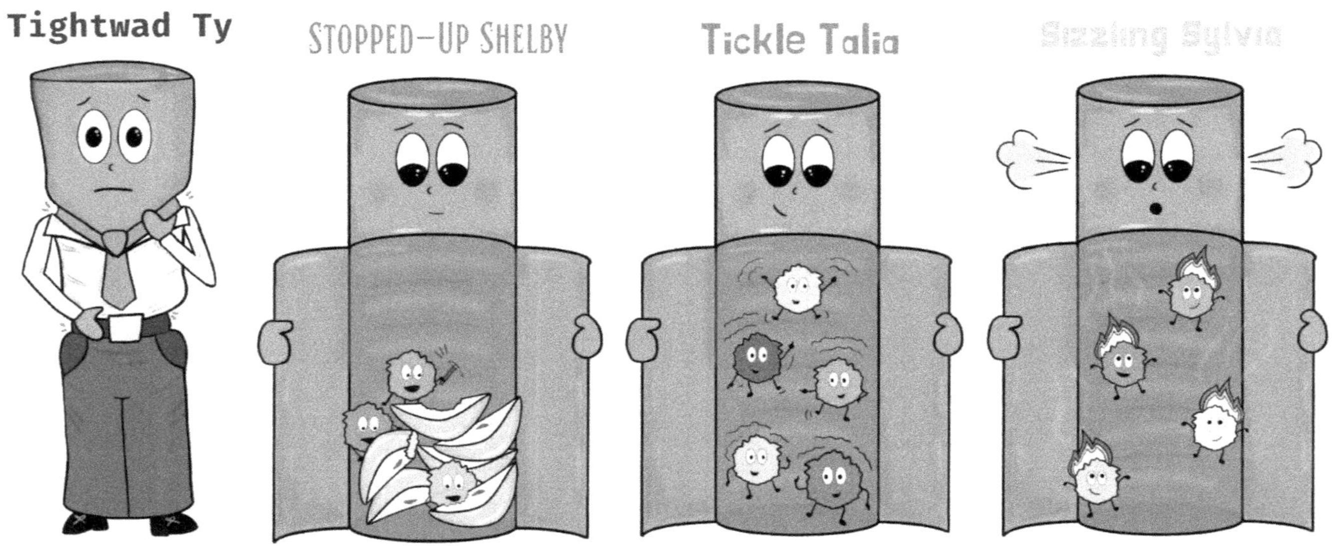

Figure 13.3 Throat sensation characters (Note: Some examples in which the initial "knee-jerk" reaction is altered to an innocuous sensation by associating this sensation with a playful character. Critically, this strategy presumes that all necessary medical evaluations have been conducted and necessary medical management has been implemented; Source: Julia Gianneschi).

experiments with eating new or feared foods by scaffolding the approach to the food. Youth are taught to build their own scaffold and approach new foods in the same curious fashion that they approach their body sensations. They may first touch the food, then smell it, then lick it, then explore taking one bite. This builds autonomy as well as teaches youth how to take action toward a desired outcome (i.e., eating a new food). Finally, youth and parents are encouraged to reflect on any challenging situations that occurred in the past to consider what they learned – again, in a nonjudgmental manner. By conducting these acceptance-based explorations of the body and foods, youth will ultimately learn to recontextualize uncomfortable sensations.

One feared experience often cited by youth is the fear of gagging (Gaggy Greg) or vomiting (Victor Vomit). Youth and their families are guided to become curious and investigative about their gag reflexes and to engage in disgusting activities that might lead to vomiting. Families are also encouraged to conduct a systematic mapping of their tongues to locate the gag reflex. Youth and parents are taught to have contingency plans in place for the worst possible outcomes, such as aprons, garbage cans, and/or decorative barf bags. Families also prepare an Aftertaste Challenge – something sure to wipe out a nasty taste. Youth and parents eat barf-flavored jelly beans and explore how our body handles it and a sensitive gag reflex is reframed as one that gets activated to unexpected sensations. Families are also taught to try to "expect the unexpected" by making predictions about what something might feel and taste like but then expect to be wrong – so that the unexpected is expected (youth love the contradictions of this). By repeating this investigation, youth learn that the unexpected does not necessarily always lead to their feared outcome, and that even if it were to result in the feared outcome they have the ability to tolerate and soothe themselves through it.

Special considerations for tube weaning

For some youth, food restriction is so severe that they must be placed on supplemental or replacement tube feeding. Given the complexity of considerations that go into the type of supplementation and subsequent weaning from tube feeding upon increased oral intake, this chapter will not attempt to delineate such procedures. However, it is notable that many of the procedures mentioned here may increase a child's motivation to approach food and thus increase intake – strategies that may help expedite the process of tube weaning. For some helpful references, including a recent position paper on best practices, see: [32–35].

Summary

Youth who come to fear their bodies may have an as-yet-untold origin story – they have sensory superpowers, abilities that allow them to feel what others cannot feel. Changing a legacy of vulnerability to one of strength is something we can try to build for all youth – but those with visceral hypersensitivity may be particularly good at it.

Pearls of wisdom

- Pleasurable memories can compete with fearful memories.
- Changing the initial perceptual framework to innocuous sensations can alter cycles of avoidance.
- Changing the quality of attention toward physical symptoms, such that it is with nonjudgmental curiosity, may be an important emphasis of treatment with youth. Youth are just

learning about their bodies and thus diverting their attention away from information that can increase their wisdom and self-trust may not be optimal.

- Creating a scaffolding around food approach that is designed by youth and includes initial "too easy" steps may build self-efficacy and confidence toward food consumption.

Recommended readings

For youth and caregivers:

- Zucker, N., Gagliano, M.E., and Loeb, K.L. (2023). *A Parent's Guide to Treating Functional Abdominal Pain in Children with Feeling and Body Investigators*. Cambridge University Press.

For mental health professionals:

- Zucker, N., Gagliano, M.E., and Loeb, K.L. (2023). *Treating Functional Abdominal Pain in Children: The Feeling and Body Investigator Intervention.* Cambridge University Press.
- Thomas, J. J., Becker, K. R., Kuhnle, M. C., Jo, J. H., Harshman, S. G., Wons, O. B., Keshishian, A. C., Hauser, K., Breithaupt, L., Liebman, R. E., Misra, M., Wilhelm, S., Lawson, E. A., & Eddy, K. T. (2020). Cognitive-behavioral therapy for avoidant/restrictive food intake disorder: Feasibility, acceptability, and proof-of-concept for children and adolescents. *The International Journal of Eating Disorders*, 53(10), 1636–1646.

References

1. Simren M, Tornblom H, Palsson OS, van Tilburg MA, Van Oudenhove L, Tack J, et al. Visceral hypersensitivity is associated with GI symptom severity in functional GI disorders: Consistent findings from five different patient cohorts. *Gut*. 2017;67(2):255–62.
2. Simren M, Tornblom H, Palsson OS, Van Oudenhove L, Whitehead WE, Tack J. Cumulative effects of psychologic distress, visceral hypersensitivity, and abnormal transit on patient-reported outcomes in irritable bowel syndrome. *Gastroenterology*. 2019;157(2):391.
3. Josefsson A, Rosendahl A, Jeristad P, Naslin G, Tornblom H, Simren M. Visceral sensitivity remains stable over time in patients with irritable bowel syndrome, but with individual fluctuations. *Neurogastroenterol Motil*. 2019;31(7).
4. Liu S, Hagiwara SI, Bhargava A. Early-life adversity, epigenetics, and visceral hypersensitivity. *Neurogastroenterol Motil*. 2017;29(9):e13170.
5. LeDoux J. *The emotional brain: The mysterious underpinnings of emotional life*. New York: Simon and Schuster; 1998.
6. Association AP. *Diagnostic and statistical manual of mental disorders (DSM-5®)*. Washington, DC: American Psychiatric Association; 2013.
7. Association AP. *Diagnostic and statistical manual of mental disorders, text revision DSM-5-TR*. Washington, DC: American Psychiatric Association; 2022.
8. Becker KR, Keshishian AC, Liebman RE, Coniglio KA, Wang SB, Franko DL, et al. Impact of expanded diagnostic criteria for avoidant/restrictive food intake disorder on clinical comparisons with anorexia nervosa. *Int J Eat Disord*. 2019;52(3):230–8.
9. Dodrill P, Gosa MM. Pediatric dysphagia: Physiology, assessment, and management. *Ann Nutr Metab*. 2015;66(Suppl. 5):24–31.
10. Fernando N, Potock M. Sights, sounds, and exploration: Understanding the sensory system raising a healthy, happy eater New York. New York: The Experiment; 2015.

11. Jadcherla S. Dysphagia in the high-risk infant: Potential factors and mechanisms. *Am J Clin Nutr*. 2016;103(2):622S–8S.
12. Morgan AT, Dodrill P, Ward EC. Interventions for oropharyngeal dysphagia in children with neurological impairment. *Cochrane Database Syst Rev*. 2012;10.
13. Suskind DL, Thompson DM, Gulati M, Huddleston P, Liu DC, Baroody FM. Improved infant swallowing after gastroesophageal reflux disease treatment: A function of improved laryngeal sensation? *The Laryngoscope*. 2006;116(8):1397–403.
14. Abadie V, Couly G. Congenital feeding and swallowing disorders. *Pediatric neurology part III. 113: Elsevier Inc. Chapters*; 2013.
15. Perry SE, Sevitz JS, Curtis JA, Kuo S-H, Troche MS. Skill training resulted in improved swallowing in a person with multiple system atrophy: An endoscopy study. *Mov Disord Clin Pract*. 2018;5(4):451–2.
16. Ko MJ, Kang MJ, Ko KJ, Ki YO, Chang HJ, Kwon J-Y. Clinical usefulness of Schedule for Oral-Motor Assessment (SOMA) in children with dysphagia. *Ann Rehabil Med*. 2011;35(4):477–84.
17. Sheppard JJ, Hochman R, Baer C. The dysphagia disorder survey: Validation of an assessment for swallowing and feeding function in developmental disability. *Res Dev Disabil*. 2014;35(5):929–42.
18. Bülow M. Videofluoroscopic swallow study: Techniques, signs and reports. *Stepping Stones to Living Well with Dysphagia*. 72: Barcelona: Karger Publishers; 2012. pp. 43–52.
19. Boseley ME, Ashland J, Hartnick CJ. The utility of the fiberoptic endoscopic evaluation of swallowing (FEES) in diagnosing and treating children with Type I laryngeal clefts. *Int J Pediatr Otorhinolaryngol*. 2006;70(2):339–43.
20. Sato Y, Fukudo S. Gastrointestinal symptoms and disorders in patients with eating disorders. *Clin J Gastroenterol*. 2015;8(5):255–63.
21. Zucker NL, Bulik CM. On bells, saliva, and abdominal pain or discomfort: Early aversive visceral conditioning and vulnerability for anorexia nervosa. *Int J Eat Disord*. 2020;53(4):508–12.
22. Brown TA, Reilly EE, Murray HB, Perry TR, Kaye WH, Wierenga CE. Validating the visceral sensitivity index in an eating disorder sample. *Int J Eat Disord*. 2021.
23. Izquierdo A, Plessow F, Becker KR, Mancuso CJ, Slattery M, Murray HB, et al. Implicit attitudes toward dieting and thinness distinguish fat-phobic and non-fat phobic anorexia nervosa from avoidant/restrictive food intake disorder in adolescents. *Int J Eat Disord*. 2019;52(4):419–27.
24. Baijens LWJ, Koetsenruijter K, Pilz W. Diagnosis and treatment of phagophobia: A review. *Dysphagia*. 2013;28(2):260–70.
25. Lopes R, Melo R, Curral R, Coelho R, Roma-Torres A. A case of choking phobia: Towards a conceptual approach. *Eat Weight Disord*. 2014;19(1):125–31.
26. Veale D, Costa A, Murphy P, Ellison N. Abnormal eating behaviour in people with a specific phobia of vomiting (emetophobia). *Eur Eat Disord Rev*. 2012;20(5):414–8.
27. Brigham KS, Manzo LD, Eddy KT, Thomas JJ. Evaluation and treatment of avoidant/restrictive food intake disorder (ARFID) in adolescents. *Curr Pediatr Rep*. 2018;6(2):107–13.
28. Craske MG, Treanor M, Conway CC, Zbozinek T, Vervliet B. Maximizing exposure therapy: An inhibitory learning approach. *Behav Res Ther*. 2014;58:10–23.
29. Hechler T. Altered interoception and its role for the co-occurrence of chronic primary pain and mental health problems in children. *Pain*. 2021;162(3):665–71.
30. Zucker NL, LaVia MC, Craske MG, Foukal M, Harris AA, Datta N, et al. Feeling and body investigators (FBI): ARFID division – An acceptance-based interoceptive exposure treatment for children with ARFID. *Int J Eat Disord*. 2019;52(4):466–72.
31. Zucker NL, Mauro C, Craske M, Wagner HR, Datta N, Hopkins H, et al. Acceptance-based interoceptive exposure for young children with functional abdominal pain. *Behav Res Ther*. 2017;97:200–12.
32. Clouzeau H, Dipasquale V, Rivard L, Lecoeur K, Lecoufle A, Le Ru-Raguénès V, et al. Weaning children from prolonged enteral nutrition: A position paper. *Eur J Clin Nutr*. 2022;76(4):505–15.
33. Krom H, de Meij TGJ, Benninga MA, van Dijk-Lokkart EM, Engels M, Kneepkens CMF, et al. Long-term efficacy of clinical hunger provocation to wean feeding tube dependent children. *Clinl Nutr*. 2020;39(9):2863–71.

34. Edwards S, Davis AM, Bruce A, Mousa H, Lyman B, Cocjin J, et al. Caring for tube-fed children: A review of management, tube weaning, and emotional considerations. *J Parenter Enteral Nutr.* 2016;40(5):616–22.
35. Gardiner AY, Fuller DG, Vuillermin PJ. Tube-weaning infants and children: A survey of Australian and international practice. *J Paediatr Child Health.* 2014;50(8):626–31.

Chapter 14

Nausea and vomiting

Sally Tarbell

Chapter aims

This chapter describes common pediatric nausea and vomiting disorders followed by recommended assessment methods to help guide treatment. Detailed descriptions of behavioral interventions are provided for gastrointestinal (GI) mental health professionals to help youth and their parents manage these conditions.

Learning points

- Characteristics of nausea and vomiting disorders and rumination.
- Assessment methods to track symptoms and optimize care.
- A framework for managing these conditions as well as specific approaches for each disorder.

Nausea and vomiting are common in GI disorders. This chapter focuses on conditions where nausea and/or vomiting are the primary diagnoses; however, guidelines for the management of these disorders can be applied to nausea and vomiting symptoms in other GI conditions. The Rome IV diagnostic criteria for nausea and vomiting disorders in children (ages 4–9) and adolescents (10 years and older) are presented in Table 14.1 [1]. Nausea and vomiting are often considered to be different symptoms of one condition; however, the child can have nausea or vomiting alone as well as in combination. Rumination, which involves bringing up undigested food, is not a vomiting disorder per se, but it will also be addressed. Contextual factors to consider when caring for these youth and their families are presented followed by treatments for specific nausea and vomiting disorders (NVD).

Compared to other GI disorders, there is limited research on underlying causes and effective treatments for NVD [2]. In fact, functional nausea and functional vomiting were not recognized as diagnostic entities until the publication of the Rome IV criteria for pediatric disorders of gut–brain interaction (DGBI; formally known as functional gastrointestinal disorders) [1]. This lack of recognition likely limited advances in clinical care and research into underlying causes and best treatment approaches. Children with NVD may see multiple specialists and undergo extensive medical work-ups to evaluate their symptoms [3, 4]. When no underlying causes are found and other conditions are ruled out, the child is diagnosed with DGBI. These disorders typically are not associated with abnormal labs, tests, or imaging. The symptoms are real; however, their pathophysiology is not well understood. After diagnosis, these children can be referred to a mental health provider to address behavioral factors that may influence symptom onset and persistence and to assist them develop strategies to cope with the symptoms and limit their impact on functioning.

DOI: 10.4324/9781003308683-16

Table 14.1 Rome IV diagnostic criteria for pediatric nausea and vomiting disorders [1]

Diagnosis	*Diagnostic criteria*
Functional nausea	Must include all of the following:[1] 1. Bothersome nausea as the predominant symptom, occurring ≥2 times per week, and generally not related to meals. 2. Not consistently associated with vomiting. 3. After appropriate evaluation, the nausea cannot be fully explained by another medical condition.
Functional vomiting	Must include all of the following:[1] 1. On average, ≥1 episodes of vomiting per week. 2. Absence of self-induced vomiting or criteria for an eating disorder or rumination. 3. After appropriate evaluation, the vomiting cannot be fully explained by another medical condition.
Cyclic vomiting syndrome	Must include all of the following:[1] 1. The occurrence of ≥2 periods of intense, unremitting nausea and paroxysmal vomiting, lasting hours to days within a 6 month period 2. Episodes are stereotypical in each patient. 3. Episodes are separated by weeks to months with return to baseline health between episodes. 4. After appropriate medical evaluation, the symptoms cannot be attributed to another condition.
Rumination	Must include all of the following:[1] 1. Repeated regurgitation and rechewing or expulsion of food that: a. Begins soon after ingestion of a meal. b. Does not occur during sleep. 2. Not preceded by retching. 3. After appropriate evaluation, the symptoms cannot be fully explained by another medical condition. 4. An eating condition and eating disorder must be ruled out.

[1]Criteria fulfilled for at least 2 months before diagnosis.

NVD are associated with several comorbidities, including other DGBI (e.g., functional constipation, and functional abdominal pain) as well as neurological conditions, postural orthostatic tachycardia syndrome (POTS), and migraine. In the case of infants (<2 years) and toddlers (2–3 years), NVD often overlaps with rumination and developmental disorders [4, 5]. Psychiatric comorbidity, particularly anxiety [4], has also been identified in youth with these disorders, with as many as 47% (40/85) meeting cut-off for an anxiety disorder in those with cyclic vomiting syndrome (CVS) as one example [6]. Nausea and/or vomiting symptoms may be aggravated or provoked by anxiety, but it would be a mistake to attribute the symptoms to psychiatric factors alone. If the child is seen by a physician who considers psychiatric factors to contribute significantly to the symptoms, the family may be left with the impression that the provider thinks the symptoms are "all in their head" and may feel their concerns are not validated. In such cases, these perceptions may interfere with families seeking out or engaging in mental health treatment. Thus, it is essential they be educated in the biopsychosocial model of DGBI to help them appreciate the rationale for the involvement of a behavioral health professional in their care (see Chapters 2 and 9).

Functional disability is common in children with nausea and vomiting. Nausea in particular is an intensely uncomfortable and often debilitating symptom. Youth with NVD have been found to miss a lot of school and to be more functionally disabled than children with other GI and other medical conditions [4–6]. For example, youth with functional abdominal pain who also have nausea have been identified as having worse short- and long-term GI and somatic symptoms as well as reduced mental health and functional outcomes, compared to those with functional abdominal pain alone [7]. Anxiety comorbidity, including the fear of having symptoms in school, can contribute to school avoidance, but for other youth it is the symptoms themselves that undermine the child's capacity to engage in normal activities. For example, the relentless nausea and vomiting associated with a CVS episode often interfere with school attendance, as most schools do not want a vomiting student to attend classes.

Assessment of youth with NVD

A biopsychosocial approach is essential to the assessment and management of NVD [8]. Assessment optimally includes a review of the youth's medical record for identification of common comorbid conditions, especially those such as migraine headaches and POTS, given their association with nausea and/or vomiting. While the mental health practitioner's role is not to differentially diagnose the NVD, it is important to consider the impact of these associated conditions on nausea and vomiting. See Box 14.1 for recommended assessment methods.

BOX 14.1 RECOMMENDED ASSESSMENT FOR NVD

Assess nausea and/or vomiting:

- The Baxter retching faces scale [9]
- Nausea severity scale [10]
- Nausea profile [11]

Screen for common comorbidities:

- PROMIS® (Patient Reported Outcomes Measurement Information System) Scales [12]: anxiety, depression, fatigue, pain, peer relationships, sleep problems

Evaluate behavioral/lifestyle factors associated with symptoms:

- Sleep hygiene
- Hydration
- Eating habits
- Overexertion
- Stress

Screen for substance use:

- Brief screening tool for alcohol and drugs (BSTAD) [13]
- Screening to brief intervention (S2B1) [14]

Evaluate the impact of symptoms on functioning:

- Functional disability inventory [15]
- PROMIS® Scales [12] e.g., pain interference, physical mobility
- Standard school attendance question from the US National Center for Health Statistics [16]

Scales that measure nausea and vomiting symptoms provide a baseline assessment of symptoms that can be readministered to review treatment impact. The Baxter retching faces scale is a self-report measure of acute nausea severity for children aged 7–18 years [9]. It consists of six faces with a rating scale of 0–10. A Spanish language version is also available [17]. The nausea severity scale was developed and validated to assess nausea severity in youth aged 11–17 with abdominal pain-related DGBI [10]. This 4-item scale assesses symptoms experienced over the past two weeks. It includes days with nausea, vomiting episodes daily, duration of nausea, and nausea intensity. As nausea is a symptom with both somatic and psychological components, much like pain, assessment, and management of these multiple dimensions can help focus treatment. The nausea profile is a 17-item questionnaire that assesses the subjective experience of nausea, providing a total and three subscale scores: somatic distress, gastrointestinal distress, and emotional distress [11]. Developed and validated in a young adult, nonclinical population, the scale has shown excellent reliability in youth aged 10 and older with chronic functional nausea [18]. Subscales have been shown to be associated with comorbid symptoms such as anxiety and orthostatic intolerance (i.e., development of symptoms such as lightheadedness and nausea upon standing that resolve when lying down) [18].

Screening for comorbid conditions such as recurrent or chronic pain, fatigue, anxiety, depression, and sleep disruption is indicated due to the potential impact of these disorders on NVD. The PROMIS® (Patient Reported Outcomes Measurement Information System) scales are recommended as an efficient method for symptom screening, as well as to assess factors that may mediate treatment outcomes such as social relations, physical functioning, coping, and self-efficacy [12]. Several of these scales are available in four- and eight-item formats, include self and parent-proxy reports, and have versions in more than one language. All provide standard scores. The scales are developed for youth aged 5–17. Information on the development and use of these scales, which are offered at no cost, is available at: www.healthmeasures.net.

Evaluation of behavioral/lifestyle factors is indicated to determine if they may contribute to symptoms and to provide insight into points of intervention for behavioral modification that can impact symptom burden. These include a brief evaluation of eating habits such as whether the child has regular meals and snacks or avoids particular foods or eating more generally due to concern about aggravation of symptoms. Although families may report specific food triggers for nausea and vomiting symptoms, there is sparse evidence that particular foods contribute to symptom onset. Fasting or irregular eating patterns and inadequate fluid intake can be associated with lightheadedness and aggravate nausea; this is especially true for adolescents (age 10+) with comorbid POTS. Sleep disruptions are common in these disorders, especially in the case of CVS, where symptom onset can disrupt sleep. Thus, assessment of sleep hygiene (e.g., regular bed time, avoidance of screens and physical activities prior to bedtime) is helpful to identify areas to intervene for symptom prevention. Stressors, including those associated with school, family and social relationships, as well as overscheduling, participation in competitive pursuits, and demanding physical activities, have the potential to aggravate and, in the case of CVS, trigger symptoms [19].

Screening for substance use is indicated in adolescents with NVD as they may use cannabis to manage symptoms. The BSTAD (brief screen for tobacco, alcohol and drugs) www.nida.nih.gov/bstad is a three-question screen for adolescents [13]. The S2BI (screening to brief intervention) www.nida.nih.gov/s2bi/#1, includes a single screening question for eight commonly misused substances [14]. Both instruments identify and categorize substance use risk level in adolescents aged 12–17 years. These screens are administered online and include self-report and clinician versions. An additional resource from the American Academy of Pediatrics provides an algorithm to help guide brief intervention for youth who are identified as having a substance use disorder [20]. Cannabis use is widely reported in CVS, especially among adolescent males, with users reporting it ameliorates their nausea and vomiting [21]. Youth may use cannabis for symptom control; however; those with weekly or greater use are at increased risk for cannabinoid hyperemesis syndrome (CHS), a disorder characterized by episodes of intense nausea, vomiting, and abdominal pain that can lead to emergency room visits for symptom control [22]. Youth with suspected CHS are advised to discontinue the use of cannabinoids. If the youth is not able or unwilling to reduce and optimally stop their marijuana use, it may be necessary to refer the youth to substance use treatment.

Given the significant functional disability reported in children and adolescents with NVD, it is important to appreciate the impact of these disorders not only on the child but on the family as a whole, as these disorders can be detrimental to parental quality of life [23]. The Functional Disability Inventory (ages 8–17) and the PROMIS measures (ages 5–17) such as the mobility and pain interference scales can be used to assess illness impact on the child [12, 15]. A validated question on illness impact on school attendance from the National Health Interview Survey [16] can be used to track this important measure of child functioning and provide population samples to compare children with other chronic illnesses. Assessment of functional disability is important upon initial evaluation, and also for tracking of treatment outcomes, particularly when symptoms may not improve but functioning can. Next, general principles to help engage youth with NVD in treatment are provided, followed by behavioral treatments for the specific disorders.

Treatment primer on NVD

The first step is to orient youth and their families to treatment, including:

- Validation of symptoms (i.e., they are not all "in your head").
- Inquire about and acknowledge the impact of the symptoms on the youth and family.
- Inspire hope that the youth can feel better and that you can help in their treatment.
- Provide education about DGBI (i.e., what we know about behavioral treatment and how it can help; see Chapters 2 and 9).
- Acknowledge any youth comorbidities identified on initial screening and how they may impact treatment (e.g., treatment of anxiety to assist with nausea and vomiting symptoms).
- Inform the family that treatment involves:
  - Collaborative youth/family participation.
  - Practice assignments or "homework" between appointments.
  - Parent involvement, such as help with symptom tracking, coaching of skills being taught to the youth, especially for young (ages 4–6) and school-aged children (7–10). Parents are also asked to encourage the youth's functioning even when symptoms persist. These efforts can help mitigate against social isolation and disengagement from normal activities, which can adversely affect mood.

After orienting the child and family to treatment, it is recommended that the GI mental health professional start with symptom tracking and mind–body interventions to focus on symptom-related distress (i.e., what is most important to the youth). The ultimate goal is to improve function and health-related quality of life, which tend to improve before symptoms, but it is helpful at the start to assure the family that you are attending to the symptoms that brought the youth to treatment in the first place.

Introduce self-monitoring. This task will vary depending on the child's age and development. For younger children and those with developmental disabilities, caretakers are tasked with symptom monitoring. Older children and adolescents can be responsible for tracking symptoms, i.e., document frequency and context of symptoms, potential triggers, and responses to treatment (see Handout 14.1). Older youth may prefer to monitor symptoms with a smartphone app.

Teach a mind–body skill. Abdominal breathing and/or other relaxation techniques to address the role of sympathetic activation in NVD. "One-size-doesn't-fit-all" when it comes to relaxation training, e.g., the youth may not respond to progressive muscle relaxation, but may respond to the use of imagery. Adolescents may also prefer an app for relaxation training and practice. Biofeedback can be especially helpful for youth who are skeptical that practicing relaxation can modify their somatic responses to stress. Younger children can be provided with props such as a picture of a flower and birthday cake and asked to "smell the flower and blow out birthday cake candles" to help them learn abdominal breathing.

Use problem-solving with the youth and family (for younger children) for lifestyle modification relevant to symptoms, as identified by symptom tracking.

Evaluate and address the role of cognitions, anxiety and mood on symptoms and functioning as per standard cognitive behavioral therapy (CBT) and/or acceptance and commitment therapy (ACT) interventions as indicated.

Ensure family involvement to support focus on function vs. only symptom control. Parents may be very distressed by their child's symptoms, especially when there are few effective medical treatments for nausea and vomiting. It is important to provide ongoing reassurance to the parent that behavioral treatments have been successful in managing these aversive symptoms. As an example, only behavioral treatments have an evidence base for rumination.

Before treatment approaches for specific NVD are addressed, it is important to acknowledge that the evidence base for behavioral treatment of these disorders is limited. Thus, the GI mental health professional is encouraged to adapt evidence-based treatment (EBT) from management of other DGBI (e.g., functional abdominal pain, irritable bowel syndrome), migraine (relevant for CVS), and psychiatric comorbidities, including anxiety and depression in the management of these conditions; see Chapter 16.

Treatment of functional nausea and functional vomiting

Clinical presentation

These disorders are typically diagnosed in older school age and adolescent children. Multifactorial etiologies are thought to contribute to these symptoms, and multisystemic comorbidities can complicate care. There are few effective medical and behavioral interventions for functional nausea and vomiting, a situation that can heighten the youth's and family distress.

Functional nausea (FN)

FN is a persistent, typically daily, distressing and often impairing symptom, noted most commonly in adolescent females [3]. Nausea has been noted to be most prominent in the morning, diminishing over the day [2]. The only evidence-based psychological treatment for pediatric

FN is hypnotherapy [24]. The impact of hypnotherapy on FN was more modest than has been shown for functional abdominal pain, with the authors suggesting that tailoring the hypnotherapy protocol specifically for FN might improve treatment response (see Chapter 17).

FN is associated with multisystem comorbidities (e.g., abdominal pain, migraine, orthostatic intolerance, and anxiety [25]). Recent research has identified subtypes of functional nausea, based on comorbidities, with one type associated with anxiety and depression [26]. Optimizing management of comorbidities with evidence-based treatments for chronic pain, anxiety, and autonomic dysregulation (e.g., increased hydration for comorbid POTS) offers opportunities to improve both nausea and functional status. Adapting the rehabilitation approach used for management of pediatric chronic pain, including decrease focus on symptom vs. function, address fear avoidance and catastrophizing, as well as collaboration with allied health (nutrition, physical therapy) in treatment, may help with the management of chronic FN (see Chapter 16).

Functional vomiting (FV)

Functional vomiting tends to be intermittent and low frequency (i.e., vomiting —one to two times per episode), as compared to the persistent, daily symptoms of functional nausea. It is important to ensure that other conditions such as rumination, eosinophilic esophagitis, or eating disorders have been ruled out as causes for the vomiting prior to intervention. There is scant literature on the psychological management of functional vomiting. However, behavioral treatments developed to address chemotherapy-related nausea and vomiting, including management of sympathetic autonomic arousal with relaxation techniques and hypnotherapy, and addressing any comorbid anxiety with EBTs, can inform approaches to FV [27]. Given the likelihood that functional vomiting may be triggered by conditioned responses to perceived stressors, symptom tracking can provide insight into factors that contribute to symptom onset and maintenance. For example, in one case the author treated, symptom tracking of FV revealed it was associated with anticipation of school presentations. The use of heart rate variability biofeedback to modify the child's stress response combined with CBT to modify cognitive distortions resulted in the resolution of the vomiting symptoms.

Treatment of cyclic vomiting syndrome (CVS)

Clinical presentation

CVS is diagnosed from infancy to adulthood, with onset most common in ages 3–5 [28]. CVS is characterized by stereotypic vomiting episodes, with each episode having the same characteristics (e.g., time of day – typically 1–3 am or upon awakening), prodromal symptoms (fatigue, excessive salivation, decreased appetite), duration (hours to days) [29]. There are four stages to a CVS episode: the prodrome, attack, and recovery period similar to migraine headaches for majority of youth, followed by an interictal period with return to baseline health between episodes [29, 30]. Due to the severity of nausea and vomiting in CVS (e.g., vomiting up to 6 times per hour, for hours or days), treatment in the attack phase can include IV hydration, sedation and pain control, limiting options for behavioral intervention. Thus, treatment focus for the GI mental health professional is on interictal periods for episode prevention.

Behavioral intervention

- The GI mental health professional provides education that CVS episodes are often preceded by identifiable triggers (e.g., excitement, anxiety/panic, specific stressors, travel, lifestyle factors such as sleep disruption, overexertion, dehydration, menses, skipping meals – factors that can "drain the body's battery" [28, 29]), see Handout 14.2.

- Youth and/or the parent (parent required for infants, toddlers, and children 4–9 years; parent involvement optional for those 10 years and older) are asked to track potential triggers (see Handout 14.1), including events that happen within 1–2 days prior to CVS episode onset. Parents and/or older youth are advised to pay special attention to: changes in sleep pattern, irregular meal times (especially fasting), lack of hydration, viral illness, and stressors (changes in schooling, social relationships). Disruptions to routines that frequently occur during holidays (travel, sleep schedule perturbations, changes in meal schedules, excitement in anticipation of a special event/occasion) can be triggers. Anything that activates the sympathetic nervous system, be it a negative stressor or positive excitement, can lower the threshold for an attack (i.e., drain the battery). In school-aged children, it is common for the child/family to report a history of the child becoming sick with a CVS episode during holidays and vacations. In such cases, gathering detailed information regarding changes in routines and stressors can identify a potential trigger that can be targeted for behavioral intervention.
- Screen for substance use in adolescents is due to the association of CVS with CHS. Provide education about the adverse impact of cannabinoids on CVS episodes. Refer youth for substance use treatment as indicated.

Once factors that may be associated with episode onset (e.g., lifestyle, stress, anxiety) are identified through the youth's symptom log (see Handout 14.1), the treatment focus turns to episode prevention by managing lifestyle risk factors and episode triggers. The GI mental health professional provides education in a relaxation technique, problem-solving for stress/trigger management, guidance in implementing lifestyle modifications, and CBT or ACT techniques as indicated to address comorbid anxiety commonly associated with CVS episodes [6]. See Box 14.2 for a case example. See also Slutsker et al. [31] for a case report of the successful treatment of CVS resulting in the sustained relief of symptoms.

BOX 14.2 CASE EXAMPLE OF CVS TREATMENT

In the evaluation of 10-year girl who had a history of CVS attacks on birthdays, her symptom log revealed that the excitement and high expectations of the special day may be potential triggers. To address this hypothesis, she was provided with training in a daily relaxation exercise, as well as the use of cognitive strategies, to address her birthday-related thoughts (e.g., "My birthday will be a fun, but it is possible to have a great day without getting 'too excited'"). She was able to engage in positive self-talk to enjoy her birthday without getting sick. For the first time in several years, she enjoyed her 10th birthday at a bowling alley and did not have a CVS attack.

Treatment of rumination

While the focus is to help the youth avoid episodes through trigger management, it is also important to support the family's efforts to obtain appropriate school accommodations. One particularly helpful modification is to have the youth's schedule for core courses modified so that they take these classes later in the day, allowing for a potential late start due to the occurrence of episodes overnight or in the early morning rather than missing the whole school day.

Clinical presentation

Rumination involves the repeated regurgitation of food during or soon after eating, which can be accompanied by rechewing, re-swallowing, or spitting out food. Rumination can occur in infants (<2 years) and toddlers (2–3 years), particularly those with developmental disabilities as well as normally developing children and teens [32]. There may be a delay in the diagnosis of rumination in older children and teens, and other conditions that may resemble rumination, such as eating disorders (e.g., bulimia), should be ruled out. There is significant functional disability identified in both young children and adolescents with rumination, including malnourishment in young children and school absences and avoidance of social activities involving eating in older children [33].

Behavioral intervention

Rumination most commonly occurs after eating, but it also can occur at other times. For early school-aged and older children, the GI mental health professional can describe rumination as a "habit" the child has developed. For example, children may engage in rumination when they experience abdominal discomfort after a meal and learn that it is relieved by the ruminative behavior.

In order to increase awareness of the rumination symptoms and to identify what factors may trigger or maintain the habit, the GI mental health professional asks the parent and/or youth to keep a detailed log of ruminative urges and behaviors and associated activities for 1–2 weeks (see Handout 14.1).

- Once triggers are identified, the GI mental health professional and youth/family engage in problem-solving together to modify suspected triggers and identify coping skills that may reduce rumination when it appears to be triggered by anxiety or other stressors.
- Next, the GI mental health professional provides education that they cannot bring food up into their mouths when they use abdominal breathing. This is because the lowering of the diaphragm in abdominal breathing is a competing response to the abdominal wall contraction that occurs in rumination. The GI mental health professional then instructs the youth in abdominal breathing.
- Have the youths put one hand on their chest and one on the abdomen. In abdominal breathing *only* the abdomen should move. The youth is encouraged to practice abdominal breathing lying down at first to help distinguish abdominal from chest breathing. GI mental health professionals can ask permission to place their hand on the child's abdomen, while encouraging the child to breathe into their hand as if they were "blowing up a balloon" to help the child grasp what abdominal breathing feels like. The GI mental health professional describes abdominal breathing as "simple but not easy" and emphasizes the need for practice to consolidate this skill.
- The GI mental health professional may suggest the app "Breathe2Relax", which has a video "Show Me How" demonstrating abdominal breathing. Parents need to coach and monitor correct practice in younger children. It is helpful for the parent to learn abdominal breathing to help supervise correct practice.

- Once youths have demonstrated the ability to do abdominal breathing, they are provided with Handout 14.3 that provides instructions on how to implement abdominal breathing to inhibit rumination after meals. Youths/parents (for younger children) are advised to track symptoms and responses to abdominal breathing.
- If feasible, have the child eat food in the GI mental health professional's office, especially any foods that are identified as potential triggers for rumination, so that the GI mental health professional can evaluate the ruminative behaviors in real time and coach the youth/parent on the use of abdominal breathing and other strategies to cope with the urge to ruminate.
- Rumination can be associated with caregiver neglect or as a self-stimulatory behavior in young children [34]. In these cases, intervention focuses on modification of the environment or caretaker–child interaction. If triggers are not readily identified through symptom charting, particularly in infants and children with development disabilities, consultation with a speech/language therapist or a behavioral analyst for functional behavioral analysis can help identify contingences influencing rumination [35].
- For refractory cases, the addition of CBT, including more intensive problem-solving related to trigger management and maintaining factors, teaching skills to cope with any discomfort associated with inhibiting the urge to ruminate, and exposures to identified triggers, has been shown to be effective in improving treatment response in adolescents and adults [36, 37].

Pearls of wisdom

- Nausea and/or vomiting symptoms may be aggravated or provoked by anxiety, but it would be a mistake to attribute the symptoms to psychiatric factors alone. Psychological treatments may be rejected due to youth feeling their symptoms are considered to be "all in their head". Therefore, approach the child and family with compassion, validate their experiences, help youth learn how psychological methods can be helpful, and inspire hope that they can feel better.
- Adapt established behavioral treatment methods for your patient. These "borrowed" treatments have an evidence base, and you are simply applying them to new disorders that have been neglected.

Summary

NVD are characterized by very aversive symptoms, multisystem comorbidities, and significant functional disability. Comprehensive initial and ongoing assessment, including symptom charting, are indicated to identify factors that influence symptom onset, persistence, and develop treatments that optimize outcomes. Psychological treatments, including hypnotherapy, abdominal breathing and other mind–body techniques, lifestyle modifications, and standard CBT interventions, have shown promise in improving symptoms and functioning in NVD.

Recommended readings

For youth and caregivers:

- Information and support for youth with CVS and families: www.cvsaonline.org
- For children aged 7–12, a primer on CBT for symptom management: Culbert, T & Kajander, R. (2007) *Be the Boss of Your Stress.* Free Spirit Publishing.

For mental health professionals:

- Williams, S.E., & Zahka, N.E. (2017). *Treating Somatic Symptoms in Children and Adolescents.* The Guilford Press.

References

1. Di Lorenzo C, Nurko S, Committee PRI. *Rome IV functional pediatric gastrointestinal disorders: Disorders of gut-brain interaction.* Drossman D, Chang L, Chey W, Kellow J, Tack J, Whitehead W, editors. Raleigh, NC: Rome Foundation; 2016:1257–61.
2. Di Lorenzo C. Functional nausea is real and makes you sick. *Front Pediatr.* 2022;10:e848659.
3. Kovacic K, Miranda A, Chelimsky G, Williams S, Simpson P, Li BU. Chronic idiopathic nausea of childhood. *J Pediatr.* 2014;164(5):1104–9.
4. Tarbell S, Sullivan E, Meegan C, Fortunato J. Children with functional nausea—Comorbidities outside the gastrointestinal tract. *J Pediatr.* 2020;225:103–8.
5. Martinez M, Rathod S, Friesen HJ, Rosen JM, Friesen CA, Schurman JV. Rumination syndrome in children and adolescents: A mini review. *Front Pediatr.* 2021;9:709326.
6. Tarbell S, Li BU. Psychiatric symptoms in children and adolescents with cyclic vomiting syndrome and their parents. *Headache.* 2008;48:259–66.
7. Russell AC, Stone AL, Walker LS. Nausea in children with functional abdominal pain predicts poor health outcomes in young adulthood. *Clin Gastroenterol Hepatol.* 2017;15(5):706–11.
8. Black CJ, Drossman DA, Talley NJ, Ruddy J, Ford AC. Functional gastrointestinal disorders: Advances in understanding and management. *Lancet.* 2020;396(10263):1664–74.
9. Baxter AL, Watcha MF, Baxter WV, Leong T, Wyatt MM. Development and validation of a pictorial nausea rating scale for children. *Pediatrics.* 2011;127:e1542–e9.
10. Russell AC, Stone AL, Wang A, Walker LS. Development and validation of a nausea severity scale for assessment of nausea in children with abdominal pain-related functional gastrointestinal disorders. *Children (Basel).* 2018;5(6):68.
11. Muth E, Stern R, Thayer J, Koch K. Assessment of the multiple dimensions of nausea: The Nausea Profile (NP). *J Psychosom Med.* 1996;40:511–20.
12. PROMIS® (Patient-Reported Outcomes Measurement Information System): Northwestern University. Available from: https://www.healthmeasures.net/explore-measurement-systems/promis.
13. Kelly S, Gryczynski J, Mitchell S, Kirk A, O'Grady K, Schwartz R. Validity of brief screening instrument for adolescent tobacco, alcohol, and drug use. *Pediatrics.* 2014;133(5):819–26.
14. Levy S, Weiss R, Sherritt L, Ziemnik R, Spalding A, Van Hook S, et al. An electronic screen for triaging adolescent substance use by risk levels. *JAMA Pediatr.* 2014;168(9):822–8.
15. Walker LS, Greene JW. The functional disability inventory: Measuring a neglected dimension of child health status. *J Pediatr Psychol.* 1991;16(1):39–58.
16. Black L, Benson V. Tables of summary health statistics for U.S. children: 2018 National health interview survey. 2019. Available from: https://www.cdc.gov/nchs/nhis/SHS/tables.htm. SOURCE: NCHS, National Health Interview Survey, 2018.
17. Watcha MF, Medellin E, Lee AD, Felberg MA, Bidani SA. Validation of the pictorial Baxter Retching Faces scale for the measurement of the severity of postoperative nausea in Spanish-speaking children. *Brit J Anaesth.* 2018;121(6):1316–22.
18. Tarbell SE, Shaltout HA, Wagoner AL, Diz DI, Fortunato JE. Relationship among nausea, anxiety, and orthostatic symptoms in pediatric patients with chronic unexplained nausea. *Exp Brain Res.* 2014;232:2645–50.
19. Thavamani A, Umapathi KK, Khatana J, Bhandari S, Kovacic K, Venkatesan T. Cyclic vomiting syndrome-related hospitalizations trends, comorbidities & health care costs in children: A population based study. *Children (Basel).* 2022;9(1):55.

20. Committee on Substance A, Levy SJ, Kokotailo PK. Substance use screening, brief intervention, and referral to treatment for pediatricians. *Pediatrics*. 2011;128(5):e1330–40.
21. Mille J, Walsh M, Patel P, Rogan M, Arnold C, Maloney M, et al. Pediatric cannabinoid hyperemesis: Two cases. *Pediatr Emerg Care* 2010;26:919–20.
22. Hasler W, Levinthal D, Venkatesan T. Clinical features of cannabinoid hyperemesis syndrome. In: Hasler W, Levinthal D, Venkatesan T, editors. *Cyclic vomiting syndrome and cannabinoid hyperemesis*. London: Academic Press; 2022. p. 141–56.
23. Wang-Hall J, Li BUK, Tarbell SE. Family health-related quality of life in pediatric cyclic vomiting syndrome. *J Pediatr Gastroenterol Nutr.* 2018;66(5):738–43.
24. Browne P, de Bruijn C, Speksnijder E, den Hollander B, van Wering H, Wessels M, et al. Skills or pills: Randomized trial comparing hypnotherapy to medical treatment in children with functional nausea. *Clin Gastroenterol Hepatol.* 2022;20:1847–56.
25. Tarbell SE, Sullivan EC, Meegan C, Fortunato JE. Children with functional nausea-comorbidities outside the gastrointestinal tract. *J Pediatr.* 2020;225:103–8.e1.
26. Sullivan E, Fortunato J, Gray E, Tarbell S. Use of cluster analysis to identify subtypes of pediatric functional nausea. *J Pediatr Gastroenterol Hepatol Nutr.* 2022;74(6):765–9.
27. Patel P, Robinson PD, Devine KA, Positano K, Cohen M, Gibson P, et al. Prevention and treatment of anticipatory chemotherapy-induced nausea and vomiting in pediatric cancer patients and hematopoietic stem cell recipients: Clinical practice guideline update. *Pediatr Blood Cancer.* 2021;68(5):e28947.
28. Li BU, Balint JP. Cyclic vomiting syndrome: Evolution in our understanding of a brain-gut disorder. *Adv Pediatr.* 2000;47:117–60.
29. Li B, Misiewicz L. Cyclic vomiting syndrome: A brain-gut disorder. *Gastroenterol Clin N Amer.* 2003;32(3):997–1019.
30. Li BU, Lefevre F, Chelimsky GG, Boles RG, Nelson SP, Lewis DW, et al. North American Society for Pediatric Gastroenterology, Hepatology, and Nutrition consensus statement on the diagnosis and management of cyclic vomiting syndrome. *J Pediatr Gastroenterol Nutr.* 2008;47(3):379–93.
31. Slutsker B, Konichezky A, Gothelf D. Breaking the cycle: Cognitive behavioral therapy and biofeedback training in a case of cyclic vomiting syndrome. *Psychol Health Med.* 2010;15(6):625–31.
32. Martinez M, Rathod S, Friesen H, Rosen J, Friesen C, Schurman J. Rumination syndrome in children and adolescents: A mini review. *Front Pediatr.* 2021;9:1–7.
33. Chial H, Camilleri M, Willaims D, Litzinger K, Perrault J. Rumination syndrome in children and adolescents: Diagnosis, treatment and prognosis. *Pediatrics.* 2003;111(1):158–62.
34. Lyons-Ruth K, Zeanah C, Benoit D, Madigan S, Mills-Koonce W. Disorder and risk for disorder during infancy and childhood. In: Mash E, Barkley R, editors. *Child Psychopathology.* 3rd ed. New York: Guilford Press; 2014. p. 673–736.
35. Woods K, Luiselli J, Tomassone S. Functional analysis and intervention for chronic rumination. *J Appl Behav Anal.* 2013;46(1):328–32.
36. Murray HB, Juarascio AS, Di Lorenzo C, Drossman DA, Thomas JJ. Diagnosis and treatment of rumination syndrome: A critical review. *Am J Gastroenterol.* 2019;114(4):562–78.
37. Schroedl R, Alioto A, Di Lorenzo C. Behavioral treatment for adolescent rumination syndrome: A case report. *Clin Pract Pediatr Psychol.* 2013;1(1):89–93.

Chapter 15

Pain disorders

Introduction, assessment, and psychophysiology

Liz Febo-Rodriguez and Miguel Saps

Chapter aims

This chapter aims to discuss types of pediatric gastrointestinal (GI) disorders that can lead to pain, as well as some of the therapeutic alternatives available to manage them.

Learning points

- Develop a basic understanding of the pathophysiology of pain.
- Being able to identify the most common GI disorders associated with pain.
- Discern the intricate link between pain and disability.
- Review medical assessment and treatment for GI pain.

Humans experience two types of pain: nociceptive (caused by noxious or potentially harmful stimulus) and neuropathic pain (pain not originating from a stimulus, often due to nerve damage). Nociceptive pain can be further subdivided into somatic and visceral pain (see Handout 15.1). Somatic pain comes from damage to muscles, bones, and skin, and thus can be identified easily. For example, if a person falls and scrapes their knee, they are able to pinpoint exactly where it hurts. Visceral pain, on the other hand, comes from internal organs, for example, due to menstrual pain or a GI infection. Abdominal pain is a form of visceral pain that is common in many GI conditions. Examples of painful conditions that frequently present in the pediatric gastroenterology practice are functional dyspepsia, celiac disease, and inflammatory bowel disease (IBD) (see Chapter 4). Identifying the exact cause of abdominal pain is important for treatment, yet given the visceral nature of this type of pain, it can be poorly localized and may be referred to other somatic and visceral structures, which challenges identification of the likely source of pain. The next section will explore the pathophysiology of abdominal pain.

Pathophysiology of abdominal pain

The underlying pathophysiology of pain is complex. Pain is not just a nociceptive signal from the gut to thc brain. Rather, these nociceptive inputs interact in complex ways with the brain, where previous experiences, cognitions, and emotions color the pain experience. Therefore, pain is always approached from a biopsychosocial model (see Chapter 2). Abdominal pain can have many different causes, including injury and inflammation. In the gut, pain can particularly be caused by changes in motility (how fast or slow the gut moves), delays in stomach emptying, as well as changes in accommodation (how much the gut wall stretches to accommodate a

DOI: 10.4324/9781003308683-17

meal). A mental health professional would rarely deal with acute abdominal pain (although see Chapter 5 for pain management related to GI procedures), yet multiple GI disorders are characterized by chronic abdominal pain and this will be the focus of the current chapter.

The role of the enteric and central nervous systems

The collection of nerves in the GI tract is referred to as the enteric nervous system. This system is complex and can regulate gut function without the help from the central nervous system (i.e., the "big brain") and is therefore sometimes dubbed "the small brain". Nociceptive and other stimuli from the enteric nervous system are relayed to the brain by the spinal cord. The central nervous system integrates other information with the nociceptive signal (e.g., What is its meaning? What is the threat value? Can we find help?), which increases or decreases our attention to the signal and determines our physiological and behavioral response. For example, if a child has pain due to being constipated and the child considers this "normal", the central nervous system may "ignore" the nociceptive signals. In a way we become unaware of the nociceptive signal. On the other hand, when youth become vigilant about the meaning of the pain – especially the worry that it may signify a disease or injury – the central nervous system may "dial up" the pain and cause the child to find help. This cross-talk between the enteric and central nervous systems, when working well, aims to not overwhelm our brain with unnecessary information (e.g., "Your stomach is churning" after you just ate), while allowing us to pay attention to signals we do need (e.g., "You are about to have diarrhea, better look for a toilet").

In some cases, pain can occur even without an injury, inflammation, or other nociceptive input. This is common for youth with painful disorders of gut–brain interaction (DGBI). These children have a disordered brain–gut axis. For example, a child may have been completely recovered from a stomach bug (gastroenteritis), but still continues to complain of stomach cramps 6 months later. The gut is healed, but the symptoms remain. This is puzzling as the pain has a high threat value and usually informs us that we are (about to be) harming ourselves. If there is no harm, why is there pain? Increased pain perception in youth with DGBI is partly related to altered central nervous system response to gut signals, combined with less descending (from central to enteric nervous system) inhibition of nociceptive signals. This means that there might be increased spinal nociceptive transmission, resulting in increased pain perception. Take the example of eating. This is a mostly nonpainful experience but a large meal consumed on Christmas can lead to stomach discomfort. The enteric and central nervous system response to a regular meal can become disordered and cause discomfort with normal-sized meals. The nervous system responds as if every meal is a feast and hence brings discomfort. This tendency to report abdominal pain at lower pain thresholds than normal is called visceral hypersensitivity.

Visceral hypersensitivity

Visceral hypersensitivity is a general increase in pain sensation experienced in internal organs. As discussed earlier, visceral hypersensitivity is caused by altered interaction between the enteric and the central nervous systems [1]. Multiple factors predispose individuals to visceral hypersensitivity, including genetic, environmental, psychosocial (early stressors in life), and diet. These factors can alter the brain–gut axis communication by altering descending inhibitory control, impairing stress response, and/or sensitizing primary sensory neurons and central spinal neurons [1]. This then leads to abnormal secretion of excitatory neurotransmitters, such as serotonin, which can result in changes in the central nervous system and trigger symptoms such as headache, abdominal pain, and discomfort [1, 2]. Brain imaging in adults has shown that those with irritable bowel syndrome (IBS) have connectivity abnormalities in emotion and sensory/motor regions [3]. Given this data, neuromodulation and psychological therapies that can alter central pathways are being increasingly used to treat DGBI [4].

Gut microbiota

Diet, stress, and early life experiences can alter the gut microbiota. This can result in abnormal GI motility, abnormal myoelectrical activity, poor antral motility and gastric emptying, and abnormal gastric accommodation. These are all pathophysiological processes underlying pain (see Chapter 2 for a more in-depth discussion on the role of microbiota on GI symptoms).

Abdominal pain in youth

DGBI and pain

Abdominal pain-predominant DGBI are highly prevalent in youth, with an overall prevalence between 25% and 29% [5, 6]. Most of the youth who seek medical advice for chronic abdominal pain are suffering from DGBI, most often functional abdominal pain disorders (FAPDs), but other disorders such as constipation can also be associated with pain [7]. FAPDs include functional dyspepsia (FD), IBS, abdominal migraine (AM), and functional abdominal pain not otherwise specified (FAP-NOS) [8]. See Table 15.1 and Chapter 3 for a more detailed description of these disorders. These disorders are characterized by abdominal pain that cannot be solely explained by organic damage or disease [9]. This often leads to the assumption that they are caused by stress

Table 15.1 FAPD subtypes

FAPDs	*Presenting symptoms*	*Proposed mechanism(s)*	*Prevalence*
FD	Postprandial fullness, early satiety, epigastric pain, burning sensation.	Visceral hypersensitivity, delayed gastric emptying, psychosocial factors, dysfunction of the central nervous system, lifestyle factors.	3–27%
IBS	Abdominal pain related to either: defecation, change in frequency of stool, change in appearance of stool.	Dysregulated brain–gut signaling, which results in visceral hyperalgesia and altered bowel habits.	2.8%
AM	Paroxysmal episodes of intense, acute periumbilical, midline, or diffuse abdominal pain; stereotypical episodes. Episodes can be associated with anorexia, nausea, vomiting, headache, photophobia, pallor.	Unclear, and thus treatment is suboptimal with avoidance of triggers and prophylactic treatment.	4%
FAPD-NOS	Episodic or continuous abdominal pain that does not occur during physiologic events (i.e., menses).	Unclear, but visceral hypersensitivity seems to play a role.	1.2–2%

or anxiety (if it is not the body, it must be the brain). Rather FAPDs are caused by changes in the brain–gut axis and can be best explained within a biopsychosocial framework (see Chapter 2).

Organic GI disorders

Organic diseases that can present with abdominal pain include but are not limited to celiac disease, IBD, eosinophilic gastroenteritis, gastritis, and gastroparesis, among others (see Chapter 3 for an explanation). In these disorders, pain is primarily caused by nociceptive processes such as inflammation. However, the severity of pain and how people respond to pain are not always directly related to the severity of the nociceptive input. Pain should be examined within a biopsychosocial framework. In these youth, pain can persist even when the inflammation has been adequately addressed. It is well described that youth with IBD have a high prevalence of IBS-type symptoms. Isgar et al. [10] were the first to report IBS-type symptoms in 33% of youth with ulcerative colitis (UC) in remission. A systematic review and meta-analysis in adults showed the prevalence of IBS in all IBD patients was 39% [11]. In youth, the prevalence of DGBI in pediatric patients with IBD in remission ranges from 9% to 26% [12, 13]. Youth with an overlap of DGBI and IBD are at increased risk for depression, fatigue, and greater impairments of quality of life [13, 14]. This may not be a condition solely affecting youth with IBD. For example, youth with celiac disease have been described to suffer from FAPDs as well [15], and youth with gastroparesis often remain symptomatic despite appropriate treatment of delayed gastric emptying. This overlap is especially problematic because both conditions can present similarly, making it difficult for the provider to discern if symptoms are related to DGBI or an exacerbation of their underlying chronic GI condition. This may result in unnecessary testing and aggressive treatments of youth with overlapping conditions.

The overlap can be frustrating for parents as well, who despite undertaking the task of managing their child's disease cannot eliminate their child's symptoms. A thorough explanation of the reason for the overlap and acknowledgment of the frustration is needed. For youth with IBD, the parent may worry the child's GI inflammation has returned and demands unnecessary testing/treatment, while for celiac disease or eosinophilic esophagitis parents may show poor adherence to dietary treatment because the child is still symptomatic. A discussion about DGBI and appropriate treatment for these symptoms needs to ensue.

Pain and disability

Pain affects all youth and may impact their lives to a large degree (see also Box 15.1). Chronic abdominal pain, no matter its origin, is associated with lower quality of life, increased psychological distress, impaired sleep, and disability [16]. In youth with IBD, rather than disease activity, the presence of pain is associated with lower quality of life and increased disability [17]. Thus, treating pain is important no matter its origin. Pain can be treated by treating the cause (harm); however, in many youth, pain can exist in excess of any biological explanation. Given the high threat value of pain, youth quickly learn to avoid situations or actions that cause or increase pain. For example, when you have broken your ankle, you avoid weight-bearing activities to allow it to heal. However, in the case of chronic pain, especially for DGBI where there is no harm, avoidance is unlikely to reduce pain. Instead of abandoning unsuccessful coping, youth often will increasingly try to control the pain by generalizing avoidance to other situations leading to intricate models of "safe" versus "unsafe" situations and foods. This can have wide impacts on the lives of youth living with pain. School avoidance due to pain is a common problem that has far-reaching consequences for youth's academic advancement. In addition, school avoidance will often increase stress (e.g., over missed work, missed tests, lower grades), which perpetuates pain. Youth also commonly avoid social situations such as attending sports practice, family gatherings, birthday parties, etc., which isolates them from peers and can further increase the occurrence, intensity, or maintenance of pain. For this reason, both pain and disability are primary targets of treatment. Even when a child presents with minor disability, strategies should be implemented to prevent avoidance from becoming more problematic over time.

BOX 15.1 CAN EVERYONE FEEL PAIN?

Pain is a ubiquitous human experience. There has been a period in which it was suggested young children (especially newborns) and people of certain backgrounds (especially Black people) could not experience pain or would feel less pain. This is pertinently untrue. Since pain levels can only be known by asking a person, identifying pain in preverbal children can be challenging. For example, to date, we do not know if infant colic is associated with abdominal pain. Crying and grimacing is a good indicator of pain, but a small child can cry without pain present. In addition, infants and toddlers may not always cry when they feel pain. It is well known that toddlers will avoid certain behaviors they associate with pain. For example, a painful bowel movement may lead to avoidance of having another one (see Chapters 18 and 19), and pain with eating may lead to avoidance of food (see Chapters 10-13).

Medical assessment and treatment of abdominal pain

Treatment of pain starts in the physician's office. Many parents and their children may come in with previous negative experiences, especially for youth with DGBI. Clinicians may have previously suggested the pain is "all in the child's head" or "the child is faking the pain". Many families also have not received appropriate explanation about why there can be pain without a medical explanation. It is important for the health professional to develop a positive therapeutic relationship with the youth and family during the first visit. Expectations as far as management and treatment outcomes should be discussed. The Rome Foundation encourages limiting invasive testing, barring any red flags (see Handout 15.2), as unnecessary procedures can place additional stress on the GI system and keep the parents hoping a "medical explanation" can be found. Once a diagnosis of abdominal pain of functional origin is established, it should be discussed as a "positive diagnosis" [18]. Engaging the family, discussing pathophysiology, and answering all questions are essential. Many families feel like their symptoms are being dismissed and that the child is "making them up"; thus, it is important to validate their feelings and make clear statements such as, "I know your pain is real" [18]. Follow-up visits should be scheduled periodically; this way, the family will feel assured that their concerns are being addressed and are not being dismissed [18]. This also allows the health professional to follow the child and make sure they are not missing a progressive disease. Thus, for any pain (organic or DGBI), it is important to reiterate that their pain is real, they are not being dismissed, and that the provider will continue to monitor them closely.

Pharmacologic management

Unfortunately, evidence supporting the use and efficacy of pharmacological treatments in youth with abdominal pain is lacking [19]. Very few randomized controlled trials exist in the pediatric world, and most of these have a small sample size, limited follow-up, inadequate concealment of treatment group allocation, lack of power, and/or use of non-validated questionnaires [8]. See Table 15.2 for a summary of therapies used for youth with FAPDs. Fortunately, there are therapeutic alternatives for youth with organic diseases, such as biologics for IBD.

Table 15.2 Pharmacologic management of abdominal pain

Form of pain medication	*Examples*	*Disease it is used for*	*Mechanism of action*
Antispasmodics	Peppermint oil	DGBI, specifically FD and IBS.	Acts directly on smooth muscle by decreasing contractions, thereby reducing cramps; relaxes lower esophageal sphincter.
	Drotaverine hydrochloride	DGBI, specifically FD and IBS	Inhibitor of phosphodiesterase isoenzyme IV.
	Mebeverine	DGBI, specifically FD and IBS	Unknown, but appears to work directly on smooth muscle within the GI tract.
Antidepressants	Amitriptyline	Abdominal pain in both organic and DGBI.	Tricyclic antidepressant; believed to have central and/or peripheral analgesic pathways properties.
	Citalopram	Abdominal pain in both organic and DGBI.	Selective serotonin reuptake inhibitor.
Antihistamines	Cyproheptadine	Abdominal pain in both organic and DGBI.	Improves fundic accommodation.
Antiseizure medications	Gabapentin, pregabalin	Abdominal pain in both organic and DGBI.	Decreases abnormal electrical activity of the brain.
Prokinetics	Domperidone, metoclopramide	Gastroparesis	Dopamine D2 receptor antagonists.
	Erythromycin	Gastroparesis	Motilin receptor agonist.
Biologics	infliximab, Adalimumab	IBD	TNF alfa inhibitor.
	Ustekinumab	IBD	IL-12 and IL-23 inhibitors.

Non-pharmacologic management

Psychological interventions have proved to be a successful intervention for abdominal pain DGBI [8, 20]. A Cochrane systematic review from 2017 concluded that cognitive behavioral therapy (CBT) and hypnotherapy, discussed in chapters 16 and 17, were promising treatments for FAPDs, although the quality of the evidence was poor [21]. Pediatric trials are notoriously difficult to perform and almost always underfunded, leading to lower quality evidence (see Chapters 16 and 17 for a discussion of these modalities). Of note, interventions are most successful when multidisciplinary care is instituted, which should include a pediatrician, specialist physician(s), mental health provider, physical therapist, nutritionist, and other stakeholders in the child's well-being [9]. This is not always feasible; however, a large number of primary care providers are integrating mental health professionals into their clinical practices and are having more success with treating mental and functional health concerns compared to those that refer out [9]. See Chapter 7 for a discussion of multidisciplinary care.

Other evidence-based nonpharmacological treatments for pain include yoga therapy [7, 8], and auricular neurostimulation (IB-Stim, Neuraxis Inc.) which modulate central pain pathways, and consequently visceral hypersensitivity [22], and a low FODMAP (fermentable oligosaccharides, disaccharides, monosaccharides, and polyols) diet lowering the consumption of fermentable carbohydrates [23]. Although diet interventions are preferred by many youth [24], adherence to the low FODMAP diet can be difficult. This diet is highly restrictive, especially removing foods youth tend to favor. This diet should preferably be recommended by a trained dietitian, as long-term use can result in nutritional deficiencies if not followed properly. A cautionary aspect of using restrictive diets is that in youth with a history of eating disorders or orthorexia, the practitioner has to make sure that the child does not interpret the diet as food being pernicious for their health. Collaboration with GI mental health professionals can be useful for this purpose.

Learning points

- The visceral nature of abdominal pain makes it increasingly difficult to manage and can be incredibly frustrating for both youth and parents. It is important to establish rapport with these families and explain the gut–brain axis and the concept of visceral pain.
- Youth with organic GI disease have a high prevalence of DGBI, making their management difficult. These should be properly screened to make sure their pain is not being caused by an exacerbation of the disease.

Pearls of wisdom

- It is important to emphasize to youth with FAPDs that their pain is real and it exists, even though all workup has thus far been normal. Explaining the brain–gut axis is extremely helpful and aids in concretizing the concept.
- Difficulties can arise when trying to identify FAPD in youth with a known organic disease, such as IBD. It is important to spend time with these families and explain that they are vulnerable to functional abdominal pain disorders.
- Pain can co-occur with other issues such as sleep problems and anxiety. These require their own treatment strategies.

Summary

Abdominal pain is a form of visceral pain that is common in diseases with and without associated anatomical or structural abnormalities. Examples of painful conditions that frequently present to pediatric gastroenterology practice are FD, IBS, IBD, and gastroparesis. Identifying the exact cause of abdominal pain is important although sometimes difficult. Given the visceral nature of this type of pain, it can be poorly localized and may be referred to other somatic and visceral structures. Somatic pain can be more easily identified, as it refers to pain in muscles, skin, or bone. Management of nonorganic abdominal pain includes pharmacological and non-pharmacological interventions. Nonpharmacological interventions include dietary modifications, auricular neurostimulation therapy, and psychological interventions such as CBT and hypnotherapy.

Recommended readings

For youth and caregivers:

- What is functional abdominal pain? (e.g., www.youtube.com/watch?v=65PeQyvQBHE).
- Functional abdominal pain (e.g., www.youtu.be/_bWfTXAgjU0).
- Understanding pain in less than 5 minutes (e.g., www.megfoundationforpain.org/2022/07/20/understanding-pain-in-less-than-5-minutes-and-what-to-do-about-it/).
- When stomachaches keep coming back (e.g., www.nytimes.com/2010/11/23/health/23klass.html).

For mental health professionals:

- Grundy, L., & Brierley, S.M. (2019). Visceral Pain. *Annual Review of Physiology* (81), 261–284.
- Hyams, J. S., Di Lorenzo, C., Saps, M., Shulman, R. J., Staiano, A., & van Tilburg, M. (2016). Functional Disorders: Children and Adolescents. *Gastroenterology*, 150.

References

1. Mani J, Madani S. Pediatric abdominal migraine: Current perspectives on a lesser known entity. *Pediatric Health Med Ther.* 2018;9:47–58.
2. Korterink J, Devanarayana NM, Rajindrajith S, Vlieger A, Benninga MA. Childhood functional abdominal pain: Mechanisms and management. *Nat Rev Gastroenterol Hepatol.* 2015;12(3):159–71.
3. Ellingson BM, Mayer E, Harris RJ, Ashe-McNally C, Naliboff BD, Labus JS, et al. Diffusion tensor imaging detects microstructural reorganization in the brain associated with chronic irritable bowel syndrome. *Pain.* 2013;154(9):1528–41.
4. Krasaelap A, Sood MR, Li BUK, Unteutsch R, Yan K, Nugent M, et al. Efficacy of auricular neurostimulation in adolescents with irritable bowel syndrome in a randomized, double-blind trial. *Clin Gastroenterol Hepatol.* 2020;18(9):1987-94.e2.
5. Robin SG, Keller C, Zwiener R, Hyman PE, Nurko S, Saps M, et al. Prevalence of pediatric functional gastrointestinal disorders utilizing the Rome IV criteria. *J Pediatr.* 2018;195:134–9.
6. Baaleman DF, Velasco-Benítez CA, Méndez-Guzmán LM, Benninga MA, Saps M. Functional gastrointestinal disorders in children: Agreement between Rome III and Rome IV diagnoses. *Eur J Pediatr.* 2021.
7. Rajindrajith S, Zeevenhooven J, Devanarayana NM, Perera BJC, Benninga MA. Functional abdominal pain disorders in children. *Expert Rev Gastroenterol Hepatol.* 2018;12(4):369–90.
8. Thapar N, Benninga MA, Crowell MD, Di Lorenzo C, Mack I, Nurko S, et al. Paediatric functional abdominal pain disorders. *Nat Rev Dis Primers.* 2020;6(1):89.
9. Puckett-Perez S, Gresl B. Psychological treatment for pediatric functional abdominal pain disorders. *Curr Opin Pediatr.* 2022;34(5):516–20.
10. Isgar B, Harman M, Kaye MD, Whorwell PJ. Symptoms of irritable bowel syndrome in ulcerative colitis in remission. *Gut.* 1983;24(3):190–2.

11. Halpin SJ, Ford AC. Prevalence of symptoms meeting criteria for irritable bowel syndrome in inflammatory bowel disease: Systematic review and meta-analysis. *Am J Gastroenterol.* 2012;107(10):1474–82.
12. Watson KL, Kim SC, Boyle BM, Saps M. Prevalence and impact of functional abdominal pain disorders in children with inflammatory bowel diseases (IBD-FAPD). *J Pediatr Gastroenterol Nutr.* 2017;65(2):212–7.
13. Zimmerman LA, Srinath AI, Goyal A, Bousvaros A, Ducharme P, Szigethy E, et al. The overlap of functional abdominal pain in pediatric Crohn's disease. *Inflamm Bowel Dis.* 2013;19(4):826–31.
14. Piche T, Ducrotté P, Sabate JM, Coffin B, Zerbib F, Dapoigny M, et al. Impact of functional bowel symptoms on quality of life and fatigue in quiescent Crohn disease and irritable bowel syndrome. *Neurogastroenterol Motil.* 2010;22(6):626–e174.
15. Saps M, Sansotta N, Bingham S, Magazzu G, Grosso C, Romano S, et al. Abdominal pain-associated functional gastrointestinal disorder prevalence in children and adolescents with celiac disease on gluten-free diet: A multinational study. *J Pediatr.* 2017;182:150–4.
16. Drewes AM, Olesen AE, Farmer AD, Szigethy E, Rebours V, Olesen SS. Gastrointestinal pain. *Nat Rev Dis Primers.* 2020;6(1):1.
17. van Tilburg MA, Claar RL, Romano JM, Langer SL, Drossman DA, Whitehead WE, et al. Psychological factors may play an important role in pediatric Crohn's disease symptoms and disability. *The Journal of pediatrics.* 2017;184:94–100. e1.
18. Schechter NL, Coakley R, Nurko S. The golden half hour in chronic pediatric pain-feedback as the first intervention. *JAMA Pediatr.* 2021;175(1):7–8.
19. de Bruijn CMA, Rexwinkel R, Gordon M, Benninga M, Tabbers MM. Antidepressants for functional abdominal pain disorders in children and adolescents. *Cochrane Database Syst Rev.* 2021;2:CD008013.
20. Gordon M, Sinopoulou V, Tabbers M, Rexwinkel R, de Bruijn C, Dovey T, et al. Psychosocial interventions for the treatment of functional abdominal pain disorders in children: A systematic review and meta-analysis. *JAMA Pediatr.* 2022;176(6):560–8.
21. Abbott RA, Martin AE, Newlove-Delgado TV, Bethel A, Thompson-Coon J, Whear R, et al. Psychosocial interventions for recurrent abdominal pain in childhood. *Cochrane Database Syst Rev.* 2017;1:CD010971.
22. Kovacic K, Hainsworth K, Sood M, Chelimsky G, Unteutsch R, Nugent M, et al. Neurostimulation for abdominal pain-related functional gastrointestinal disorders in adolescents: A randomised, double-blind, sham-controlled trial. *Lancet Gastroenterol Hepatol.* 2017;2(10):727–37.
23. Dogan G, Yavuz S, Aslantas H, Ozyurt BC, Kasirga E. Is low FODMAP diet effective in children with irritable bowel syndrome? *North Clin Istanb.* 2020;7(5):433–7.
24. Sturkenboom R, Keszthelyi D, Masclee AA, Essers BA. Discrete choice experiment reveals strong preference for dietary treatment among patients with irritable bowel syndrome. *Clin Gastroenterol Hepatol.* 2022;20(11):2628–37.

Chapter 16

Pain disorder interventions

Cognitive behavior therapy and acceptance and commitment therapy

Tasha Murphy, Miranda A.L. van Tilburg, and Rona L. Levy

Learning points

- Discussion of psychosocial aspects of pediatric abdominal pain.
- Review of common maladaptive cognitions in youth with abdominal pain and their parents.
- Overview of common assessment and treatment approaches for youth with abdominal pain.
- Practical recommendations for the use of cognitive behavior therapy (CBT), acceptance and commitment therapy (ACT), and exposure-based strategies in youth living with gastrointestinal (GI) conditions.

Chapter aims

This chapter will provide practical approaches to the assessment and treatment of youth abdominal pain using CBT, ACT, and exposure approaches.

Pediatric GI pain overview

GI disorders in youth are associated with a myriad of physical symptoms, of which abdominal pain is perhaps the most frequent target for psychological interventions. Abdominal pain is the most common symptom in youth with many GI disorders, particularly disorders of gut–brain interaction (DGBI; formally referred to as functional gastrointestinal disorders, FGIDs) [1–4]. Many children with persistent abdominal pain meet the criteria for functional abdominal pain disorder (FAPD), defined as episodic or continuous abdominal pain without evidence of physiological etiology [5]. FAPD can even coexist with other medical disorders such as inflammatory bowel disease (see Chapter 15). FAPD accounts for more than 50% of referrals to GI clinics [6] and is the main reason for GI emergency room visits among youth [16]. Children with FAPD have significantly lower health-related quality of life (HRQoL), greater anxiety and depression, and more frequent school absences than healthy peers [7–12].

This chapter will cover psychosocial treatments for youth with abdominal pain, with a focus on CBT, ACT, and exposure therapy. These treatments have been shown to decrease pain and disability and increase the quality of life [13–15]. While the chapter will use FAPD as a primary example condition, the outlined treatments can be applied in many situations to help youth manage pain in conjunction with other accepted medical treatments as appropriate. The chapter will also review assessment strategies to inform treatment and provide recommendations for using these approaches in the clinical setting.

DOI: 10.4324/9781003308683-18

Psychosocial aspects of pediatric GI pain

Emotional distress

Youth with chronic abdominal pain, including FAPD, have significantly higher rates of anxiety and depression and lower HRQoL compared to their healthy peers [16–23]. Elements of CBT such as guided imagery, progressive muscle relaxation, and cognitive restructuring have shown to be especially helpful for treating anxiety symptoms in youth with abdominal pain [24, 25], whereas distraction, goal-setting, deep breathing, and cognitive restructuring are helpful for youth with abdominal pain who also have depression symptoms [13, 26, 27]. Treating general anxiety and depression is important but not the major goal of psychogastroenterology treatment. Rather, psychogastroenterology treatment is usually focused on anxiety specific to pain. In fact, studies have shown that general anxiety does not mediate the outcomes of CBT for abdominal pain in youth [28, 29].

Common cognitions associated with pediatric GI pain

Psychological approaches to treating youth with chronic GI pain often focus on maladaptive, or unhelpful, cognitions. Two common unhelpful cognitions are catastrophizing and "hurt vs. harm".

Catastrophizing

Catastrophizing can amplify pain when a person ruminates about their symptoms and views themselves as helpless to change them [30]. It is a common cognition in youth with chronic pain as well as their parents. When a child catastrophizes about their pain (e.g., "it will never get better", or "am I going to die?"), they often seek help or comfort from a caregiver, focusing on their pain instead of schoolwork or other activities. Youth catastrophizing has been associated with greater pain intensity and functional disability and increased emotional distress [31–33]. Catastrophizing has also been found to mediate the relationship between pediatric abdominal pain and anxiety and other adverse outcomes [34], and it has also been shown to mediate treatment effects in youth with FAPD [35].

Parents catastrophize about their own health and symptoms *as well as* about their child's pain. As Figure 16.1 shows, parental catastrophizing is associated with increased pain, pain behaviors (actions that show discomfort, for example, pain complaints, grimacing, groaning, asking for help, or crying), and functional disability in their children [12, 36, 37]. Thus, treatments aimed at reducing catastrophizing in both the parent and child can be helpful in the management of pediatric GI pain [38].

Hurt vs. harm

When a person is injured, pain serves as a warning sign that something bad has happened. However, the experience of pain can continue without continued physical injury due to a variety of factors, including central nervous system action, anxiety, stress, and the reactions of others. Cognitions, in particular emotional and contextual factors, thoughts, feelings, beliefs, and past experiences, can all play a role in how we experience pain. If we are having a good day or are busy, we may not notice any sensations of pain. But if we are feeling stressed or anxious, we might feel a pain sensation and interpret it as being more severe and long-lasting,

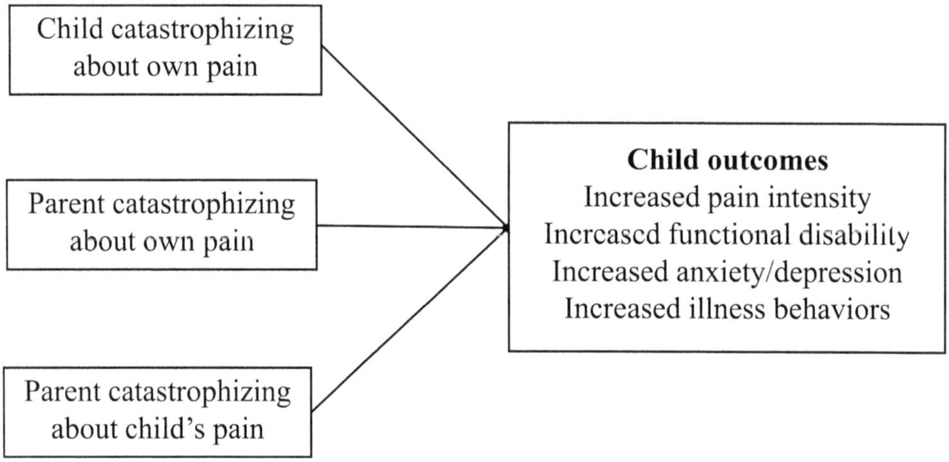

Figure 16.1 Impact of child and parent catastrophizing on child and health outcomes (Source: Authors).

or that there is a serious cause. When this happens, we might believe that pain equals harm or damage.

Children with abdominal pain and their parents often confuse hurt with harm. Parents may interpret child pain as a sign that their child is physically harmed. As a result, the parent may become anxious and protective [37, 39], seeking ways to alleviate their child's pain. They may become solicitous (giving extra attention or sympathy) [39, 40], inadvertently reinforcing illness behaviors by encouraging rest and avoidance of regular activities, keeping their child home from school, and seeking out medical care unnecessarily [41].

Other pain cognitions

Other cognitions can also be associated with pain, particularly "I can't" or "I ought" or "I should" statements. For example, "I can't go to school with a stomachache" or "I should not be in this much pain". These kinds of thoughts can communicate feelings of helplessness. Thoughts that typical activities are only possible once pain is resolved, e.g., "I can't see my friends or play soccer if I have any stomach pain" can be particularly disabling. Such black-and-white thinking can lead to high levels of functional disability and delays in returning to potentially enjoyable activities that likely would be possible, even if attenuated, despite the presence of some level of abdominal pain.

Social influences on pediatric GI pain

Social learning theory provides a strong conceptual framework for understanding the development and maintenance of illness behaviors in youth with abdominal pain [13–15]. Two critical social learning theory constructs are modeling and reinforcement.

Modeling

Youth learn, in part, by watching what others do and listening to what they say (social learning). They then repeat the behaviors that they have observed (modeling). When a child has pain or any illness, they learn from their parents and others how they should respond to their discomfort (e.g., resting, avoiding activities), even if these responses are not particularly helpful. This is especially true for youth whose parents themselves have chronic pain or a DGBI, as what children learn from their parents may make a greater contribution to the risk of developing a DGBI than genetics [42].

Several studies provide support for this idea. In one study, children of mothers with irritable bowel syndrome (IBS) reported significantly more GI symptoms, more frequent stomach aches, and more school absences and doctor visits for GI symptoms than control children [43]. Another study of youth with recurrent abdominal pain found a significant relationship between somatic symptom severity and similar symptoms in their parents [44]. Additionally, Stone et al. [45] found that adolescents' observations of parental pain behaviors significantly predicted adolescents' pain severity, pain bother, and a number of daily pain locations, suggesting that observations of parent pain behaviors contributed to the child's pain experience.

These findings suggest that engaging parents to identify and modify their own illness behaviors may be useful to reduce child pain. One parent-focused social learning and cognitive behavioral treatment protocol developed by Levy et al. [41] showed improvements in several outcomes, including parental solicitousness, pain catastrophizing, quality of life, and fewer healthcare visits and missed school days.

Reinforcement paradigms

Parents naturally want to protect and help their children when they don't feel well. Even with the best of intentions, however, parents can inadvertently emphasize illness instead of wellness by reacting to child pain behaviors with parental attention, comfort (e.g., hugs), treats, freedom from chores, etc. These solicitous (rewarding) responses then reinforce pain behaviors, making it more likely that they will continue. Suggesting that pain merits rest (e.g., mom or dad are worried) also communicates to the child that they perhaps should become more vigilant about any discomfort, increasing pain complaints over time.

Studies have found that parental solicitousness increases symptom complaints in youth with abdominal pain. Levy et al. [43] found that youth with higher school absenteeism for GI symptoms were more likely to have parents who were more solicitous in response to their child's symptoms [43]. In another study, youth with solicitous mothers experienced more severe stomach aches and more school absences than other youth [44].

Psychosocial assessment for youth with abdominal pain

Prior to beginning treatment, conducting a psychosocial assessment is recommended to inform treatment of youth with abdominal pain. Clinical assessments are more thoroughly discussed in Chapter 6, but there are domains of particular interest to treatment, including pain behaviors, parental response, pain cognitions, emotional distress, life stressors, and coping style. See Handout 16.1 for a list and description of recommended pretreatment assessments for each of these domains.

Treatment approaches

Cognitive behavioral therapy (CBT)

CBT is perhaps the most widely studied psychosocial treatment for youth with DGBI, with studies showing efficacy in pediatric IBS), FAPD, functional dyspepsia, and others [46–53].

CBT is a short-term intervention that aims to (1) alter maladaptive thoughts, (2) engage in problem-solving [54, 55], and (3) promote engagement in positive coping [55]. It has been suggested that CBT is most effective when it includes both parents and children, so therapeutic approaches should endeavor to include both when possible [56, 57]. Behavioral treatment components include changing illness behaviors to wellness behaviors, relaxation strategies, distraction techniques, and teaching parents how to reinforce adaptive rather than maladaptive child pain coping behaviors [37]. The following are summaries of elements of CBT that mental health professionals can use in treating youth with abdominal pain. See Handout 16.2 for an overview of CBT treatment strategies.

Cognitive restructuring and problem-solving

Cognitive restructuring is a technique designed to modify thinking errors that bias information processing as well as maladaptive thoughts (e.g., catastrophizing and hurt vs. harm). Mental health professionals can work with youth and their parents to identify maladaptive cognitions around pain, and then examine and challenge them. As more logical and adaptive ways of thinking are learned, the child's pain symptoms can decrease and functioning can improve.

Cognitive restructuring for pain should center on maladaptive cognitions related to pain. Addressing general maladaptive cognitions not only does not address the pain but also communicates to youth and their family that treatment is for their general anxiety, depression, or other mental health issue, rather than pain. This can alienate them from treatment.

Problem-solving is an important cognitive strategy that is incorporated into cognitive restructuring. Maladaptive or ineffective problem-solving is believed to lead to a variety of negative outcomes, including depression, anger, anxiety, interpersonal problems, and somatic complaints [11]. A goal of treatment is to define the problem, outline possible solutions, try the "best" one, evaluate, and refine the approach if needed.

While cognitive restructuring is helpful in reducing maladaptive thoughts and improving problem-solving, this technique may be difficult for younger youth. Although CBT has been utilized in youth living with DGBI as young as 5–8 years of age [56–58], younger youth may not yet have the cognitive development to think logically or problem-solve; these skills typically develop starting around 8 years of age. When working with younger youth, mental health professionals should aim to use simple language and consider play therapy, role-play, or modeling adaptive responses. In addition, since parents or other caregivers have a significant influence on the experiences of younger youth, it is preferable to involve them heavily in their treatment. See Handout 16.3 for recommendations relating to cognitive restructuring.

Relaxation training

Relaxation techniques have long been a staple of psychological treatments for chronic pain conditions, including DGBI. These strategies are designed to directly address the tension–pain cycle where stress creates muscle tension and autonomic arousal that leads to increased pain. Pain then creates more stress, creating a cycle (see Figure 16.2). Relaxation techniques help to reduce tension and thus break the cycle, decreasing pain sensations.

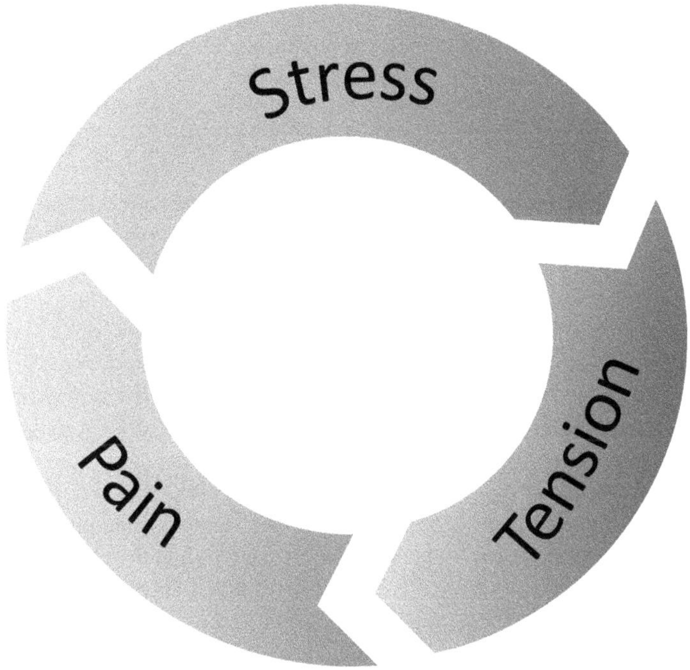

Figure 16.2 Tension–pain cycle (Source: Authors).

Several types of relaxation methods have been featured in the DGBI literature. These include diaphragmatic breathing, guided imagery, progressive muscle relaxation, biofeedback, and mindfulness meditation. The relaxation techniques applied are usually not specifically focused on pain, but rather general relaxation. The one exception can be guided imagery, which can include pain-specific suggestions for improvement. In this case, guided imagery is not different from self-hypnosis and more details on pain-specific imagery can be found in Chapter 17.

Some studies have delivered relaxation exercises as stand-alone treatments. Biofeedback has been studied in pediatric recurrent abdominal pain and IBS in youth as young as 6 years of age [59, 60]. These studies have found consistent reduction in pain and other GI symptoms. Guided imagery also has been found to be effective in reducing pain and disability in youth with abdominal pain [61, 62]. More research is needed if relaxation exercises alone, as opposed to applying them as part of CBT, is helpful.

Distraction

Engaging in thoughts or activities that distract attention away from pain is one of the most commonly used and highly endorsed strategies for controlling youth abdominal pain [63]. Distraction can be a helpful strategy because it takes focus away from pain and promotes engagement in regular activities (e.g., going to school, playing sports, or activities with family and friends).

It is well accepted that parental distraction (vs. attention) can reduce child symptom severity [64]. When encouraging parents to introduce distraction to their child, however, it is possible that parents will resist, thinking it is important to give attention (reassurance and sympathy) to their child. GI mental health professionals should thus emphasize that distraction does not mean disregarding a child's needs or minimizing their symptoms; rather, it is a way to help youth cope with their pain and reduce disability.

Exposure therapy

Exposure therapy, sometimes considered as a variant of CBT, focuses on reducing pain and fear of bodily sensations and increasing emotional awareness and self-regulation. Whereas CBT for child abdominal pain focuses on maladaptive cognitions and teaches coping skills and relaxation to relieve symptoms, exposure therapy emphasizes in vivo, imagined, or virtual reality exposure to a feared stimulus to reduce fear and avoidance behaviors [65–67]. It has been utilized extensively in adult populations to treat IBS [68, 69]. Two studies exist in the pediatric population. Exposure-based CBT was used in a pilot study of 20 youth with pain-related DGBI. Youth improved significantly in pain intensity, pain frequency, GI symptoms, quality of life, depression, anxiety, school absenteeism, and somatic symptoms [70]. Another pilot study of an internet-delivered exposure-based CBT for adolescents with FAPD or functional dyspepsia [71] found significant improvement in pain intensity, GI symptoms, and quality of life. Handout 16.4 provides guidance for the use of exposure therapy for youth with abdominal pain. Exposure therapy is especially helpful in youth who report high levels of pain anxiety and avoidance behaviors/seeking safety.

Acceptance and commitment therapy (ACT)

ACT is a relatively new (conceptualized in the early 2000s) psychological intervention that comprises acceptance and mindfulness procedures, along with commitment and behavior change strategies, to increase psychological flexibility (being open, aware, and present, and engaging in behaviors which facilitate life goals) and reduce stress [72]. While there is some overlap between CBT and ACT for pain management, ACT differs in that it does not attempt to eliminate or change beliefs (e.g., trying to replace irrational or maladaptive thoughts about the pain experience with more adaptive ones), nor does it emphasize reduction or control of symptoms. Rather, ACT sees distress, including the distress associated with physical pain, as a natural consequence of being human; the experience of suffering, self-doubt, fear, uncertainty, self-criticism, negative thinking, etc., are normal human experiences. ACT treatment thus eschews interventions to reduce pain; instead, it consists of accepting negative thoughts, emotions, and sensations and encourages engaging in activities that are meaningful although possibly painful or fear-provoking [72, 73]. This process motivates a person to distance themselves from pain and distress in order to decrease the impact of these experiences on behavior [73].

Systematic reviews of chronic pain in adults have supported the effectiveness of ACT, showing improvements in physical functioning, anxiety, depression, and emotional distress [74, 75]. In youth, ACT has shown efficacy with parent and child interventions in chronic pain [73, 76–80]. For GI conditions (including abdominal pain) specifically, ACT studies are lacking. Nevertheless, lessons from studies in other clinical populations can be adapted for youth with abdominal pain. Handout 16.5 outlines the core principles of ACT and provides examples of how mental health practitioners can utilize ACT with youth suffering from abdominal pain.

Pearls of wisdom

- Psychological treatment of youth with abdominal pain requires a flexible approach while considering developmental context; it is important to tailor treatment, especially those involving cognitive restructuring, to the age and language of the child.
- Parents, extended family, teachers, and others are important contributors to a child's pain experience; including these individuals in interventions and/or psychoeducation can support treatment success.
- General anxiety is not a treatment target for abdominal pain. Rather pain-specific anxiety and pain avoidance/safety behaviors should be targeted.

Summary

Pain is a common experience for youth and adolescents with GI disorders and often results in missed school and reduced activities. Youth with abdominal pain can experience emotional distress, and they and their parents may exhibit maladaptive cognitions such as catastrophizing and hurt vs. harm. Because parents' responses to their child's pain can contribute to the expression of pain behaviors, it is important to include parents in treatment. Psychological treatment approaches include CBT, ACT, and exposure therapies. CBT is the most studied approach, and is a highly effective, short-term, GI-symptom-focused intervention that is well suited to a range of GI symptoms and disorders. ACT and exposure therapy can also be helpful approaches, though the research and their use in pediatric GI disorders are limited.

Recommended readings

For youth and caregivers:

- UNC hospitals video: What is functional abdominal pain: www.youtube.com/watch?v=65PeQyvQBHE.
- Meg Foundation: Understanding pain in less than 5 minutes: www.megfoundationforpain.org/2022/07/20/understanding-pain-in-less-than-5-minutes-and-what-to-do-about-it/.
- Nationwide hospital: Treating abdominal pain: www.youtu.be/bWfTXAgjU0.
- New York Times: When stomachache keeps coming back www.nytimes.com/2010/11/23/health/23klass.html.

For mental health professionals:

- van Tilburg, M.A.L. (2023). Cognitive behavior therapy for functional gastrointestinal disorders and functional disorders in children. In: C. Faure, N. Thapar, C. DiLorenzo. *Pediatric Neurogastroentrology*. New York, NY: Springer.
- Santucci, N.R.; Saps, M.; van Tilburg, M. (2020). New advances in the treatment of paediatric functional abdominal pain disorders. *Lancet Gastroenterol Hepatol*, *5*, 316–328.
- Levy, R.L. (2011). Exploring the intergenerational transmission of illness behavior: From observations to experimental intervention. *Annals of Behavioral Medicine*, *41*, 174–182.
- Friesen, C.; Colombo, J.M.; Deacy, A.; Schurman, J.V. (2021). An update on the assessment and management of pediatric abdominal pain. *Pediatric Health, Medicine, and Therapeutics*, 12, 373–393.

References

1. Jones MP, Faresjo A, Beath A, Faresjo T, Ludvigsson J. Abdominal pain in children develops with age and increases with psychosocial factors. *Clin Gastroenterol Hepatol.* 2020;18(2):360–7.
2. Limbri LF, Wilson TG, Oliver MR. Prevalence of irritable bowel syndrome and functional abdominal pain disorders in children with inflammatory bowel disease in remission. *JGH Open.* 2022;6(12):818–23.
3. Saps M, Adams P, Bonilla S, Chogle A, Nichols-Vinueza D. Parental report of abdominal pain and abdominal pain-related functional gastrointestinal disorders from a community survey. *J Pediat Gastroenterol Nutr.* 2012;55(6):707–10.
4. Merskey HM, Bogduk N. *Classification of chronic pain: Descriptions of chronic pain syndromes and definition of pain terms*. Seattle: IASP Press; 1994.
5. Hyams JS, Di Lorenzo C, Saps M, Shulman RJ, Staiano A, van Tilburg M. Functional disorders: Children and adolescents. *Gastroenterol.* 2016;150(6):1456-68.e2.
6. Rouster AS, Karpinski AC, Silver D, Monagas J, Hyman PE. Functional gastrointestinal disorders dominate pediatric gastroenterology outpatient practice. *J Pediatr Gastroenterol Nutr.* 2015;62(6):847–51.
7. Youssef NN, Murphy TG, Langseder AL, Rosh JR. Quality of life for children with functional abdominal pain: A comparison study of patients' and parents' perceptions. *Pediatrics.* 2006;117(1):54–9.
8. Assa A, Ish-Tov A, Rinawi F, Shamir R. School attendence in children with functional abdominal pain and inflammatory bowel diseases. *J Pediatr Gastroenterol Nutr.* 2015;61(5):553–7.
9. von Gontard A, Moritz A-M, Thorme-Granz S, Equit M. Abdominal pain symptoms are associated with anxiety and depression in young children. *Acta Paediatr.* 2015;104(11):1156–63.
10. Varni JW, Bendo CB, Nurko S, Shulman RJ, Self MM, Franciosi JP, et al. Health-related quality of life in pediatric patients with functional and organic gastrointestinal diseases. *J Pediatr.* 2015;166(1):85–90.
11. Robin SG, Keller C, Zwiener R, Hyman PE, Nurko S, Saps M, et al. Prevalence of pediatric functional gastrointestinal disorders according to the Rome IV criteria. *J Pediatr.* 2018; in press(195):134–9.
12. Newton E, Schosheim A, Patel S, Chitkara DK, van Tilburg MAL. The role of psychological factors in pediatric functional abdominal pain disorders. *Neurogastroenterol Motil.* 2019;31(6):e13538.
13. Levy RL, Langer SL, Walker LS, Romano JM, Christie DL, Youssef N, et al. Cognitive-behavioral therapy for children with functional abdominal pain and their parents decreases pain and other symptoms. *Am J Gastroenterol.* 2010;105:946–56.
14. van Tilburg MAL, Carter CA. Integration of biomedical and psychosocial treatments in pediatrics functional gastrointestinal disorders. *Gastroenterol Clin North Am.* 2018;47(4):863–75.
15. Abbott RA, Martin AE, Newlove-Delgado TV, Bethel A, Thompson-Coon J, Whear R, et al. Psychosocial interventions for recurrent abdominal pain in childhood. *Cochrane Database Syst Rev.* 2017;1:Cd010971.
16. Korterink JJ, Diederen K, Benninga MA, Tabbers MM. Epidemiology of pediatric functional abdominal pain disorders: A meta-analysis. *PLoS One*. 2015;10:e0126982.
17. Helgeland H, Sandvik L, Mathiesen KS, Kristensen H. Childhood predictors of recurrent abdominal pain in adolescence: A 13-year population-based prospective study. *J Psychosom Res.* 2010;68(4):359–67.
18. Gulewitsch MD, Enck P, Schwille-Kiuntke J, Weimer K, Schlarb AA. Rome III criteria in parents' hands: Pain-related functional gastrointestinal disorders in community children and associations with somatic complaints and mental health. *Eur J Gastroenterol Hepatol.* 2013;25(10):1223–9.
19. Luntamo T, Sourander A, Rihko M, Aromaa M, Helenius H, Koskelainen M, et al. Psychosocial determinants of headache, abdominal pain, and sleep problems in a community sample of Finnish adolescents. *Eur Child Adolesc Psychiatry*. 2012;21(6):301–13.

20. Youssef NN, Atienza K, Langseder AL, Strauss RS. Chronic abdominal pain and depressive symptoms: Analysis of the National Longitudinal Study of Adolescent Health. *Clin Gastroenterol Hepatol.* 2008;6(3):329–32.
21. Zernikow B, Wager J, Hechler T, Hasan C, Rohr U, Dobe M, et al. Characteristics of highly impaired children with severe chronic pain: A 5-year retrospective study on 2249 pediatric pain patients. *BMC Pediatr.* 2012;12:54.
22. Cunningham NR, Cohen MB, Farrell MK, Mezoff AG, Lynch-Jordan A, Kashikar-Zuck S. Concordant parent-child reports of anxiety predict impairment in youth with functional abdominal pain. *J Pediatr Gastroenterol Nutr.* 2015;60(3):312–7.
23. Schurman JV, Danda CE, Friesen CA, Hyman PE, Simon SD, Cocjin JT. Variations in psychological profile among children with recurrent abdominal pain. *J Clin Psychol Med Settings.* 2008;15(3):241–51.
24. Cunningham NR, Nelson S, Jagpal A, Moorman E, Farrell MK, Pentiuk S, et al. Development of the Aim to Decrease Anxiety and Pain Treatment (ADAPT) for pediatric functional abdominal pain disorders. *J Pediatr.* 2018;66(1):16–20.
25. Cunningham N, Kalomiris A, Peugh J, Farrell M, Pentiuk S, Mallon D, et al. Cognitive behavior therapy tailored to anxiety symptoms improves pediatric functional abdominal pain outcomes: A randomized clinical trial. *J Pediatr.* 2021;230:62–70.
26. Nieto R, Boixados M, Ruiz G, Hernandez E, Huguet A. Effects and experiences of families following a web-based psychosocial intervention for children with functional abdominal pain and their parents: A mixed-methods pilot randomized controlled trial. *J Pain Res.* 2019;12:3395–412.
27. Saini S, Narang M, Srivastava S, Shah D. Behavioral intervention in children with functional abdominal pain disorders: A promising option. *Turk J Gastroenterol.* 2021;32(5):443–50.
28. Lalouni M, Hesser H, Bonnert M, Hedman-Lagerlöf E, Serlachius E, Olén O, et al. Breaking the vicious circle of fear and avoidance in children with abdominal pain: A mediation analysis. *J Psychosom Res.* 2021;140:110287.
29. van Tilburg MA, Levy RL, Stoner S, Romano JM, Murphy TB, Abdullah B, et al. Mediation of outcomes for cognitive behavioral therapy targeted to parents of children with functional abdominal pain disorders. *J Psychosom Res.* 2021;150:110618.
30. Levy RL, Crowell MD, Drossman DA, Halpert AD, Keefer L, Lackner JM, et al. Biopsychosocial aspects of functional gastrointestinal disorders: How central and environmental processes contribute to the development and expression of the FGIDs. In: Drossman DA, et al., editors. *ROME IV: The functional gastrointestinal disorders. McLean.* The Rome Foundation, Degnon Associates, Inc.; 2016.
31. Warschburger P, Hanig J, Friedt M, Posovszky C, Schier M, Calvano C. Health-related quality of life in children with abdominal pain due to functional or organic gastrointestinal disorders. *J Pediatr Psychol.* 2014;39(1):45–54.
32. Kaminsky L, Robertson M, Dewey D. Psychological correlates of depression in children with recurrent abdominal pain. *J Pediatr Psychol.* 2006;31:956–66.
33. van Tilburg MA, Claar RL, Romano JM, Langer SL, Walker LS, Whitehead WE, et al. Role of coping with symptoms in depression and disability: Comparison between inflammatory bowel disease and abdominal pain. *J Pediatr Gastroenterol Nutr.* 2015;61(4):431–6.
34. Feldman ECH, Lampert-Okin SL, Greenley RN. Relationships between abdominal pain, mental health, and functional disability in youth with inflammatory bowel diseases: Pain catastrophizing as a longitudinal mediator. *Clin J Pain.* 2022;38(12):711–20.
35. Levy RL, Langer SL, Romano JM, Labus J, Walker LS, Murphy TB, et al. Cognitive mediators of treatment outcomes in pediatric functional abdominal pain. *Clin J Pain.* 2014;30(12):1033–43.
36. Langer SL, Romano JM, Levy RL, Walker LS, Whitehead WE. Catastrophizing and parental response to child symptom complaints. *Child Health Care.* 2009;38(3):169–84.
37. Palermo TM, Valrie CR, Karlson CW. Family and parent influences on pediatric chronic pain: A developmental perspective. *Am Psychol.* 2014;69(2):142–52.

38. Levy RL, Langer SL, Romano JM, Labus J, Walker LS, Murphy TB, et al. Cognitive mediators of treatment outcomes in pediatric functional abdominal pain. *Clin J Pain*. 2014:Epub ahead of print.
39. van Tilburg MA, Chitkara DK, Palsson OS, Levy RL, Whitehead WE. Parental worries and beliefs about abdominal pain. *J Pediatr Gastroenterol Nutr*. 2009;48(3):311–7.
40. DuPen MM, van Tilburg MAL, Langer SL, Murphy TB, Romano JM, Levy RL. Parental protectiveness mediates the association between parent-perceived child self-efficacy and health outcomes in pediatric functional abdominal pain disorder. *Children (Basel)*. 2016;3(3):15.
41. Levy RL, Langer SL, van Tilburg MA, Romano JM, Murphy TB, Walker LS, et al. Brief telephone-delivered cognitive behavioral therapy targeted to parents of children with functional abdominal pain: A Randomized Controlled Trial. *Pain*. 2017;158(4):618–28.
42. Levy RL, Jones KR, Whitehead WE, Feld SI, Talley NJ, Corey LA. Irritable bowel syndrome in twins: Heredity and social learning both contribute to etiology. *Gastroenterology*. 2001;121(4):799–804.
43. Levy RL, Whitehead WE, Walker LS, Von KM, Feld AD, Garner M, et al. Increased somatic complaints and health-care utilization in children: Effects of parent IBS status and parent response to gastrointestinal symptoms. *AmJGastroenterol*. 2004;99(12):2442–51.
44. Walker LS, Greene JW. Children with recurrent abdominal pain and their parents: More somatic complaints, anxiety, and depression than other patient families? *J Pediatr Psychol*. 1989;14(2):231–43.
45. Stone AL, Walker LS. Adolescents' observations of parent pain behaviors: Preliminary measure validation and test of social learning theory in pediatric chronic pain. *J Pediatr Psychol*. 2017;42(1):65–74.
46. Kinsinger SW. Cognitive-behavioral therapy for patients with irritable bowel syndrome: Current insights. *Res Behav Manag*. 2017;10:231–7.
47. Galdston MR, John RM. Mind over gut: Psychosocial management of pediatric functional abdominal pain. *J Pediatr Health Care*. 2016;30(6):535–45.
48. Bonnert M, Olen O, Bjureberg J, Lalouni M, Hedman-Lagerlof E, Serlachius E, et al. The role of avoidance behavior in the treatment of adolescents with irritable bowel syndrome: A mediation analysis. *Behav Res Ther*. 2018;105:27–35.
49. Levy R, Langer S, Walker L, Romano J, Christie D, Youssef N, et al. Twelve month follow-up of cognitive behavioral therapy for children with functional abdominal pain. *JAMA Pediatr*. 2013;167(178–184).
50. Freeman KA, Riley A, Duke DC, Fu R. Systematic review and meta analysis of behavioral interventions for fecal incontinence with constipation. *J Pediatr Psychol*. 2014;39(8):887–902.
51. Slutsker B, Konichezky A, Gothelf D. Breaking the cycle: Cognitive behavioral therapy and biofeedback training in a case of cyclic vomiting syndrome. *Psychol Health Med*. 2010;15(6):625–31.
52. van Tilburg MAL. Cognitive behavioral therapy for functional gastrointestinal disorders. In: Faure C, Thapar N, DiLorenzo C, editors. *Neurogastroenterology: Gastrointestinal Motility and Functional Disorders in Children*. New York: Springer; 2017.
53. Lalouni M, Ljotsson B, Bonnert M, Ssegonja R, Benninga M, Bjureberg J, et al. Clinical and cost effectiveness of online cognitive behavioral therapy in children with functional abdominal pain disorders. *Clin Gastroenterol Hepatol*. 2019;17:2236–44.
54. Reed B, Buzenski J, van Tilburg MAL. Implementing psychological therapies for gastrointestinal disorders in pediatrics. *Expert rev Gastroenterol Hepatol*. 2020;14(11):1061–7.
55. Person H, Keefer L. Brain-Gut therapies for pediatric functional gastrointestinal disorders and inflammatory bowel disease. *Curr Gastroenterol Rep*. 2019;21(4):12.
56. Sanders MR, Shepherd RW, Cleghorn G, Woolford H. The treatment of recurrent abdominal pain in children: A controlled comparison of cognitive-behavioral family intervention and standard pediatric care. *J Consult Clin Psychol*. 1994;62(2):306–14.
57. Duarte MA, Penna FJ, Andrade EMG, Cancela CSP, Neto JCA, Barbosa TF. Treatment of nonorganic recurrent abdominal pain: Cognitive-behavioral family intervention. *J Pediatr Gastroenterol Nutr*. 2006;43(1):59–64.

58. Finney JW, Lemanek KL, Cataldo MF, Katz HP, Fuqua RW. Pediatric psychology in primary health care: Brief targeted therapy for recurrent abdominal pain. *Behav Ther.* 1989;20(2):283–91.
59. Humphreys PA, Gevirtz RN. Treatment of recurrent abdominal pain: Components analysis of four treatment protocols. *J Pediatr Gastroenterol Nutr.* 2000;31(1):47–51.
60. Stern MJ, Guiles RAF, Gevirtz R. HRV biofeedback for pediatric irritable bowel syndrome and functional abdominal pain: A clinical replication series. *Appl Psychophysiol Biofeedback.* 2014;39:287–91.
61. van Tilburg MA, Chitkara DK, Palsson OS, Turner M, Blois-Martin N, Ulshen M, et al. Audio-recorded guided imagery treatment reduces functional abdominal pain in children: A pilot study. *Pediatrics.* 2009;124(5):e890–e7.
62. Weydert JA, Shapiro DE, Acra SA, Monheim CJ, Chambers AS, Ball TM. Evaluation of guided imagery as treatment for recurrent abdominal pain in children: A randomized controlled trial. *BMC Pediatr.* 2006;6:1–10.
63. Johnson MH. How does distraction work in the management of pain? *Curr Pain Headache Rep.* 2005;9(2):90–5.
64. Walker LS, Williams SE, Smith CA, Garber J, Van Slyke DA, Lipani TA. Parent attention versus distraction: Impact on symptom complaints by children with and without chronic functional abdominal pain. *Pain.* 2006;122(1–2):43–52.
65. Sprenger L, Gerhards F, Goldbeeck L. Effects of psychological treatment on recurrent abdominal pain in children – a meta-analysis. *Clin Psychol Rev.* 2011;31(7):1192–7.
66. Abramowitz JS. The practice of exposure therapy: Relevance of cognitive-behavioral theory and extinction theory. *Behav Ther.* 2013;44(4):548–58.
67. Huang Q, Lin J, Han R, Peng C, Huang A. Using virtual reality exposure therapy in pain management: A systematic review and meta-analysis of randomized controlled trials. *Value Health.* 2022;25(2):288–301.
68. Craske MG, Wolitzky-Taylor KB, Labus J, Wu S, Frese M, Mayer EA, et al. A cognitive-behavioral treatment for irritable bowel syndrome using interoceptive exposure to visceral sensations. *Behav Res Ther.* 2011;49(6–7):413–21.
69. Ljotsson B, Hesser H, Andersson E, Lindfors P, Hursti T, Ruck C, et al. Mechanisms of change in an exposure-based treatment for irritable bowel syndrome. *J Consult Clin Psychol.* 2013;81(6):1113–26.
70. Lalouni M, Olen O, Bonnert M, Hedman E, Serlachius E, Ljotsson B. Exposure-based cognitive behavior therapy for children with abdominal pain: A pilot trial. *PLoS One.* 2016;11(10):e0164647.
71. Bonnert M, Olen O, Lalouni M, Hedman-Lagerlof E, Sarnholm J, Serlachius E, et al. Internet-delivered exposure-based cognitive-behavioral therapy for adolescents with functional abdominal pain or functional dyspepsia: A feasibility study. *Behav Ther.* 2019;50(1):177–88.
72. Wynne B, McHugh L, Gao W, Keegan D, Byrne K, Rowan C, et al. Acceptance and commitment therapy reduces psychological stress in patients with inflammatory bowel diseases. *Gastroenterology.* 2019;156(4):935–45.
73. Wicksell RK, Melin L, Lekander M, Olsson GL. Evaluating the effectiveness of exposure and acceptance strategies to improve functioning and quality of life in longstanding pediatric pain- A randomized controlled trial. *Pain.* 2009;141(3):248–57.
74. Veehof MM, Trompetter HR, Bohlmeijer ET. Acceptance and mindfulness-based interventions for the treatment of chronic pain: A meta-analytic review. *Cognitive Behav Ther.* 2016;45(1):5–31.
75. Hann KE, McCracken LM. A systematic review of randomized controlled trials of acceptance and commitment therapy for adults with chronic pain: Outcome domains, design quality, and efficacy. *J Context Behav Sci.* 2014;3(4):217–27.
76. Balter LJT, Lipsker CW, Wicksell RK, Lekander M. Neuropsychiatric symptoms in pediatric chronic pain and outcome of acceptance and commitment therapy. *Front Psychol.* 2021;12:576943.

77. Zetterqvist V, Gentili C, Rickardsson J, Sorensen I, Wicksell RK. Internet-delivered acceptance and commitment Therapy for adolescents with chronic pain and their parents: A nonrandomized trial. *J Pediatr Psychol.* 2020;45(9):990–1004.
78. Gauntlett-Gilbert J, Connell H, Clinch J, McCracken LM. Acceptance and values-based treatment of adolescents with chronic pain: Outcomes and their relationship to acceptance. *J Pediatr Psychol.* 2013;38(1):72–81.
79. Kanstrup M, Jordan A, Kemani MK. Adolescent and parent experiences of acceptance and commitment therapy for pediatric chronic pain: An interpretative phenomenological analysis. *Children (Basel)*. 2019;6(9):101.
80. Pielech M, Vowles KE, Wicksell RK. Acceptance and commitment therapy for pediatric chronic pain: Theory and application. *Children (Basel)*. 2017;4(2):10.

Chapter 17

Pain disorder interventions

Hypnotherapy

Arine M. Vlieger

Chapter aims

This chapter aims to provide information on the efficacy of hypnotherapy in children with brain–gut disorders like irritable bowel syndrome (IBS) or chronic nausea. The reader is provided with protocols and tips on applying hypnosis and explaining its use to youth living with a gastrointestinal (GI) condition.

Learning points

- Learn what gut-directed hypnotherapy is, and how effective this treatment can be in youth with abdominal complaints like pain or nausea.
- How to explain the nature of hypnosis to youth living with a GI condition?
- How to provide this safe and well-accepted therapy to children using standard protocols?

Gut-directed hypnotherapy is increasingly used to treat pediatric disorders of gut–brain interaction (DGBI). During this treatment, mental health professionals (or other trained professionals including physicians and nurses) induce a trance while providing suggestions to normalize the youths' gut–brain dysregulation. It is, therefore, also defined as one of the brain–gut behavior therapies. This chapter explains what hypnosis is and who should provide this treatment. The current evidence for the efficacy of gut-directed hypnosis in pain-predominant DGBI like IBS and functional abdominal pain (FAP), as well as for chronic nausea and inflammatory bowel disease (IBD), is discussed. Hypnotherapy protocols for youth with DGBI are provided in the handouts.

What is hypnotherapy?

Hypnotherapy is defined as the use of hypnosis in the treatment of a medical or psychological disorder. It can be used as a stand-alone treatment or in combination with other therapies. During hypnotherapy, an individual is induced into a hypnotic trance, characterized by focused attention on thoughts or images and openness to suggestions. Although movies and stage hypnosis may suggest otherwise, this hypnotic trance is a normal and frequently occurring phenomenon. It is, for example, comparable to the trance youth experience while daydreaming when they become absorbed by images or thoughts.

This hypnotic trance is used to provide repetitive, hypnotic suggestions for changes in sensations, emotions, thoughts, or behavior. One should realize that youth do not follow suggestions if

DOI: 10.4324/9781003308683-19

they don't suit them. So, in contrast to what is suggested during stage hypnosis, a hypnotherapist does not control the subject. A traditional hypnotherapy session follows a fixed pattern (see Table 17.1). First, the GI mental health professional induces a hypnotic trance (e.g., by inviting the child to focus on a fixed point on the wall or their breathing). Then the child is usually encouraged to close their eyes, followed by deepening the trance using techniques like counting from ten to one. The youngest age group for hypnotherapy (5–7 years) may not close their eyes, which is entirely acceptable. Numerous techniques can be employed during the therapeutic phase, all using repetitive suggestions for change. These suggestions can be linked to images, such as being on a beach, but it can also be a monotonous, soothing, and sometimes confusing verbal repetition of all kinds of suggestions. Suggestions can be formulated for the here-and-now and also the future. The latter are called post-hypnotic suggestions (e.g., "*You will notice after this session that every time you are at school, you will feel more relaxed and more confident about your school performances*").

Table 17.1 Stages of hypnosis in gut-directed hypnotherapy

Stages of hypnosis	*Recommended strategies for youth*
Induction	• Magnetic finger technique is a fun and fast method. • Eye fixation on a toy or coin is a straightforward technique to introduce focus with a decreased awareness of the surroundings. • Conversational induction by starting a conversation about, for example, their favorite hobby and then slowly introducing a trance is a more modern form of induction, making hypnosis less of a "technique" and more of an art.
Deepening	• In primary school children, deepening is less critical because they easily switch between reality and hypnotic trance. In adolescents, deepening can be necessary, especially during the first session. Trance induction becomes easier the second time. • Progressive muscle relaxation, counting down ten steps, or imagining a safe place is pleasant and well-accepted deepening techniques.
Therapeutic suggestions	• Suggestions are often coupled to images; see Handout 17.1 for examples. • Utilize suggestions aiming at control of GI functions, improving feelings of happiness and confidence, and relaxation.
Return to usual alertness	• Invite the child to turn the attention back to the room at their own pace. • Repeat post-hypnotic suggestions. • Suggest that every time the child listens to this exercise or repeats it by themself (self-hypnosis), it will be easier to do and the effects will be stronger.

After the therapeutic phase, the child is invited to return to his/her usual alertness. Youth generally respond very well to hypnotherapy since their suggestibility is higher than that of adults [1]. They enjoy listening to the exercises and creating their own stories with their vivid imaginations. It is a very safe therapy. Sometimes dizziness is reported, which can be prevented by lying down during the hypnotherapy sessions. In case reports, other adverse events, like increased anxiety, have been described, but they are rare [2]. In a study of 34 children, only one child developed a side effect (mild transient headaches) [3]. It is not uncommon for youth to experience some sadness evoked by the relaxation of the mind and the body or by images linked to past events. In those cases, the trance doesn't have to be ended, but the GI mental health professional can say something like "how good it is for the tears to flow until they stop since they know that you are safe, and you know it is okay".

A particular form of hypnosis is self-hypnosis, in which children go into trance by themselves, creating images while repeating suggestions for their goals. Teaching self-hypnosis provides them with the skill to regulate and control their emotions, behavior, and mind–body reactions. Many report still using self-hypnosis years after treatment (e.g., to improve sleep or concentration). Hypnosis is very comparable to guided imagery, which is usually defined as guiding another person or oneself in imagining sensations and especially in visualizing images to bring about a desired physical response (as a reduction in stress, anxiety, or pain). During guided imagery, suggestions for the desired outcome are also provided, making it almost impossible to discriminate between the two techniques. Some health professionals even prefer the term guided imagery, given the many misconceptions people may still have about hypnotherapy.

Who should provide gut-directed hypnotherapy in youth?

Requirements for becoming a skilled and licensed hypnotherapist for youth are different worldwide and will, therefore, will not be discussed extensively. In general, it is recommended that pediatric hypnotherapy is provided by a healthcare professional already trained in working with youth, such as pediatricians, general practitioners, psychologists, nurses, and play therapists. A rule of thumb is that if you don't treat the child with tools other than hypnosis, you shouldn't do so with hypnotherapy. Several countries offer trainings in general pediatric hypnotherapy. Probably the best known are the annual workshops organized by the National Pediatric Hypnosis Training Institute in the United States (www.NPHTI.org).

Empirical support for hypnotherapy in pediatric GI disorders

To date, four randomized controlled trials (RCTs), with a total of 146 participants <18 years, have evaluated the effect of hypnotherapy/guided imagery in children with IBS or FAP. A Cochrane review concluded that hypnotherapy has a substantial effect on pain scores. Still, the GRADE quality of this conclusion was regarded as low due to the small number of participants across the studies and bias caused by unblinded allocation [4]. Apart from its effect on abdominal pain, hypnotherapy also improves noncolonic symptoms, feelings of anxiety and depression, and quality of life. Positive results of hypnotherapy are long-lasting, with 85% of patients being symptom-free at 1-year follow-up after receiving treatment, and 68% after 5 years follow-up. In the control group, these outcomes were only 25% and 20%, respectively [5].

The precise mechanisms by which hypnotherapy impacts pain-predominant DGBI are poorly understood. It is likely through a combination of effects on GI motility, visceral hypersensitivity, and psychological factors. A study using functional magnetic resonance imaging to measure cortical activation patterns during rectal distensions in adult IBS patients indicated that hypnotherapy could normalize the central processing of visceral signals [6]. Improvement in IBS symptoms after hypnotherapy often parallels improvement in psychological symptoms [7, 8]. Whether these psychological changes cause pain improvement or are the consequence remains to be elucidated.

Hypnotherapy is also used for other pediatric GI disorders. An RCT in 100 children recently demonstrated that hypnotherapy was slightly more effective than medication in functional nausea, with adequate relief rates of up to 80% in the hypnotherapy group [9]. Furthermore, it was demonstrated in adolescents with Crohn's disease that hypnotherapy is a feasible adjunct to treatment, improving quality of life and abdominal pain [10]. Studies on other GI disorders in youth are lacking, but adult data [11, 12] and the author's experience suggest that hypnotherapy can also be used for gastro-oesophageal reflux or globus sensations.

When and how to use hypnotherapy in youth with pain-related GI disorders?

Both hypnotherapy and cognitive behavioral therapy (CBT) are effective in treating youth with IBS or FAP. No studies, however, have compared these two modalities regarding efficacy and outcome predictors. Therefore, few recommendations can be given on which brain–gut therapy should be offered to each child.

When considering hypnotherapy as a treatment for youth with a pain-related brain–gut disorder, there are several issues to take into account. First, most research on hypnotherapy for pediatric IBS/FAP has been performed in secondary or tertiary care. So, to date, it is unknown if youth in primary care should also receive hypnotherapy. Many of them likely experience spontaneous improvement in time. For these youth, a wait-and-see policy in combination with education may suffice. On the other hand, hypnotherapy should not be postponed too long, as it has been shown in a group of youth with an average symptom duration of 2.5 years that a relatively shorter duration was associated with higher treatment success [8]. Youth with many negative pain beliefs respond less to hypnotherapy, which suggests that these youth may benefit more from CBT [8]. High baseline scores for anxiety or depression, on the other hand, are not a contraindication for hypnotherapy; in fact, anxiety and depression often improve significantly after hypnotherapy [8]. Also, skepticism in parents or the child is not a contradiction: low expectations before the start of hypnotherapy were not associated with worse outcomes [8]. It is, however, important to discuss these doubts since they may interfere with the child's daily listening to the exercises. Finally, suggestibility is not an issue, with most youth being highly suggestible.

Box 17.1 provides an example of how hypnotherapy can be explained to parents and their children. The rationale for hypnotherapy should be presented to the parents as using the brain to control and normalize gut functions since the brain and the gut are constantly communicating with each other. Moreover, one can add that hypnotherapy treatment will enable youth to learn new skills: not only to develop control over the GI tract, but also over emotions like sadness or anxiety. It is recommended to provide the child with a simple explanation of the current understanding of the pathophysiological mechanisms at play in brain–gut disorders. For example, the nerves in the gut have become overly sensitive due to a previous GI infection or stressful life events. At the same time, the brain misinterprets these signals coming from the gut. The communication between the brain and the gut needs to be normalized, and the nerves in the belly need to relax again. This will also improve gut functions, resulting in a normal transport of gas and poop. For further information and metaphors relating to the brain–gut axis, see Chapter 2.

BOX 17.1 HOW TO DISCUSS HYPNOTHERAPY WITH YOUTH AND PARENTS

Hypnotherapy for abdominal pain is an effective and well-studied therapy that helps you to normalize the pain signals from your belly. It is a treatment you can do alone, with a little help from a therapist.

Many youth who hear the word hypnosis may think of a scary guy with a watch going back and forth, making them do funny things, that is, *stage hypnosis* and has nothing to do with medical hypnotherapy.

Medical hypnotherapy is more like daydreaming. You likely have experienced this before. You are sitting in the classroom, thinking of your favorite sport or a nice vacation, and you forget that you are at school because you are entirely absorbed in your imagination.

Hypnotherapy is daydreaming with the purpose of making you feel better! During hypnotherapy, you focus your imagination on something you want to improve – for example, going to sleep easier, or training your belly to be happier, relaxed, and more comfortable. And the good news is that everyone can do it, and the more you do it, the better you get and the better it works.

Some people think hypnosis is losing control, but that is not true! In fact, when it is properly used in medicine, you get even more control over your body and your feelings. It is like learning a new sport; the more you practice, the better you will become.

In gut-directed hypnotherapy, suggestions are usually directed toward controlling and normalizing gut functions. Examples of these suggestions are provided in Handout 17.1. Therapists often apply metaphors during treatment, for instance, suggesting that an alarm in the brain has become too sensitive and needs to reset. Since stress plays an essential bidirectional role in pain, suggestions for relaxation are a standard part of hypnotherapy. Also, many youth suffer from anxiety or depression, so hypnotherapy sessions can focus on creating happy feelings with ego-strengthening suggestions.

The Dutch protocol (see Handout 17.2) has been adapted from the adult Manchester protocol and involves five to six 45- to 50-minute sessions delivered within 2–3 months [8, 13]. In between sessions, patients are provided with either a recording of the previous session or a standardized recording, which they should listen to at least 5 times per week. When there is no effect after the fifth session, a sixth session can be scheduled to perform hypnoanalysis to look for possible unrecognized psychological issues.

Individual hypnotherapy versus home-based treatment

The lack of well-trained hypnotherapists, waiting lists, and inadequate coverage by commercial health insurance are possible shortcomings of hypnotherapy. Therefore, three trials have examined using a cheaper, home-based treatment with standardized hypnotherapy exercises on compact discs (CDs) in youth with IBS or FAP. The first study, using the North Carolina protocol (see Handout 17.3), compared this modality with a waitlist in 34 youth, aged 6–15 years [3]. Two-thirds of youth responded favorably compared to only 27% in the control group. The effects were maintained for at least six months. A second small study in 32 youth (6–17 years) compared two forms of treatment with CDs, either with gut-directed hypnotherapy exercises or with more general exercises aiming at relaxation and increased well-being, and showed an improvement in 75% of youth, with no differences between groups [14]. The third study by Rutten et al., involving 260 youth aged 8–18, compared home-based treatment to individual hypnotherapy provided by a therapist [8]. Treatment success rates and the number of youth reporting adequate relief (70–80%) after treatment were comparable, but costs were significantly lower in the CD group.

A recent follow-up study showed that this home-based treatment had persisting positive results in more than 80% of the youth six years after treatment [15]. Therefore, audio-recorded self-hypnosis can be an attractive therapy for youth with FAP or IBS because of its efficacy, low costs, and direct availability. An online version of the Dutch hypnotherapy audio recordings [13] is available in English, Spanish, and Dutch [16]. A mobile app with the North Carolina protocol (see Handout 17.3) is being developed [17], and the authors share their scripts with trained therapists.

Advantages of these standardized, recorded hypnotherapy exercises are obvious, but some disadvantages also need to be addressed. Standardized scripts don't use hypnoanalytic techniques and underlying psychological issues can be overlooked. Moreover, suggestions and images are not adjusted to the child's interests, creating the possibility that the child doesn't like listening to the exercises. Also, the child becomes fully responsible for daily listening without reinforcement by the therapist. Finally, the child doesn't learn how to use self-hypnosis for future problems. Most issues can be tackled by keeping in touch with the child during the period they use these standard exercises and/or scheduling one or two individual sessions.

Identifying and managing challenges associated with hypnotherapy in GI youth

Hypnosis is very relaxing and most youth will gladly practice. However, some youth lack interest in regularly practicing self-hypnosis, which decreases symptom improvement. Lack of time should not be an issue since hypnosis exercises usually last 15–20 minutes. The best time to do self-hypnosis or listen to audio recordings is probably before bedtime. Some youth may say they don't like listening to the recordings. It is possible that due to relaxation during the hypnosis, emotions come up that these children are eager to suppress. It may be helpful to explore this possibility. You can tell the child, for example,

> In the word "emotion", one can already find what needs to be done with it. E-motions need to "move to the exit". Hence, getting tears or feelings of anger during the exercises is a good thing because it creates space inside for nicer feelings like happiness or relaxation.

Another challenge may be ongoing problems at home or school the child can't or won't talk about, like ongoing sexual abuse. When this is suspected, referral to an experienced child psychologist is strongly advised.

In conclusion, gut-directed hypnotherapy is a very effective treatment for GI problems in youth, especially for abdominal pain. Treatment can be provided individually by a therapist or by standardized audio recordings.

Pearls of wisdom

- Explain to youth, especially those who have had complaints for many years without the effect of other therapies, that hypnotherapy is one of the most effective therapies for chronic abdominal pain. It is, however, not a magic tool with adequate relief after just one hypnotherapy session. It will require youth's investment in time, meaning they must commit to practicing at least 5 times a week for 3 months. Also, it is vital to explain to youth that response to treatment differs per person: some already improve after one session, while others may need more time and experience improvement after 3 months or more.

- In families with perpetuating misconceptions about hypnosis or in very religious ones, it is advised to use terms like *guided imagery*, *mindpower*, *gut–brain therapy*, or *medical daydreaming*. To them, you can explain that our mind has difficulty discerning an image or a thought from the truth. It is like thinking about lice: as soon as you talk about them and see them in your mind, the skin of your head starts to feel itchy. So, you are using images to influence the body.
- Professionals who just started using hypnotherapy tend to weaken their suggestions as if they are already afraid their hypnosis won't work. For example, instead of saying: "*the more you do this, the better you will feel*", they say: "*if you do this, you may be feeling a bit better*". So, before you start a hypnotherapy session with a child, examine your own expectations about the process and outcome.

Summary

Children generally like gut-directed hypnotherapy, given their vivid imagination and suggestibility. It is highly effective for children with pain-predominant DGBI, like IBS and FAP. It also significantly improves anxiety and depression, non-colonic symptoms, and quality of life. Gut-directed hypnotherapy can also be applied for other GI disorders, like functional nausea or IBD, and more research is needed for other GI indications. Several treatment protocols are provided in this chapter, either for individual hypnotherapy by a therapist or for a home-based treatment with recorded hypnosis exercises.

Recommended readings

For youth and caregivers:

- Hypnotherapy for children and teenagers: www.firstwayforward.com/children-and-teenagers/.
- Understanding hypnosis: www.psychologytoday.com/us/blog/understanding-hypnosis/202209/using-hypnosis-help-manage-physical-ailments.
- Hypnosis for abdominal pain: www.hypnosis4abdominalpain.com.

For health professionals:

- Kohen, D.P. & Olness K. (2011). *Hypnosis and Hypnotherapy with Children* (4th edition). Routledge.
- Lyons, L. (2015). *Using Hypnosis with Children. Creating and delivering effective interventions.* W.W. Norton & Company.
- Anbar, R.A. (2021). *Changing Children's Lives with Hypnosis: A Journey to the Center.* Rowman & Littlefield.
- Yapko, M.D. (2014). *Essentials of Hypnosis.* Taylor & Francis Ltd.

References

1. London P. Hypnosis in children: An experimental approach. *Int J Clin Exp Hypn*. 1962;10(2):79–91.
2. Lyszczyk M, Karkhaneh M, Gladwin KK, Funabashi M, Zorzela L, Vohra S. Adverse events of mind-body interventions in children: A systematic review. *Children*. 2021;8(5):358.
3. van Tilburg MA, Chitkara DK, Palsson OS, Turner M, Blois-Martin N, Ulshen M, et al. Audio-recorded guided imagery treatment reduces functional abdominal pain in children: A pilot study. *Pediatrics*. 2009;124(5):e890–e7.
4. Abbott RA, Martin AE, Newlove-Delgado TV, Bethel A, Thompson-Coon J, Whear R, et al. Psychosocial interventions for recurrent abdominal pain in childhood. *Cochrane Database Syst Rev*. 2017(1).
5. Vlieger AM, Rutten JM, Govers AM, Frankenhuis C, Benninga MA. Long-term follow-up of gut-directed hypnotherapy vs. standard care in children with functional abdominal pain or irritable bowel syndrome. *Am J Gastroenterol*.| ACG. 2012;107(4):627–31.
6. Lowén MB, Mayer EA, Sjöberg M, Tillisch K, Naliboff B, Labus J, et al. Effect of hypnotherapy and educational intervention on brain response to visceral stimulus in the irritable bowel syndrome. *Aliment Pharmacol Ther*. 2013;37(12):1184–97.
7. Palsson OS, Turner MJ, Johnson DA, Burnett CK, Whitehead WE. Hypnosis treatment for severe irritable bowel syndrome: Investigation of mechanism and effects on symptoms. *Dig Dis Sci*. 2002;47(11):2605–14.
8. Rutten JM, Vlieger AM, Frankenhuis C, George EK, Groeneweg M, Norbruis OF, et al. Home-based hypnotherapy self-exercises vs individual hypnotherapy with a therapist for treatment of pediatric irritable bowel syndrome, functional abdominal pain, or functional abdominal pain syndrome: A randomized clinical trial. *JAMA Pediatr*. 2017;171(5):470–7.
9. Browne PD, de Bruijn CM, Speksnijder EM, den Hollander B, van Wering HM, Wessels MM, et al. Skills or pills: Randomized trial comparing hypnotherapy to medical treatment in children with functional nausea. *Clin Gastroenterol Hepatol*. 2022;20(8):1847–56. e6.
10. Lee A, Moulton D, Mckernan L, Russell A, Slaughter JC, Acra S, et al. Clinical hypnosis in pediatric Crohn's disease: A randomized controlled pilot study. *J Pediatr Gastroenterol Nutr*. 2021;72(3):e63–e70.
11. Jones H, Cooper P, Miller V, Brooks N, Whorwell PJ. Treatment of non-cardiac chest pain: A controlled trial of hypnotherapy. *Gut*. 2006;55(10):1403–8.
12. Kinsinger SW, Joyce C, Venu M, Palsson OS. Pilot study of a self-administered hypnosis intervention for functional dyspepsia. *Dig Dis Sci*. 2022;67(7):3017–25.
13. Rutten JM, Vlieger AM, Frankenhuis C, George EK, Groeneweg M, Norbruis OF, et al. Gut-directed hypnotherapy in children with irritable bowel syndrome or functional abdominal pain (syndrome): A randomized controlled trial on self exercises at home using CD versus individual therapy by qualified therapists. *BMC Pediatr*. 2014;14(1):1–8.
14. Gulewitsch MD, Schlarb AA. Comparison of gut-directed hypnotherapy and unspecific hypnotherapy as self-help format in children and adolescents with functional abdominal pain or irritable bowel syndrome: A randomized pilot study. *Eur J Gastroenterol Hepatol*. 2017;29(12):1351–60.
15. Rexwinkel R, Bovendeert JF, Rutten JM, Frankenhuis C, Benninga MA, Vlieger AM. Long-term follow-up of individual therapist delivered and standardized hypnotherapy recordings in pediatric irritable bowel syndrome or functional abdominal pain. *J Pediatr Gastroenterol Nutr*. 2022;75(1):24.
16. The dutch foundation for hypnosis in children. Available from: https://hypnosis4abdominalpain.com/; https://hipnosisparadolorabdominal.com; https://hypnosebeibauchschmerzen.de; https://hypnosebijbuikpijn.nl.
17. Hollier JM, Vaughan AO, Liu Y, van Tilburg MA, Shulman RJ, Thompson DI. Maternal and child acceptability of a proposed guided imagery therapy mobile app designed to treat functional abdominal pain disorders in children: Mixed-methods predevelopment formative research. *JMIR Pediatr Parent*. 2018;1(1):e8535.

Chapter 18

Constipation and soiling

Infant/toddler

Christina Low Kapalu and John M. Rosen

Chapter aims

The aim of this chapter is to introduce practical evaluation and treatment strategies for constipation and soiling in infants and toddlers, with a specific focus on typical child development as well as behavioral interventions that complement dietary and pharmacologic treatments.

Learning points

- Constipation is the most common disorder of gut–brain interaction (DGBI) in toddlers, and diagnostic testing is rarely needed.
- Constipation must be adequately treated before toilet training.
- Soiling is normal in children under age 4 or the developmental equivalent.
- Toilet training should proceed based on readiness, not age.

Infant and toddler constipation is a common symptom with a prevalence of approximately 9% [1]. Generally, constipation is defined as difficulty with the passage of stool and may include excessively large, hard, or infrequent bowel movements but is not limited to a specific size, consistency, or frequency. Specific disease states such as Hirschsprung disease (a birth defect in which some nerve cells are missing in the large intestine) and celiac disease (gluten autoimmunity) can also present with constipation in infants and toddlers. An underrecognized diagnosis important to consider in infants presenting with constipation is infant dyschezia, occurring in approximately 2% of children. Rome IV criteria [2] define this disorder as excessive straining or crying in an infant under 9 months of age who is attempting to defecate. These children usually produce soft stools, and the straining is due to the child not yet being able to coordinate abdominal and pelvic floor muscles to have a bowel movement. As the child's coordination of these muscles is expected to develop over time, this is a self-resolving disorder that is not harmful to the child but can be distressing for parents.

In the vast majority of toddlers, constipation is a disorder called functional constipation. Functional constipation, a DGBI, is defined by specific symptom-based criteria (Rome IV) [2] that include infrequent, hard, and/or large-diameter stools occurring repeatedly over time. For this reason, this chapter will mostly focus on functional constipation, though other reasons for constipation will also be briefly addressed.

DOI: 10.4324/9781003308683-20

The cycle of constipation

When toilet training, many toddlers begin to voluntarily withhold their stool when they notice the urge to defecate. Withholding may occur for various reasons including discomfort with stooling on available toilets or passage of a hard stool that makes stooling uncomfortable. The longer the stool stays in the colon, the more water is drawn out of the stool, creating harder and larger stools that become painful to pass. Since stooling now hurts, a young child tries not to do it as often and may develop a fear of defecating which paradoxically makes the constipation worse. As the size and hardness of the stool increases, it becomes difficult to pass and a child may not have a bowel movement for several days or sometimes even weeks. Unformed stool can leak around this hard mass and can cause accidents. This may give the impression that the child has diarrhea when in fact they are constipated. The passage of overflow stool is called fecal incontinence or encopresis (see Handout 18.1). This is particularly burdensome for families who deal with multiple changes of dirty underwear every day.

To break the cycle of constipation (see Figure 18.1), youth have to learn through the repeated passage of soft stools that stooling is no longer a painful experience to avoid. This can take months to years and many youth relapse before they permanently improve. More on the long-term effects of constipation for children and adolescents can be found in Chapter 19.

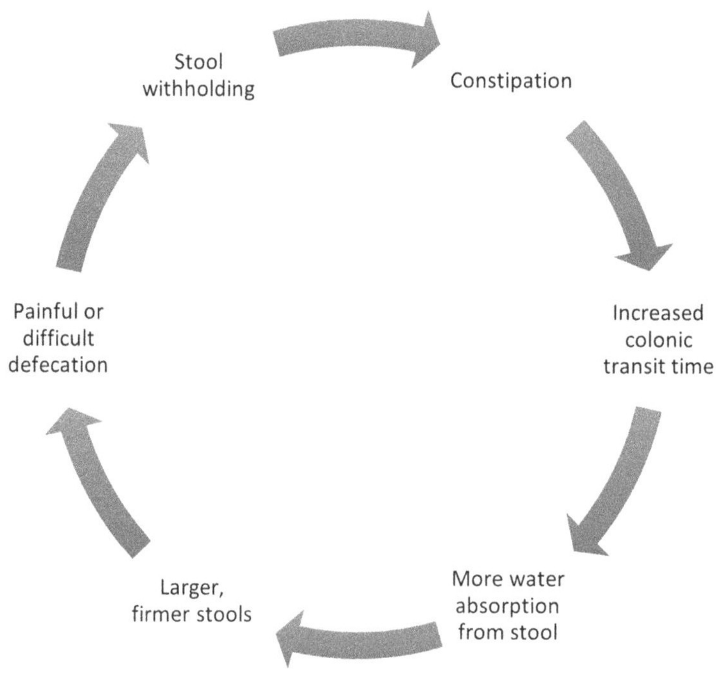

Figure 18.1 A vicious cycle: constipation (Source: Authors).

Medical assessment

A typical medical exam would include a detailed history of symptoms of stooling, growth patterns, dietary history, urologic symptoms, diagnostic testing performed, and prior treatment strategies [3]. A health professional usually also performs a physical examination including:

- Abdominal palpation: to feel for presence/absence of stool including consistency and volume, and to determine if there is pain that could signify an alternate disease.
- Visual assessment of the spine and gross motor assessment: to look for spinal cord and muscle tone/strength abnormality that signals a neuromuscular disease.
- Visual external anal exam: to assess for anorectal anatomic malformation.

Abdominal X-rays are sometimes performed to assess how much stool is in a child's colon/rectum. Yet these tests are not recommended. Interpretation of X-ray for stool burden is inconsistent and can lead to both false-positive and false-negative results [4].

Other symptoms can be indicative of underlying constipation such as unexplained abdominal pain (the pressure of large stools can be painful), fecal or urinary accidents after achieving continence (overflow leakage of unformed stool around the large hard mass in the rectum), low appetite, inadequate weight gain, and nausea/vomiting (due to the cologastric brake, a filled colon makes children feel "full").

Most infants and toddlers can be adequately managed in primary care and no testing is needed. Consultation from a gastrointestinal (GI) specialist may be considered when constipation and related symptoms do not improve despite first-line medical intervention, or when "red flag" symptoms are present (see Box 18.1).

BOX 18.1 RED FLAGS INDICATING THE NEED FOR FURTHER EVALUATION [3]

- Hematochezia (blood in stool).
- Sacral tuft or dimple.
- Inadequate weight gain or weight loss.
- Severe abdominal distension.
- Abnormal perianal exam.
- Delayed passage of meconium (the first stool of a newborn).

Medical treatment

Medical treatment is adequate for most youth. Treatment of constipation begins with a specific diagnosis and education to the family that no further testing is required. It is important to set expectations and identify shared goals for treatment, including that long-term symptoms likely require long-term management (there is no quick fix). Parents often feel their child should be pooping every day, when "normal" can be pooping every 3 days for toddlers and every 5–7 days for infants.

For infants with difficulty defecating (dyschezia), family reassurance and education are all that is needed. This is a self-limited condition. Infant constipation with decreased stool frequency or firmer consistency may develop after changes in diet (e.g., introducing formula, or starting solid foods). Formula-fed infants may be treated by ensuring appropriate formula mixing recipe or with a trial of an extensively hydrolyzed formula in which protein is partially digested.

For toddlers with functional constipation, treatment usually consists of three components:

(1) Toddlers with large masses of stool that they cannot evacuate on their own will need a bowel cleanout, using oral or rectal laxatives. This is sometimes performed in the hospital.
(2) Maintenance laxative treatments focused on keeping bowels soft. Over time a child will no longer associate an urge with pain.
(3) Toilet sitting. Due to the gastrocolic reflex, most youth will feel an urge to defecate about 15–20 minutes after a meal. Youth of toilet training age will be asked to sit on a toilet after a meal to help them recognize and act on this urge. No defecation is required at that time, and a toddler's sitting behavior should be reinforced (praise, stickers, etc.) rather than focus on having a bowel movement.

Two primary classes of laxatives are osmotic and stimulant laxatives. Osmotic laxatives hold fluid in stool, softening its consistency. Common examples include lactulose (particularly used for newborns), magnesium hydroxide, and polyethylene glycol 3350 (PEG3350). The latter is often preferred since it is tasteless and odorless and can be added to a toddler's favorite clear drink. Although concerns have been raised about PEG3350's neuropsychiatric effects and long-term stimulant laxative use dependency, neither has been validated and both have scientific (laboratory and clinical) evidence to the contrary [5–8]. Stimulant laxatives such as sennosides and bisacodyl cause contraction of colonic smooth muscle making the urge to stool easier to detect and more difficult to ignore.

Rectal therapy with suppositories or enemas may also be used to treat constipation. Stimulation secondary to insertion of a suppository or enema may result in colon contraction and bowel movement, or the specific medication used (e.g., glycerine, bisacodyl, water, saline) may assist through physical or physiologic action. Rectal therapy provides the advantage of stimulus and response, leading to the predictability of stool output, which may benefit the child and caregiver. Parental concerns about safety and comfort should be addressed. Other treatments are used in the management of infant and toddler constipation including prune juice, abdominal massage, magnesium supplements, traditional medications (i.e., Ayurvedic, Chinese), probiotics, prebiotics, and anal botulinum toxin injection. For each treatment, benefits and risks should be weighed. Dietary interventions for constipation in toddlers are popular but rarely helpful [3]. Increased fiber intake can even increase gas production and distension and may be a stressful goal with limited benefit.

Although many children experience symptom relief with the initiation of a bowel management program, early identification of constipation and ongoing reassessment is important – constipation does not frequently resolve without intervention and up to 25% of youth continue to experience constipation as adults [9].

Behavioral assessment

For the typically developing infant/toddler, minimal assessment beyond a clinical history and possibly a broadband behavioral screener is needed to treat constipation and/or soiling. Consider gathering information about developmental milestones, current developmental level, history of painful bowel movements or negative toileting experiences (see Box 18.2), as well as fear of toileting. Additionally, inquire about the living situation, caregiver beliefs about constipation and treatment, medical history, and current bowel management plan (see Handout 18.2 for constipation/toileting intake questions). Behavioral screeners such as the behavioral assessment system for children (3rd Ed.) [10] can be useful in identifying any externalizing (e.g., hitting, noncompliance) or internalizing (e.g., anxiety, withdrawal) behavioral challenges that may impact medical and/or behavioral management.

BOX 18.2 IS TOILET TRAINING A CONTRIBUTOR TO CONSTIPATION?

Toilet training is a major developmental milestone for toddlers, initiated between the ages of 18 months and 4 years. Toileting is a learned skill like walking and talking, and each child develops at their own pace. The American Academy of Pediatrics states that it is not the child's age, but readiness to toilet train that should prompt toilet training [11]. Toilet training readiness is indicated by several skills/behaviors such as the ability to sit on the toilet or notice they are wet/dry (see Handout 18.3 for toilet training readiness skills). Starting toilet training prior to readiness often leads to frustration for caregiver and toddler, can worsen constipation, and may cause delayed attainment of continence.

If a child has a recent history of passing large or painful stools, aggressive medical management of constipation is needed prior to pursuing toilet training. Caregivers should be encouraged to delay toilet training until their child has had weeks or months of soft and easy-to-pass stools, so that they desensitize to fears about stooling, making toilet training easier (see Handout 18.4 for toilet training tips for caregivers).

Daycare/preschool toilet training requirements at age 3 block educational access for some toddlers. Consider writing a letter outlining the steps being taken to treat constipation and establish continence and ask that the school consider accepting an otherwise school-ready child.

Behavioral treatment

Although constipation in toddlers is often functional, it is recommended that GI mental health professionals require a family to seek medical evaluation first. Referral to a mental healthcare provider for pediatric constipation is indicated when a child does not respond to standard medical management and can be very helpful for families struggling with medical treatment adherence due to either parent and/or child factors. Behavioral treatment in toddlers entails three main components: (1) education, (2) behavioral modification, and (3) relapse prevention.

Education

Although most families will have already received education about the constipation cycle and the importance of laxative treatment and toilet sitting, many families may still struggle with understanding or accepting this explanation of their child's symptoms. Education on the cycle of constipation should be repeated. Furthermore, a GI mental health professional should normalize constipation, e.g., explaining that it occurs in between 5% and 27% of infants and toddlers, and is rarely indicative of a serious medical problem [2]. The median age of onset of constipation is estimated to be 2.3 years [2] and estimates suggest that 17–40% of youth will experience constipation starting within the first year of life [12]. Sharing these statistics can quell caregiver fears.

Adherence with medical treatment

Laxative treatment can last months and sometimes years. Medication adherence can be a challenge due to both child (e.g., refusing to take medication) and parent factors (e.g., stopping medication when child is symptom-free). Mental health professionals are vital to the promotion of adherence by assessing barriers and collaboratively problem-solving. It is recommended to evaluate medication adherence in an open-ended manner (e.g., "How many times a week does your child miss one or more prescribed medications?") with a nonjudgmental tone at every appointment. See Handout 18.5 for a summary of common barriers to medication adherence and related solutions.

Behavioral modification

Toileting intervention for toddlers is grounded in behavioral therapy principles. Parents are taught how to use reinforcement and consequences to shape their child's toileting behaviors, based on their child's specific behavioral deficits/needs. A brief description of behavioral intervention is provided below. See Handout 18.6 for toileting behaviors and related intervention options for toddlers, and Handout 18.7 for behavioral troubleshooting tips.

Behavioral modification may include promoting their child's comfort with stooling, encouraging evacuation of stool in youth with a history of withholding, and supporting the development of toilet training readiness skills. Caregivers should be actively discouraged from using punishment or shaming as responses to stool withholding or soiling. A low-pressure toileting environment is encouraged, and parents should be reassured that the medications will help their child to stool more often/easily.

If toddlers have a fear of stooling, parents can provide gentle encouragement and praise for "letting the poop out" or "listening to their bodies". Concerned caregivers may become hypervigilant to their child's stooling patterns and place undue pressure on the child to stool, which can be counterproductive. Caregivers are encouraged to provide lots of attention and encouragement for stooling and perhaps a single redirection (i.e., "your body is telling you to poop") or active ignoring for stool withholding.

Treatment goals for toddlers include increasing stooling frequency (thus decreasing withholding), allowing diaper changes if diapered, taking medications, developing toilet training readiness skills, and sitting on or eliminating in the toilet. Skills are broken down into smaller component skills and caregivers provide reinforcement for approximations of target behaviors. For example, children may start by sitting on the toilet for 10 seconds, then 20 seconds, then 30 seconds, working up to 3 minutes eventually. Parents provide attention, praise, and perhaps tangible reinforcement (e.g., piece of candy, small toy) for completing each task, creating behavioral momentum, and increasing child engagement.

In some cases, caregivers may need to address the fear of stooling. To decondition the fear of stooling, a toddler must have lots of opportunities for pain-free stooling over periods of weeks or months. In some cases, caregivers should be encouraged to help their child increase stool output regardless of whether it is passed into the toilet or a diaper. This can be difficult for caregivers eager to toilet train or for those with previously continent children. Dexterity issues, balance concerns, or age-typical fears (see Box 18.3) can also cause toileting-related anxiety. The use of step stools, adaptive toileting supports, and parent presence can be helpful.

BOX 18.3 "HELP! I'LL FALL IN THE TOILET"

In addition to pain with stooling, it is common for toddlers to have fears around the toilet itself. They may fear falling in, flushing a part of themselves away, or monsters coming through the toilet. Assessing and addressing these fears are important. Strategies involve: (1) talking about the fear (e.g., the pipes are too small for a monster to come through), (2) improving comfort (e.g., using a toilet seat insert, step stool, or potty), and (3) distraction (e.g., blowing bubbles or playing games while toilet sitting). Some children may need stepped exposure therapy starting with just simply being in the toilet space or sitting dressed on a potty, before gradually moving to more feared situations.

Relapse prevention

Once a toddler has achieved good soiling control, medical and behavioral interventions may need to remain in place for some time. Many caregivers are eager to stop medications or toilet sittings soon after goals are reached, which can result in return of constipation and soiling. Encourage families to continue toileting interventions for approximately 1–6 months (or longer) or as guided by their medical provider. Continued use of these supports helps with skill building and habit formation. Constipation exacerbation should be normalized, and relapse prevention discussed. Common reasons for increases in constipation in infants/toddlers include transition to solid foods, toilet training, changes in routine, exposure to stressors, changes in diet common in toddlers, illness, or travel. These reasons are likely associated with changes in toileting schedule, introduction of unfamiliar toilets/facilities, changes in fluid and/or fiber intake, and stool postponement. Tools, such as the constipation action plan can help to provide families with increased self-efficacy and decreased need for medical follow-up [13].

Pearls of wisdom

- Clearly define the constipation criteria for families as it is often underrecognized and therefore undertreated. If inadequately treated, behavioral intervention is less beneficial.
- A key task for GI mental health providers in treatment of constipation/soiling is promoting medication adherence, including educating when misinformation is present. Start here!
- Medical and behavioral intervention is often terminated too quickly, leading to the recurrence of symptoms and family frustration.

Summary

Constipation is common in infants and toddlers and is treatable. Difficult or painful defecation may lead to stool withholding, which potentiates constipation and disrupts toilet training. It is important for mental health professionals to have a basic understanding of the physiology of constipation and related medical treatments when providing behavioral intervention to this group. Treatment for infants will often involve medication management of constipation as they are not yet expected to be continent. In toddlers, combined medical and behavioral intervention is the gold standard treatment. Behavioral intervention can increase readiness, decrease stool withholding, and improve toileting skills. Shame, blame, and punishment have no place in the treatment of constipation/soiling and will make the problem worse. Toilet training should proceed when the child shows readiness and not be solely based on age.

Recommended readings

For youth and caregivers:

- The complete constipation care package – available in English, Spanish, and French: www.gikids.org/constipation/complete-constipation-care-package/.

For mental health professionals:

- Uniformed services constipation action plan – available in English and Spanish: www.wrnmmc.libguides.com/ld.php?content_id=57110850.
- NASPGHAN constipation care package: www. naspghan.org/files/documents/pdfs/medical-resources/Constipation_Care_Package.pdf.

References

1. Velasco-Benitez CA, Collazos-Saa LI, Garcia-Perdomo HA. Functional gastrointestinal disorders in neonates and toddlers according to the Rome IV criteria: A systematic review and meta-analysis. *Pediatr Gastroenterol Hepatol Nutr.* 2022;25(5):376–86.
2. Benninga MA, Faure C, Hyman PE, St James Roberts I, Schechter NL, Nurko S. Childhood functional gastrointestinal disorders: Neonate/toddler. *Gastroenterology.* 2016 Feb 15:S0016-5085(16)00182-7.
3. Tabbers MM, DiLorenzo C, Berger MY, Faure Ç, Langendam MW, Nurko S, et al. Evaluation and treatment of functional constipation in infants and children: Evidence-based recommendations from ESPGHAN and NASPGHAN. *J Pediatr Gastroenterol Nutr.* 2014;58(2):258–74.
4. Benninga MA, Tabbers MM, van Rijn RR. How to use a plain abdominal radiograph in children with functional defecation disorders. *Arch Dis Child Educ Pract Ed.* 2016;101(4):187–93.
5. Williams KC, Rogers LK, Hill I, Barnard J, Di Lorenzo C. PEG 3350 Administration is not associated with sustained elevation of glycol levels. *J Pediatr.* 2018;195:148–53 e1.
6. Rachel H, Griffith AF, Teague WJ, Hutson JM, Gibb S, Goldfeld S, et al. Polyethylene glycol dosing for constipation in children younger than 24 MONTHS: A systematic review. *J Pediatr Gastroenterol Nutr.* 2020;71(2):171–5.
7. Salman SS, Williams KC, Marte-Ortiz P, Rumpf W, Mashburn-Warren L, Lauber CL, et al. Polyethylene glycol 3350 changes stool consistency and the microbiome but not behavior of CD1 Mice. *J Pediatr Gastroenterol Nutr.* 2021;73(4):499–506.
8. Worona-Dibner L, Vazquez-Frias R, Valdez-Chavez L, Verdiguel-Oyola M. Efficacy, safety, and acceptability of polyethylene glycol 3350 without electrolytes vs magnesium hydroxide in functional constipation in children from six months to eighteen years of age: A controlled clinical trial. *Rev Gastroenterol Mex (Engl Ed).* 2023 Apr-Jun; 88(2):107–117.
9. Bongers ME, van Wijk MP, Reitsma JB, Benninga MA. Long-term prognosis for childhood constipation: Clinical outcomes in adulthood. *Pediatrics.* 2010;126(1):e156–62.
10. Reynolds C, Kamphaus R. *Behavior assessment system for children–Third Edition* (BASC-3). Bloomington, MN: Pearson; 2015.

11. Toilet training guidelines: Parents-the role of the parents in toilet training. *Pediatrics*. June 1999;103(6 Pt 2):1362–3.
12. Loening-Baucke V. Constipation in early childhood: Patient characteristics, treatment, and longterm follow up. *Gut*. 1993;34(10):1400–4.
13. Reeves PT, Jack BO, Rogers PL, Kolasinski NT, Burklow CS, Min SB, et al. The uniformed services constipation action plan: An effective tool for the management of children with functional constipation. *J Pediatr.*. 2023 Feb; 253:46–54.e1.

Chapter 19

Constipation and soiling

Children and adolescents

Jaclyn A. Shepard and Alex C. Nyquist

Chapter aims

This chapter provides an overview of diagnosis, assessment, and management of constipation and soiling in childhood and adolescence. Treatment emphasizes behavioral principles familiar to gastrointestinal (GI) mental health professionals.

Learning points

- Diagnostic criteria and prevalence of constipation and soiling in children and adolescents.
- Clinical assessment of constipation and soiling.
- Collaborative care treatment models for the management of constipation and soiling.
- Future directions in clinical research and interprofessional training in evidence-based treatments for constipation and soiling.

Overview of constipation and soiling

Constipation is characterized by infrequent bowel movements that are hard, sometimes large, and difficult or painful to pass. Based on the Rome IV criteria for disorders of gut–brain interaction (DGBI; formally known as functional GI disorders), functional constipation involves at least 1 month of at least two of the following with insufficient criteria for a diagnosis of irritable bowel syndrome: 2 or fewer stools in the toilet per week in a child of a developmental age of at least 4 years; at least one episode of fecal incontinence per week; history of retentive posturing or excessive volitional stool retention; history of painful or hard bowel movements; presence of a large fecal mass in the rectum; and history of large diameter stools [1]. It is important to highlight that in children and adolescents with functional constipation, fecal incontinence or soiling is a symptom of the diagnosis, and not a separate condition.

Although soiling is associated with constipation in most cases, there is a subset of youth who experience soiling without constipation or another underlying medical cause, termed nonretentive fecal incontinence (NFI) [1]. For a child to meet Rome IV criteria for NFI, they must be older than 4 years of age or the developmental equivalent, exhibit at least a 1-month history of defecating in inappropriate places (e.g., clothing, floor), exhibit lack of fecal retention, and experience soiling that is not explained by another medical condition. NFI is far less common than functional constipation and represents one in every ten cases of fecal incontinence [2].

DOI: 10.4324/9781003308683-21

Clinical presentation

Although functional constipation peaks in incidence at the time of toilet training, older children and adolescents are frequently affected as well. For many youth, functional constipation is triggered when defecation is avoided due to pain or other reasons such as discomfort with stooling at school, while traveling, or in an unfamiliar setting. Once the stool is withheld, water is increasingly absorbed from the stool by the colon, resulting in increasingly firm stools that are difficult or painful to evacuate. Consequently, the youth becomes even less likely to expel the stool, causing the rectum to become distended and a larger stool mass to accumulate. Liquid stool can leak around this hard stool mass, resulting in overflow fecal incontinence and fecal soiling. Over time, a distended rectum will lose sensation resulting in the loss of the normal urge to defecate. Youth will also likely develop upper GI symptoms including loss of appetite, abdominal distention, and pain.

Other factors that may contribute to the development of functional constipation in youth include specific phobias, such as fear of public or unfamiliar toilets, and generalized fear of all toilets and/or bathrooms, which again leads to stool holding until preferred toilets/situations become available. Although parents often interpret functional constipation and subsequent fecal incontinence as their children being obstinate or preferring to soil their pants instead of stopping a preferred activity (e.g., a video game), this is not commonly true unless the child has a co-occurring neurodevelopmental condition, such as attention-deficit/hyperactivity disorder [3, 4]. Over time, stool withholding can result in acquired megacolon, a condition characterized by a colon that has become stretched and displays increased diameter and length in the absence of organic disease. Though typically reversible, treatment of acquired megacolon involves a strict bowel management program at a minimum.

Children with constipation and soiling tend to have higher rates of internalizing symptoms, disruptive behaviors, and attention problems compared to healthy children, though these are most often clinically subthreshold concerns and not necessarily predictive, as behavioral symptoms can emerge as a result of symptoms and/or stigma of constipation [5]. Although it has been surmised that chronic constipation with soiling is associated with or even predictive of past sexual abuse, fecal soiling is not a useful predictor of sexual abuse status in children [6].

Assessment of constipation and soiling

According to the biopsychosocial model of DGBI (see Chapter 2), multiple factors contribute to the etiology, maintenance, and treatment of constipation. At the outset, it is important to assess and understand the biological, sociocultural, psychological, and behavioral factors in a child's presentation of constipation and soiling.

Medical assessment

Medical evaluation is warranted to rule out any organic etiology of constipation and soiling before proceeding with behavioral interventions. Many children with functional constipation will respond to laxative therapy and a regular toilet sitting plan as recommended by their pediatrician with no further intervention required. For youth who initiate medical interventions such as laxative therapy for constipation and soiling but who fail to respond satisfactorily, or who struggle with adherence to the laxative and toilet sitting regimen, simultaneous and collaborative treatment from a GI mental health professional may be indicated [7].

Psychosocial assessment

Sufficient clinical information can be gathered using a combination of clinical interview and psychometrically sound parent- and/or teacher-report measures. The profile of toileting issues (POTI) [8] can be used to gauge levels of difficulty with toileting and accidents. Broad-based behavioral and emotional assessment scales such as the behavior assessment system for children, third edition (BASC-3) [9], offer self-, parent-, and teacher-report forms to measure adaptive and problem behaviors (see Chapter 6 for more detailed information on screeners and validated measures specific to constipation and soiling).

The GI mental health professional will meet with the caregiver(s) and child to gather a complete toileting history. For adolescents, it is helpful to dedicate a portion of the interview without the caregiver present for privacy considerations. The clinical interview should focus on information about toilet training; any developmental delays or sensory differences; history of constipation and associated treatment; current bowel and bladder patterns, including onset, frequency, location (home, school, public); and response related to withholding behaviors and, if relevant, soiling. Previous behavioral interventions, such as a toilet sit schedule, use of rewards and/or consequences, and contributing factors should also be assessed. Regarding co-occurring emotional or behavioral concerns, the GI mental health professional should gather information about the frequency, intensity, cues (triggers), and resolution of symptoms to guide treatment planning and recommendations.

Given the role of withholding in maintaining the cycle of functional constipation, factors serving to potentially maintain withholding are especially important to assess. These may include fear of experiencing pain when stooling, fear of hearing or the possibility that others will hear the sounds associated with stooling, or discomfort with using toilets outside the home. In order to systematically treat anxious cognitions that are contributing to the withholding behaviors, it is necessary to identify and build a behavioral hierarchy around these cognitions.

Management of constipation and soiling

Youth with chronic constipation and soiling who fail to respond to initial medical management and who have access to a pediatric medical center may benefit from referral to a bowel management program designed to provide multidisciplinary treatment. In such programs, medical specialty providers, including gastroenterology, urology, and developmental pediatrics, lend expertise in medical assessment and medication management of constipation. Allied health providers, such as physical therapists and occupational therapists, offer unique interventions (e.g., pelvic floor training or rehabilitation) that complement the efforts of GI mental health professionals, who bring expertise in child behavior. Communication and collaboration among these specialists and with the family is essential to the management of constipation. Effective management for constipation includes three components: (1) education, (2) bowel management, and (3) behavioral intervention to improve toileting behaviors.

Education

Education is provided to caregivers, including age-appropriate and brief explanations to the child as well, often with visual aids (see Chapter 18). This vital treatment component clarifies for parents that (in a majority of cases) their child is not soiling out of spite or laziness (see Handout 19.1). At the start of treatment, it is essential that the GI mental health professional form a collaborative relationship with the caregiver(s). Education aims to orient parenting strategies to the child's behavior (i.e., taking medications daily, sitting on the toilet when prompted, responding to the urge to defecate, cleaning up an accident) rather than whether the child produces stool in the toilet. For NFI, parent education aims to clarify that the child's incontinence stems from emotional distress and is not solely due to bad behavior.

Bowel management

Bowel management includes a bowel cleanout and maintenance laxation regimen. The cleanout involves fecal disimpaction, allowing for routine bowel movements before initiating maintenance therapy. This component is managed primarily by a medical specialist. Once the cleanout is complete, maintenance laxation therapy is typically prescribed by the medical specialist. The goal of the bowel regimen is to eliminate painful bowel movements through the use of laxatives and/or stool softeners, paired with a toilet sit schedule [10]. Toilet sits are typically scheduled 20–30 minutes following meals to capitalize on the gastrocolic reflex [3]; see Handout 19.1 for more information. Maintenance laxative therapy aims to ensure regular, soft, and painless bowel movements so that treatment progress does not regress following a painful stooling experience. The maintenance laxative regimen frequently is prescribed for months or years to maintain a pattern of regular bowel movements and will require regular follow-up and monitoring by the medical specialist.

Behavioral strategies

Behavioral strategies are needed if families struggle with medication adherence, behavior tracking, and general compliance training around the toilet sit schedule. The specific combination of strategies will vary depending on the child's unique needs (see Table 19.1). Behavior tracking is a useful strategy for any health behavior change because this information can help the family and GI mental health professional monitor treatment progress as well as inform adjustments to the treatment plan (see Handout 19.2 for children and Handout 19.3 for adolescents).

Of note, punishment is *not* an effective or recommended strategy for adherence or general compliance training. GI mental health professionals also help caregivers work with teachers on setting accommodations to manage constipation at school (see Box 19.1).

BOX 19.1 EXAMPLES OF SCHOOL ACCOMMODATIONS

School accommodations for students with constipation

- Prompt student to take scheduled bathroom breaks, such as after lunch or before recess or physical education class.
- Allow student to visit the school nurse for cleanup following soiling accidents.
- Allow student use or private (single-occupancy) bathroom at school.

Most often the GI mental health professional will focus on compliance training for the toilet sit schedule. Some children may have phobic reactions to the toilet and/or bathroom, which should be treated with graduated exposures (for more detailed information see Whiteside et al. [11]).

Table 19.1 Summary table of behavioral issues and suggested interventions

Common issue: Fear and avoidance of sitting on the toilet (or public toilets)

Suggested assessment: Determine whether there is a sensory component (e.g., sound of toilet flush or touch of the toilet seat). Assess the child's willingness to use toilets at home, school, public, friend's house, etc.

Suggested intervention: Shaping protocol (graduated exposures) whereby the child is prompted and coached to face the avoided circumstance incrementally. For example, if a child refuses to poop in other bathrooms, the initial exposure might be to poop in another bathroom in their home. Next might be to use the bathroom at a grandparent's (or other trusted friend's) home.

Common issue: Fear of painful bowel movements

Suggested assessment: Does the child make comments about pain? Is there any history of painful stooling?

Suggested intervention: Maintenance therapy (i.e., laxation) is essential to breaking the child's association of bowel movements and pain. Along with practicing daily toilet sits, the child will unlearn the belief that bowel movements are always painful.

Common issue: Nonadherence to laxative regimen

Suggested assessment: When is medication given? Who prompts the child and administers the medication? Does the child dislike the taste or texture? What happens before and after the child takes medication?

Suggested interventions: Allow sufficient time in the daily routine. Utilize incentives that the child is willing to work for, such as preferred breakfast foods or after-school snacks. Sometimes, it is possible to mix medication with drinks or foods.

Common issue: Nonadherence to toilet sits

Suggested assessment: When do the toilet sits fit into the child's routine? What happens when the child is prompted? How long or intense are tantrums?

Suggested interventions: Teach caregivers to use effective commands. Help caregivers establish behavioral contingencies (e.g., prize, token, privilege, or other reward) for toilet sits. Remove alternate reinforcers (e.g., toys and electronics). Teach caregivers to use planned ignoring.

The GI mental health professional will work with the family to create an exposure hierarchy and coach the parents to implement exposure at home. For some children, the toilet sit is not feared but is a non-preferred task, in which case the GI mental health professional should employ behavioral strategies such as contingency management similar to other non-preferred tasks, like chores or homework (see Table 19.1). Youth typically respond well to earning a reward they would not otherwise have access to for compliance with each scheduled toilet sit, such as 15 minutes of electronics time after exiting the bathroom.

Working with caregivers

Caregivers benefit from validation of their frustration, especially for those who have children who soil, and reassurance that constipation is not their fault. They should be informed that constipation is very treatable, which also helps build a collaborative relationship between the GI mental health professional and caregiver as well as bolster parental motivation for the treatment plan. Setting small goals that are quickly attainable (e.g., placing all clean underwear and supplies for cleaning accidents in the bathroom so that the youth becomes accustomed to using the bathroom for stooling, and charting each administration of laxative and toilet sit to provide immediate visual feedback) can increase buy-in to behavioral treatment. Regular praise and encouragement of the caregivers' follow-through also goes a long way in maintaining their motivation for treatment adherence. See Chapter 8 for further recommendations relating to working with caregivers.

Special considerations for adolescents

Constipation with soiling typically resolves before puberty, whether spontaneously or with treatment [10]; thus, treatment referrals for adolescents are less common than for school-aged children. Treating adolescents with soiling can be challenging, in part due to a longer learning history for the cycle of withholding and chronic constipation. Adolescents with treatment refractory constipation with soiling should be referred to a gastroenterologist to rule out dyssynergic defecation, a condition in which the pelvic floor muscles fail to communicate normally with the surrounding muscles and nerves to produce a coordinated bowel movement. If so, the adolescent may benefit most from pelvic floor biofeedback to learn through visual and auditory feedback how to relax and contract the necessary muscles in a coordinated fashion to produce a normal bowel movement [12]. Although biofeedback is not indicated for children, teens are more like adults, in whom evidence for pelvic floor physical therapy (PFPT) and biofeedback for chronic constipation has been demonstrated [13].

Adolescents seeking treatment for constipation and soiling may present with comorbid depressive symptoms and shame or embarrassment. Treatment should address these concerns simultaneously by increasing the adolescent's self-confidence, such as behavioral activation for mood (for more detailed information see McCauley et al. [14]), or self-regulation strategies, such as structure, daily schedules, and routines for attention and executive function concerns.

Special considerations for autism spectrum disorder (ASD)

Children with ASD often exhibit a delay in toilet training and have higher rates of soiling than typically developing peers, likely due to an increased prevalence of constipation in this population [15]. Similar to neurotypical youth, there is emerging evidence for the feasibility and efficacy of combined medical and behavioral treatment strategies, though they may require longer and more intensive management [16, 17]. It is best to refer youth with constipation and ASD to specialist teams focused on this population.

Evidence-based interventions

Although there are no "gold standard" treatment packages for constipation and soiling, based on several reviews (e.g., Freeman et al. and Shepard et al. [7, 18]), two behavioral treatments have demonstrated the most efficacy: enhanced toilet training (ETT) and pelvic floor biofeedback. Though not feasible in all practice settings, there are promising clinical outcomes for interdisciplinary group interventions (e.g., Lamparyk et al. [19]), which deliver the same essential treatment components described above.

Enhanced toilet training (ETT)

ETT is a behavioral treatment protocol for constipation and soiling, that, in conjunction with medical treatment, applies reinforcement and scheduling to promote response to urges to defecate, education, and behavioral training components [20]. In a comparison study of ETT to intensive medical therapy and anal sphincter biofeedback therapy, all treatments produced comparable decreases in the frequency of soiling, though ETT significantly benefited more youth with soiling while using less laxative therapy [21]. Results demonstrating the effectiveness of ETT serve to support protocolized, behavioral intervention as a core treatment component for functional constipation.

A note on treatment for NFI: While stool withholding and constipation do not contribute to NFI, behavioral treatment is highly similar. Axelrod and Fontaini-Axelrod [22] demonstrated good clinical outcomes for ETT with the addition of a cleanup procedure for soiling.

Pelvic floor physical therapy and biofeedback

Chronic constipation and soiling can lead to or exacerbate abnormal dynamics of defecation, such that pelvic floor muscles contract instead of relax when the child tries to defecate [3]. Pelvic floor physical therapy (PFPT) is a well-established, evidence-based intervention used in the management of abdominal and pelvic floor dysfunction in adults [23]. It consists of patient education, behavioral strategies, functional exercise training – including effective muscle contraction and increased muscle and body awareness, coordination, and control – biofeedback, and electrotherapy [24]. In pediatrics, PFPT is an emerging field and was adapted from adult intervention to include pediatric-specific needs and parental support and education [12]. Biofeedback, a component of PFPT, is a promising intervention that has demonstrated some efficacy in pediatric constipation treatment [5]. It aims to improve the ease and efficiency of bowel movements by teaching children to tighten and relax their anorectal muscles and is often implemented in conjunction with various medical and behavioral treatments. Given the limitations of early pediatric studies on long-term benefits, PFPT and biofeedback are not yet considered a standard of care for constipation, but may offer benefits in conjunction with laxative therapy, particularly for adolescents with treatment refractory constipation [25].

Pearls of wisdom

- Parents often delay care-seeking for constipation due to misattribution of soiling to their child's "bad behavior". This reinforces the pain-stool withholding cycle. To decondition youth, painless and stressless bowel movements may be needed for as long as they had undiagnosed constipation.
- Although 70% of youth will do well with medical treatment alone, most will relapse at some point. One should develop appropriate treatment plans for relapses and avoid talking about these with shame (for either the child or family).
- Psychoeducation is critical for the way parents think about the problem *and* their "buy-in" or follow-through with behavior management strategies.
- The child's limited diet may be a "stuck point" for parents. There is more support in the literature for the effectiveness of modification of toilet-related behaviors and biofeedback than diet modification.
- The mental health professional is not expected to be an expert in the medical management of constipation and fecal incontinence. Their unique contribution to the team is their knowledge and application of behavioral principles, such as shaping and positive reinforcement, to manage factors that maintain soiling.

Summary

Functional constipation and soiling are commonly occurring conditions in pediatrics, and many youth will present with co-occurring internalizing or externalizing symptoms. Youth with ASD and developmental delays have higher rates of constipation and soiling compared to neurotypical youth. Treatment with the best outcome data involves a combination of medical and behavioral interventions. Psychoeducation is a critical component of treatment. Behavioral treatment always involves caregivers and focuses on adherence to the medical regimen and the child's behaviors around toileting using familiar psychological strategies, including behavioral shaping, positive reinforcement, and exposures. Adolescents may benefit from individual therapy to promote a sense of self-efficacy and to address shame around difficulties with constipation and soiling. Adolescents may also benefit from an evaluation with a trained physical therapist to assess whether pelvic floor biofeedback would be indicated. Collaboration with medical subspecialists and other allied health professionals is key to delivering evidence-based treatment for constipation and soiling.

Recommended readings

For youth and caregivers:

- Information and treatment overview: www.healthychildren.org/English/health-issues/conditions/abdominal/Pages/constipation.aspx.
- Information on constipation, soiling, and treatment: www.kidshealth.org/en/parents/encopresis.html and www.encopresistreatment.com.

For mental health professionals:

- Colombo, J. M., Wassom, M. C., & Rosen, J. M. (2015). Constipation and encopresis in childhood. *Pediatrics in Review*, *36*(9), 392–402.
- Low Kapalu, C., & Christophersen, E. (2022). Elimination disorders in children and adolescents. *Comprehensive Clinical Psychology* (2nd Ed.), 5, 435–452.
- Shepard, J.A., Poler Jr., J.E., & Grabman, J.H. (2017). Evidence-based psychosocial treatments for pediatric elimination disorders. *Journal of Clinical Child & Adolescent Psychology, 46*, 767–797.

References

1. Hyams JS, Di Lorenzo C, Saps M, Shulman RJ, Staiano A, van Tilburg M. Childhood functional gastrointestinal disorders: Child/adolescent. *Gastroenterology*. 2016;150(6):1456–68. e2.
2. Hyman P. *Childhood defecation disorders: Constipation and soiling*. New Orleans, Louisiana: International Foundation for Functional Gastrointestinal Disorders; 2009.
3. Colombo JM, Wassom MC, Rosen JM. Constipation and encopresis in childhood. *Pediatr Rev*. 2015;36(9):392–402.
4. McKeown C, Hisle-Gorman E, Eide M, Gorman GH, Nylund CM. Association of constipation and fecal incontinence with attention-deficit/hyperactivity disorder. *Pediatrics*. 2013;132(5):e1210–e5.
5. Cox DJ, Morris Jr JB, Borowitz SM, Sutphen JL. Psychological differences between children with and without chronic encopresis. *J Pediatr Psychol*. 2002;27(7):585–91.

6. Mellon MW, Whiteside SP, Friedrich WN. The relevance of fecal soiling as an indicator of child sexual abuse: A preliminary analysis. *J Dev Behav Pediatr*. 2006;27(1):25–32.
7. Shepard JA, Poler Jr JE, Grabman JH. Evidence-based psychosocial treatments for pediatric elimination disorders. *J Clin Child Adolesc Psychol*. 2017;46(6):767–97.
8. Matson J, Dempsey T, Fodstad J. *The profile of toileting issues (POTI)*. Baton Rouge, LA: *Disability Consultants*, LLC; 2010.
9. Kamphaus RW, & Reynolds, CR. *BASC-3 behavioral and emotional screening system*. Bloomington: NCS Pearson Inc; 2015.
10. Field CE, Friman PC. *Encopresis. Practitioner's guide to evidence-based psychotherapy*. Springer; 2006. Pp. 277–83.
11. Whiteside SP, Ollendick TH, Biggs BK. *Exposure therapy for child and adolescent anxiety and OCD*. New York, New York: Oxford University Press; 2020.
12. Zar-Kessler C, Kuo B, Cole E, Benedix A, Belkind-Gerson J. Benefit of pelvic floor physical therapy in pediatric patients with dyssynergic defecation constipation. *Digestive Diseases*. 2019;37(6):478–85.
13. Bharucha AE, Lacy BE. Mechanisms, evaluation, and management of chronic constipation. *Gastroenterology*. 2020;158(5):1232–49. e3.
14. McCauley E, Gudmundsen G, Schloredt K, Martell C, Rhew I, Hubley S, et al. The adolescent behavioral activation program: Adapting behavioral activation as a treatment for depression in adolescence. *J Clin Child Adolesc Psychol*. 2016;45(3):291–304.
15. McElhanon BO, McCracken C, Karpen S, Sharp WG. Gastrointestinal symptoms in autism spectrum disorder: A Meta-analysis. *Pediatrics*. 2014;133(5):872–83.
16. Axelrod MI, Tornehl M, Fontanini-Axelrod A. Co-occurring autism and intellectual disability: A treatment for encopresis using a behavioral intervention plus laxative across settings. *Clin Pract Pediatr Psychol*. 2016;4(1):1.
17. Lomas Mevers J, Call NA, Gerencser KR, Scheithauer M, Miller SJ, Muething C, et al. A pilot randomized clinical trial of a multidisciplinary intervention for encopresis in children with autism spectrum disorder. *J Autism Dev Disord*. 2020;50(3):757–65.
18. Freeman KA, Riley A, Duke DC, Fu R. Systematic review and meta-analysis of behavioral interventions for fecal incontinence with constipation. *J Pediatr Psychol*. 2014;39(8):887–902.
19. Lamparyk K, Mathis M, Piorkowski L, Polasky S, Gross M, Feinberg L. Development and evaluation of an interdisciplinary group intervention for pediatric functional constipation. *Clin Pract Pediatr Psychol*. 2022;11(1):74–83.
20. Cox DJ, Sutphen J, Borowitz S, Kovatchev B, Ling W. Contribution of behavior therapy and biofeedback to laxative therapy in the treatment of pediatric encopresis. *Ann Behav Med*. 1998;20(2):70–6.
21. Borowitz SM, Cox DJ, Sutphen JL, Kovatchev B. Treatment of childhood encopresis: A randomized trial comparing three treatment protocols. *J Pediatr Gastroenterol Nutr*. 2002;34(4):378–84.
22. Axelrod MI, Fontanini-Axelrod A. Treating functional nonretentive fecal incontinence using a comprehensive behavioral treatment across settings. *Clin Pract Pediatr Psychol*. 2022;10(2):180.
23. Rao SS, Valestin J, Brown CK, Zimmerman B, Schulze K. Long-term efficacy of biofeedback therapy for dyssynergic defecation: Randomized controlled trial. *Am J Gastroenterol*. 2010;105(4):890.
24. Ladi-Seyedian S-S, Sharifi-Rad L, Nabavizadeh B, Kajbafzadeh A-M. Traditional biofeedback vs. pelvic floor physical therapy – Is one clearly superior? *Curr Urol Rep*. 2019;20(7):1–9.
25. Tabbers M, DiLorenzo C, Berger M, Faure C, Langendam M, Nurko S, et al. Evaluation and treatment of functional constipation in infants and children: Evidence-based recommendations from ESPGHAN and NASPGHAN. *J Pediatr Gastroenterol Nutr*. 2014;58(2):258–74.

Part 3

Transition and future challenges in pediatric Psychogastroenterology

Chapter 20

Chronic illness adjustment and transition

Sara L. Lampert-Okin, Meghan M. Howe, Angela Yu, Kim Grzesek, and Rachel Neff Greenley

Chapter aims

This chapter reviews the literature pertaining to adjustment to illness, self-management, and transition to adult care for youth living with gastrointestinal (GI) disorders. It also provides recommendations on evidence-based assessment and intervention to enhance functioning in the aforementioned domains.

Learning points

- Describe psychosocial adjustment considerations uniquely relevant to youth living with chronic GI conditions.
- Describe disease self-management and transition challenges for youth living with chronic GI conditions.
- Provide practical, evidence-based recommendations to enhance adjustment to illness, treatment adherence, and transition readiness.

Chronic pediatric GI conditions vary in terms of physiological mechanisms, disease course, and treatment regimen, yet overlap in symptom presentation exists, and all are best conceptualized via a biopsychosocial perspective [1]. Moreover, commonalities exist in disease self-management and transition challenges. This chapter summarizes condition adjustment, self-management, and transition readiness challenges experienced by youth living with chronic GI conditions and provides practical, evidence-based advice for clinical assessment and intervention.

Psychosocial functioning in chronic GI conditions

Emotional and behavioral functioning

Youth living with chronic GI conditions are at risk for internalizing symptoms (i.e., anxiety and depressive symptoms), and in some cases display higher levels of internalizing disorders compared to their peers without chronic health conditions [2–5]. Risk factors, studied primarily in inflammatory bowel disease (IBD), include lower socioeconomic status (SES), older age at diagnosis, greater disease severity, corticosteroid treatment, and parental distress [6, 7]. Depressive symptoms correlate with higher levels of pain, functional impairment, and anxiety [8], highlighting the importance of clinical assessment and treatment of internalizing symptoms. See Chapter 2 for additional coverage of psychological factors and their association with the brain–gut axis.

DOI: 10.4324/9781003308683-23

Clinically significant behavioral issues occur no more frequently in youth living with chronic GI conditions than in healthy youth [3]. No consistent data support a link between celiac disease and attention deficit hyperactivity disorder (ADHD) [9, 10], and there is no evidence that a gluten-free diet resolves ADHD symptoms [9].

Social and school functioning

Youth living with chronic GI conditions report lower levels of social competence, poorer social functioning, and greater levels of isolation and peer victimization compared with healthy youth [3, 5, 11–13]. Males may experience more social difficulties than female youth [14, 15]. Among those with celiac disease, dietary restrictions are a barrier to social participation [16]. Moreover, the embarrassing or impairing nature of GI symptoms may make youth reluctant to disclose symptoms to peers and may interfere with participation in social activities, dating, and romantic relationships [17, 18]. GI symptoms and their treatment may also adversely impact school attendance [19] and participation in extracurricular activities [15, 19]. School absences, in turn, can interfere with social opportunities and social skill development. The impact of GI symptoms on social functioning is particularly detrimental for adolescents who spend more time with peers than younger youth [14, 20] and because peer acceptance is paramount during adolescence [21].

Health-related quality of life (HRQoL)

HRQoL reflects one's subjective sense of the impact of health status on their physical and psychosocial well-being [22]. HRQoL may be more influenced by disease symptoms than other measures of psychosocial functioning, particularly among adolescents [23]. Youth with GI conditions report lower HRQoL than healthy youth, but their HRQoL is comparable to other chronic illness groups [1, 7, 24, 25]. Risk factors for impaired HRQoL include more disease symptoms [7], poorer psychological functioning, [26], and family dysfunction [7]. Impaired HRQoL, in turn, is linked with a variety of adverse psychosocial and disease outcomes [16, 25].

Other adjustment considerations

Youth living with GI conditions must manage several additional challenges to psychosocial functioning uniquely relevant to those with chronic health conditions including illness uncertainty (i.e., uncertainty related to disease symptoms and course), illness intrusiveness (i.e., extent to which one's health condition disrupts various daily life activities), and perceived stigma (i.e., the experience of or concern about being evaluated negatively or treated differently due to one's health condition). Greater perceived stigma and illness uncertainty are associated with more depressive symptoms [18, 27, 28], calling attention to the importance of these cognitions as targets for clinical intervention.

Additionally, youth may experience illness-specific anxiety, or worries specific to their symptoms, medical treatment, and/or the impact of their condition on important life domains. Such worries can be present in the absence of disease symptoms and are disproportionate to the broader disease context [29]. Illness-specific anxiety has been mostly studied in IBD [29], is distinct from more general anxiety symptoms, and is more strongly associated with HRQoL than the general measures of anxiety and depression [30]. Moreover, higher illness-specific anxiety is associated with adverse outcomes including greater healthcare utilization and impaired social functioning [29].

Finally, among certain GI conditions, such as IBD, body image may be affected [31]. Among those with IBD, females, older adolescents, and those older at diagnosis had higher body image dissatisfaction, as did those with active disease and those currently prescribed steroids. Body image dissatisfaction, in turn, is significantly associated with greater depressive and anxiety symptoms [31].

Recommendations to promote adjustment to illness

Chapter 6 provides a thorough overview of the assessment of psychosocial functioning and case conceptualization in youth living with a GI condition. Evidence suggests that HRQoL measures are more sensitive to the impact of disease symptoms on functioning than more general measures of psychological symptoms [23]. Disease-specific and general HRQoL measures are widely available, and several GI-specific HRQoL measures assess body image (e.g., IMPACT scales for IBD). Similarly, validated measures of illness-specific anxiety [30] and illness uncertainty [18, 27] have been used in research contexts and are applicable clinically. Since psychosocial functioning is dynamic, routine assessment is important and assessment may be particularly beneficial during times of major transition (e.g., starting at a new school) and when disease symptoms or regimens change.

When clinically significant symptoms exist, research points to several useful intervention modalities. Cognitive behavioral therapy (CBT) is helpful for depression, anxiety, and HRQoL, among other outcomes in pediatric IBD [32–34]. Chapter 16 summarizes the efficacy of CBT for pain-based GI disorders. Mindfulness-based interventions [35, 36], problem-solving skills training [37], multicomponent interventions [38], and peer support interventions [16, 39–42] also show promise in enhancing select domains of psychosocial functioning. See Table 20.1 for additional details on these interventions.

GI mental health professionals can also proactively facilitate adjustments. At diagnosis, families may benefit from education about the disease and regimen and help in developing adaptive coping skills to deal with illness uncertainty, illness-specific anxiety, and disease management demands. Relatedly, encouraging families to become involved with disease-specific foundations or local support groups may enhance social support, which benefits psychosocial adjustment. Fostering open communication about frustrations and challenges is important, and GI mental health professionals can help families develop adaptive problem-solving skills, which may also contribute to better disease management. Helping families develop developmentally appropriate boundaries related to adolescent symptom disclosure, along with identifying age-appropriate condition-management responsibilities, is important. For younger children or recently diagnosed youth, explicit discussion about what information they will share with teachers and peers about their diagnosis and how they will talk about their condition may be beneficial. Finally, GI mental health professionals can help families develop skills to effectively communicate and advocate with their medical team. Helping families develop a system for organizing their questions and role-playing challenging interactions with providers may improve communication skills and disease outcomes.

Self-management of chronic GI conditions

Self-management is challenging for youth and families, as evidenced by suboptimal adherence and adverse disease outcomes associated with nonadherence [43]. Self-management of most chronic GI conditions includes some or all of the following: (1) taking medications [44], (2)

Table 20.1 Evidence-based interventions to enhance psychosocial functioning, adherence, and transition readiness

Domain and reference	*Intervention type*	*Intervention components*	*Pediatric group of focus*	*Major findings*
Psychosocial functioning [33]	CBT with IBD- specific anxiety additions	13 individual weekly in-person sessions + 2 post-treatment booster sessions	IBD	Significant reduction in IBD-specific anxiety compared to control.
Psychosocial functioning [38]	Multicomponent intervention	6 in-person group sessions	IBD	Intervention group (but not control group) reported improvement in optimism and self-perception scores.
Psychosocial functioning [16]	Peer support/camp	In-person camp attendance (length varied)	Celiac disease	Camp attendance associated with: (1) higher HRQoL and mediated by more friends with celiac disease, (2) higher illness acceptance, and (3) lower anxiety.
Psychosocial functioning [41]	Peer support/camp	Weeklong in-person camp	Celiac disease	Camp attendees noted no longer feeling different from peers.
Psychosocial functioning [32]	CBT and social learning	3 weekly in-person individual sessions	IBD	Fewer school absences 6 months post-treatment.
Psychosocial functioning [42]	Peer support	6 biweekly peer group sessions	Celiac disease	Higher HRQoL scores post-treatment in intervention group compared to control group.
Psychosocial functioning [40]	Peer support/camp	Weeklong in-person camp	IBD	Improvement in HRQoL.
Psychosocial functioning [39]	Peer support/camp	Weeklong in-person camp followed by 2 months of active participation in Facebook group	IBD	Improvement in HRQoL.
Psychosocial Functioning [36]	Virtual reality application	6-minute one-time mindfulness practice via an application	IBD	Reduction in anxiety after using application.
Psychosocial functioning [35]	Mindfulness	8 in-person group-based weekly sessions	IBD	Improvements in depression and anxiety scores for intervention group.

Psychosocial functioning and medication adherence [37]	Problem-solving skills training	4 phone-based, family training sessions	IBD	Improvement in HRQoL and oral medication adherence for those with imperfect baseline adherence.
Dietary adherence [83]	Behavioral intervention	6 in-person group sessions over 8 weeks for youth and parents	IBD	Greater increases in calcium intake for intervention group compared to control.
Medication adherence [84]	Multicomponent	4 individual in-person weekly sessions	IBD	Increase in medication adherence.
Transition readiness [80]	Psychoeducation	Individual 30-minute in-person meeting with educator Provided with IBD pocket guide	IBD	Improved disease knowledge in treatment group compared to control group.
Transition readiness [82]	Technology-based social cognitive intervention	8 months of receiving content on disease management 3–5 text messages per week with reminders and queries about content	IBD	Improvements in health-related self-efficacy, disease management, and transition readiness compared to controls.
Transition readiness [81]	Multicomponent	One in-person group session + 4 individualized telehealth sessions with a transition coach over 4–5 months	IBD	Improvements in transition readiness.

attending medical appointments [44], (3) implementing dietary or lifestyle modifications (e.g., improving sleep hygiene, eating at regular intervals, avoiding dietary allergens), (4) developing effective problem-solving and decision-making skills related to managing symptoms, and (5) learning to interface effectively with the healthcare system [45, 46].

Nonadherence is common among pediatric GI samples [47–49]. Rates vary depending on the regimen and sample surveyed, but perfect adherence is rare. Adherence to dietary regimens and multicomponent regimens is more challenging than adherence to simple (e.g., once daily) regimens. For example, adherence to a gluten-free diet is the primary self-management task in celiac disease, and nonadherence is as high as 56% [50]. In contrast, adherence to scheduled infusion appointments for patients with IBD is above 90% [51]. Importantly, nearly every youth living with a chronic GI condition must follow a multicomponent regimen or follow dietary restrictions. Thus, nonadherence is expected, and clinical efforts to evaluate and improve adherence are important.

Adolescents display greater nonadherence than children [52] due, in part, to developmental shifts in the allocation of condition-management responsibilities (i.e., caregivers decreasing their involvement). Scholars have differentiated between accidental nonadherence (e.g., forgetting to take medication) and volitional nonadherence (e.g., choosing to discontinue medication because of undesirable side effects) [53], and each is linked with different barriers and requires different intervention approaches [47]. Adherence barriers are common and vary by developmental level [47]. Whereas adolescents commonly report disease frustration [48] and concern about disclosure/taking medication around peers [17], ingestion difficulties, and medication refusal are more common in younger youth [54]. Given greater nonadherence among adolescents, interventions to support self-management during this developmental period are particularly important [47].

Modi and colleagues [55] published a comprehensive model of influences on pediatric self-management that highlights the complex set of individual, family, community, and health system factors that influence the process of disease self-management and self-management outcomes. In youth living with GI conditions, individual factors (e.g., fewer active disease symptoms, adolescent age, lower self-efficacy), family factors (e.g., lack of caregiver knowledge and/or involvement in the regimen), community factors (e.g., lack of peer support), and healthcare system factors (e.g., lack of multidisciplinary care, suboptimal relationship with provider) have all been associated with nonadherence [43–45, 52, 56].

Recommendations to promote adherence

Evidence-based assessments of medication adherence include self-report, pill counts, and objective monitoring via electronic monitors [57]; however, the latter is less feasible in clinical than in research contexts. Self-report accuracy is enhanced when nonadherence is normalized and when individuals report on the recent past. Since visual analog ratings correlate well with more elaborate self-report measures [58], these may have particular clinical utility. Dietary recalls are commonly used to assess dietary adherence [57]. Comprehensive assessment of adherence barriers is important and several existing measures tap into barriers experienced by youth living with GI conditions (e.g., Adolescent Medication Barriers Scale [59]). GI mental health professionals should assess adherence and adherence barriers in each appointment, given that variability in adherence exists over time. Interviewing adolescents individually is suggested to increase the truthfulness of reporting, and using a combination of brief self-report instruments (e.g., visual analog ratings and adherence barriers checklists) may be of value in identifying actionable next steps. See Handouts 20.1 for practical recommendations for adherence assessment, and Handout 20.2 for a summary of common barriers to adherence for youth living with chronic GI conditions.

As summarized in Table 20.1, interventions focused on teaching family problem-solving skills and/or multicomponent interventions that include a combination of psychoeducation, skills training, and CBT may improve medication adherence [37]. Family-based interventions may be especially useful when nonadherence is related to diffuse roles in condition management or with younger youth. See Chapter 8 for a discussion of working with parents to promote adherence. Among adults, dose simplification, visual reminder systems, and pill organizers improve accidental nonadherence, and these may also be useful among pediatric samples [47, 60]. For young children, incentivizing adherence via rewards may be useful, particularly when there is an adverse aspect to the regimen (e.g., pain related to an injection). Regarding dietary adherence promotion, working with families to help limit food that is inconsistent with dietary restrictions in the home, making plans for situations in which it may be difficult to adhere to the restrictions (e.g., bringing a snack that meets dietary guidelines to a party), and helping adolescents gain skills and comfort in inquiring about food ingredients are useful adherence promotion strategies. Incentivizing adherence to dietary or lifestyle modifications and using diaries to track patterns of nonadherence may also be beneficial. Handout 20.3 provides practical recommendations to promote adherence.

Transition to adult care in the context of chronic GI conditions

Transition to adult care reflects the planned movement of adolescents and young adults (AYA) from their pediatric healthcare team to a provider/team with expertise in treating adult patients [61]. The North American Society for Pediatric Gastroenterology, Hepatology, & Nutrition (NASPGHAN) recommends that pediatric healthcare teams systematically evaluate and plan for transition to adult care, beginning in early adolescence. Specific recommendations for care during this transition period include: (1) meeting with the patient without caregivers (for at least a portion of each visit) to build independence and self-reliance, (2) repeated, open discussions of the benefits of transition, (3) collaborative selection of an adult gastroenterologist with expertise in AYA needs, and (4) sharing of medical records in advance of the transfer to instill confidence that the pediatric and adult providers are working together [62]. Additionally, joint visits between pediatric and adult providers and systematic assessment of transition readiness knowledge and skills during medical appointments can facilitate transition readiness.

Many institutions have established transition clinics that do some/all of the above in an effort to facilitate an effective transition to adult care [63]. Patients with IBD who participate in formal transition clinics have fewer disease flares, fewer emergency department visits, and less steroid use post-transfer to adult care compared to those not participating in transition programs [64]. Similarly, Eros [65] reports that structured transition protocols may also enhance adherence, disease knowledge, willingness to attend clinical visits, self-efficacy, and patient satisfaction for those with IBD.

Development of transition readiness skills is a critical task for AYA, and GI mental health professionals are well-equipped to evaluate and promote transition readiness. This is a critical task given that significant variability in transition readiness skills exists and because many youth lack the necessary skills to self-manage their condition until after age 18 [44, 66–70]. Condition-specific benchmarks for successful transition exist for IBD [71] and celiac disease [67]. Models of transition readiness [72] are similar to models of self-management in highlighting the importance of factors across a variety of domains in influencing transition readiness. Factors associated with transition readiness are well studied in pediatric IBD and include better self-management skills, self-efficacy, older age at transfer to adult care, female sex, and white race [66, 73, 74]. Factors associated with successful transition to adult care in pediatric celiac disease patients include older age at diagnosis and greater symptom scores [75].

Recommendations to promote transition readiness

GI mental health professionals should regularly assess transition readiness skills since the transition period is a vulnerable time in AYA's disease management, during which increases in nonadherence have been documented [76]. Several existing measures are applicable to pediatric GI groups including the TRAQ [77] and the UNC TRxANSITION Index [78]. Parfeniuk [79] reviews other transition readiness measures. Assessment of transition readiness should begin during late childhood and continue throughout adolescence [67]. When skills or knowledge deficiencies are identified, GI mental health professionals should address these issues prior to transfer. GI mental health professionals may be uniquely suited to helping youth and their families address and navigate emotional barriers to transition readiness. AYA living with chronic GI conditions frequently express fear and hesitation to leave pediatric providers who have cared for them, oftentimes for many years. These emotions can be validated and normalized as an anticipated part of growing up, much like the mixed emotions that may come with graduating high school and starting college or a career.

GI mental health professionals should help families develop written goals related to adolescent skill and knowledge acquisition, so that progress can be tracked and goals updated over time. Parents will likely benefit from guidance on how best to scaffold support so that youth can take on increasing disease-related responsibility as parents reduce responsibility while remaining as engaged supervisors. Encouraging adolescents to participate in peer mentoring programs may also be a useful method of skill-building and knowledge acquisition. See Handout 20.4 for additional practical recommendations for promoting a successful transition.

Several interventions have attempted to enhance transition readiness skills via psychoeducation, but results are mixed [80]. Gray [81] implemented a 4–5-month program for AYA with IBD (including psychoeducation, skill-building, and behavioral contracting) and found improved self-management skills, transition readiness, and disease knowledge. Similarly, Huang [82] evaluated an 8-month technology-based intervention (MD2Me) based on social cognitive theory in a group of AYA with various conditions including IBD and found improvements in disease self-efficacy and self-management. See Table 20.1 for details about these interventions.

Pearls of wisdom

- GI mental health professionals should assess adjustment to illness with particular emphasis on internalizing symptoms, social functioning, and HRQoL given bidirectional associations between disease symptoms and psychosocial adjustment, and because optimal psychosocial functioning facilitates adherence and transition readiness.
- GI mental health professionals should normalize nonadherence and routinely assess adherence barriers to inform the choice of intervention strategy.
- GI mental health professionals should assess transition readiness skills and knowledge, develop plans to address areas of deficit, and talk openly about transition timelines and expectations. Structured transition programs that involve meeting the adult provider are recommended.

Summary

Youth with chronic GI conditions are at risk for internalizing symptoms, impairments in social functioning, and suboptimal HRQoL, though most function well. Certain unique psychosocial challenges also exist including managing illness uncertainty. GI mental health professionals can promote psychosocial adjustment and self-management via ongoing assessment of psychosocial, self-management, and transition readiness. Those with symptom elevations may benefit from CBT, problem-solving, or multicomponent interventions. However, even in the absence of clinically significant distress, youth benefit from interventions to enhance self-efficacy, to improve condition knowledge and skills, and to build social support. GI mental health professionals can also work with healthcare teams to implement structured transition protocols to facilitate a successful transition to adult care. Since the preponderance of work in this area has focused on IBD, research with additional GI patient groups is needed.

Recommended readings

For youth and caregivers:

- Resource for creating a "health passport" document to store disease and treatment information: www.wapps.sickkids.ca/myhealthpassport/.
- Compilation of resources for families related to the development of self-care and transition readiness skills: www.chop.edu/centers-programs/transition-adulthood-services/health-resources.

For mental health professionals:

- Provider training module on transition to adult care: www.adolescenthealth.org/Training-and-CME/Adolescent-Medicine-Resident-Curriculum/Adolescent-Medicine-Resident-Curriculum-(9).aspx#Chronic.
- Provider resources on transition readiness assessment and transition planning: www.chop.edu/centers-programs/transition-adulthood-services/health-resources.

References

1. Reed-Knight B, Mackner LM, Crandall WV. Psychological aspects of inflammatory bowel disease in children and adolescents. *Pediatr Inflamm Bowel Dis*. 2017:615–23.
2. Coburn S, Rose M, Sady M, Parker M, Suslovic W, Weisbrod V, et al. Mental health disorders and psychosocial distress in pediatric celiac disease. *J Pediatr Gastroenterol Nutr*. 2020;70(5):608–14.
3. Greenley RN, Hommel KA, Nebel J, Raboin T, Li SH, Simpson P, et al. A meta-analytic review of the psychosocial adjustment of youth with inflammatory bowel disease. *J Pediatr Psychol*. 2010;35(8):857–69.
4. Loftus EV, Guérin A, Yu AP, Wu EQ, Yang M, Chao J, et al. Increased risks of developing anxiety and depression in young patients with Crohn's disease. *Am J Gastroenterol*. 2011;106(9):1670–7.
5. MacKner LM, Greenley RN, Szigethy E, Herzer M, Deer K, Hommel KA. Psychosocial issues in pediatric inflammatory bowel disease: Report of the north american society for pediatric gastroenterology, hepatology, and nutrition. *J Pediatr Gastroenterol Nutr*. 2013;56:449–58.
6. Brooks AJ, Rowse G, Ryder A, Peach EJ, Corfe BM, Lobo AJ. Systematic review: Psychological morbidity in young people with inflammatory bowel disease – Risk factors and impacts. *Aliment Pharmacol Ther*. 2016;44:3–15.
7. Touma N, Varay C, Baeza-Velasco C. Determinants of quality of life and psychosocial adjustment to pediatric inflammatory bowel disease: A systematic review focused on Crohn's disease. *J Psychosom Res*. 2021;142.
8. Murphy LK, De La Vega R, Kohut SA, Kawamura JS, Levy RL, Palermo TM. Systematic review: Psychosocial correlates of pain in pediatric inflammatory bowel disease. *Inflamm Bowel Dis*. 2021;27:697–710.

9. Ertürk E, Wouters S, Imeraj L, Lampo A. Association of ADHD and celiac disease: What is the evidence? A systematic review of the literature. *J Atten Disord.* 2020;24(10):1371–6.
10. Gaur S. The association between ADHD and celiac disease in children. *Children.* 2022;9(6):781.
11. Donovan E, Martin SR, Lung K, Evans S, Seidman LC, Cousineau TM, et al. Pediatric irritable bowel syndrome: Perspectives on pain and adolescent social functioning. *Pain Medicine.* 2019;20(2):213–22.
12. Martinez W, Carter JS, Legato LJ. Social competence in children with chronic illness: A meta-analytic review. *J Pediatr Psychol.* 2011;36(8):878–90.
13. Varni JW, Bendo CB, Nurko S, Shulman RJ, Self MM, Franciosi JP, et al. Health-related quality of life in pediatric patients with functional and organic gastrointestinal diseases. *J Pediatr.* 2015;166(1):85–90.e2.
14. MacKner LM, Greenley RN, Szigethy E, Herzer M, Deer K, Hommel KA. Psychosocial issues in pediatric inflammatory bowel disease: Report of the north american society for pediatric gastroenterology, hepatology, and nutrition. *J Pediatr Gastroenterol Nutr.* 2013;56(4):449–58.
15. Shull MH, Ediger TR, Hill ID, Schroedl RL. Health-related quality of life in newly diagnosed pediatric patients with celiac disease. *J Pediatr Gastroenterol Nutr.* 2019;69(6):690–5.
16. Shani M, Kraft L, Müller M, Boehnke K. The potential benefits of camps for children and adolescents with celiac disease on social support, illness acceptance, and health-related quality of life. *J Health Psychol.* 2022;27(7):1635–45.
17. Barned C, Stinzi A, Mack D, O'Doherty KC. To tell or not to tell: A qualitative interview study on disclosure decisions among children with inflammatory bowel disease. *Soc Sci Med.* 2016;162:115–23.
18. Gamwell KL, Baudino MN, Bakula DM, Sharkey CM, Roberts CM, Grunow JE, et al. Perceived illness stigma, thwarted belongingness, and depressive symptoms in youth with inflammatory bowel disease (IBD). *Inflamm Bowel Dis.* 2018;24(5):960–5.
19. Assa A, Ish-Tov A, Rinawi F, Shamir R. School attendance in children with functional abdominal pain and inflammatory bowel diseases. *J Pediatr Gastroenterol Nutr.* 2015;61(5):553–7.
20. Larson R, Richards MH. Daily companionship in late childhood and early adolescence: Changing developmental contexts. *Child Dev.* 1991;62(2):284.
21. Berndt TJ. Friendship quality and social development. *Curr Dir Psychol Sci.* 2002;11(1):7–10.
22. Eiser C, Morse R. The measurement of quality of life in children: past and future perspectives. *J Dev Behav Pediatr.* 2001;22(4):248–56.
23. Loonen HJ, Grootenhuis MA, Last BF, Koopman HM, Derkx HHF. Quality of life in paediatric inflammatory bowel disease measured by a generic and a disease-specific questionnaire. *Acta Paediatr.* 2007;91(3):348–54.
24. Herzer M, Denson LA, Baldassano RN, Hommel KA. Patient and parent psychosocial factors associated with health-related quality of life in pediatric inflammatory bowel disease. *J Pediatr Gastroenterol Nutr.* 2011;52(3):295–9.
25. Varni JW, Lane MM, Burwinkle TM, Fontaine EN, Schwimmer JB, Pardee PE, et al. Health-related quality of life in pediatric patients with irritable bowel syndrome: A comparative analysis. 2006.
26. De Carlo C, Bramuzzo M, Canaletti C, Udina C, Cozzi G, Pavanello PM, et al. The role of distress and pain catastrophizing on the health-related quality of life of children with inflammatory bowel disease. *J Pediatr Gastroenterol Nutr.* 2019;69(4):E99–E104.
27. Baudino MN, Gamwell KL, Roberts CM, Grunow JE, Jacobs NJ, Gillaspy SR, et al. Disease severity and depressive symptoms in adolescents with inflammatory bowel disease: The mediating role of parent and youth illness uncertainty. *J Pediatr Psychol.* 2019;44(4):490–8.
28. Roberts CM, Gamwell KL, Baudino MN, Perez MN, Delozier AM, Sharkey CM, et al. Youth and parent illness appraisals and adjustment in pediatric inflammatory bowel disease. *J Dev Phys Disabil.* 2019;31(6):777–90.
29. Reigada LC, Bruzzese JM, Benkov KJ, Levy J, Waxman AR, Petkova E, et al. Illness-specific anxiety: Implications for functioning and utilization of medical services in adolescents with inflammatory bowel disease. *J Spec Pediatr Nurs.* 2011;16(3):207–15.

30. Reigada LC, Moore MT, Martin CF, Kappelman MD. Psychometric evaluation of the IBD-specific anxiety scale: A novel measure of disease-related anxiety for adolescents with IBD. *J Pediatr Psychol.* 2018;43(4):413–22.
31. Claytor JD, Kochar B, Kappelman MD, Long MD. Body image dissatisfaction among pediatric patients with inflammatory bowel disease. *J Pediatr.* 2020;223:68–72. e1.
32. Levy RL, Van Tilburg MAL, Langer SL, Romano JM, Walker LS, Mancl LA, et al. Effects of a cognitive behavioral therapy intervention trial to improve disease outcomes in children with inflammatory bowel disease. *Inflamm Bowel Dis.* 2016;22(9):2134–48.
33. Reigada LC, Polokowski AR, Walder DJ, Szigethy EM, Benkov KJ, Bruzzese JM, et al. Treatment for comorbid pediatric gastrointestinal and anxiety disorders: A pilot study of a flexible health sensitive cognitive-behavioral therapy program. *Clin Pract Pediatr Psychol.* 2015;3(4):314–26.
34. Szigethy E, Kenney E, Carpenter J, Hardy DM, Fairclough D, Bousvaros A, et al. Cognitive-behavioral therapy for adolescents with inflammatory bowel disease and subsyndromal depression. *J Am Acad Child Adolesc Psychiatry.* 2007;46(10):1290–8.
35. Ahola Kohut S, Stinson J, Jelen A, Ruskin D. Feasibility and acceptability of a mindfulness-based group intervention for adolescents with inflammatory bowel disease. *J Clin Psychol Med Settings.* 2020;27(1):68–78.
36. Wren AA, Neiman N, Caruso TJ, Rodriguez S, Taylor K, Madill M, et al. Mindfulness-based virtual reality intervention for children and young adults with inflammatory bowel disease: A pilot feasibility and acceptability study. *Children.* 2021;8(5):368.
37. Greenley RN, Gumidyala AP, Nguyen E, Plevinsky JM, Poulopoulos N, Thomason MM, et al. Can you teach a teen new tricks? Problem solving skills training improves oral medication adherence in pediatric patients with inflammatory bowel disease participating in a randomized trial. *Inflamm Bowel Dis.* 2015;21(11):2649–57.
38. Grootenhuis MA, Maurice-Stam H, Derkx BH, Last BF. Evaluation of a psychoeducational intervention for adolescents with inflammatory bowel disease. *Eur J Gastroenterol Hepatol.* 2009;21(4):340–5.
39. Plevinsky JM, Greenley RN. Exploring health-related quality of life and social functioning in adolescents with inflammatory bowel diseases after attending camp oasis and participating in a facebook group. *Inflamm Bowel Dis.* 2014;20(9):1611–7.
40. Shepanski MA, Hurd LB, Culton K, Markowitz JE, Mamula P, Baldassano RN. Health-related quality of life improves in children and adolescents with inflammatory bowel disease after attending a camp sponsored by the Crohn's and colitis foundation of America. 2005.
41. Simon Bongiovanni TR, Clark AL, Garnett EA, Wojcicki JM, Heyman MB. Impact of gluten-free camp on quality of life of children and adolescents with celiac disease. *Pediatrics.* 2010;125(3):e525–9.
42. Taşdelen Baş M, Çavuşoğlu H, Bükülmez A. Peer-interaction group support in adolescents with celiac disease: A randomized controlled study in Turkey. *Child and Youth Care Forum.* 2021.
43. Fishman LN, Houtman D, Van Groningen J, Arnold J, Ziniel S. Medication knowledge: An initial step in self-management for youth with inflammatory bowel disease. *J Pediatr Gastroenterol Nutr.* 2011;53(6):641–5.
44. Fishman LN, Barendse RM, Hait E, Burdick C, Arnold J. Self-management of older adolescents with inflammatory bowel disease: A pilot study of behavior and knowledge as prelude to transition. *Clin Pediatr.* 2010;49(12):1129–33.
45. Meyer S, Rosenblum S. Development and validation of the celiac disease-children's activities report (CD-chart) for promoting self-management among children and adolescents. *Nutrients.* 2017;9(10):1130.
46. Plevinsky JM, Greenley RN, Fishman LN. Self-management in patients with inflammatory bowel disease: Strategies, outcomes, and integration into clinical care. *Clin Exp Gastroenterol.* 2016;9:259–67.
47. Greenley RN, Kunz JH, Walter J, Hommel KA. Practical strategies for enhancing adherence to treatment regimen in inflammatory bowel disease. *Inflamm Bowel Dis.* 2013;19:1534–45.

48. Greenley RN, Reed-Knight B, Wojtowicz AA, Plevinsky JM, Lewis JD, Kahn SA. A bitter pill to swallow: Medication adherence barriers in adolescents and young adults with inflammatory bowel diseases. *Children's Health Care*. 2018;47(4):416–31.
49. Schurman JV, Friesen CA. Integrative treatment approaches: Family satisfaction with a multidisciplinary paediatric abdominal pain clinic. *Int J Integr Care*. 2010;10:1–9.
50. Meyer S, Rosenblum S. Examining core self-management skills among adolescents with celiac disease. *J Health Psychol*. 2021;26(13):2592–602.
51. Vitale DS, Greenley RN, Lerner DG, Mavis AM, Werlin SL. Adherence to infliximab treatment in a pediatric inflammatory bowel disease cohort. *J Pediatr Gastroenterol Nutr*. 2015;61(4):408–10.
52. LeLeiko NS, Lobato D, Hagin S, McQuaid E, Seifer R, Kopel SJ, et al. Rates and predictors of oral medication adherence in pediatric patients with IBD. *Inflamm Bowel Dis*. 2013;19(4):832–9.
53. Schurman JV, Cushing CC, Carpenter E, Christenson K. Volitional and accidental nonadherence to pediatric inflammatory bowel disease treatment plans: Initial investigation of associations with quality of life and disease activity. *J Pediatr Psychol*. 2010;36(1):116–25.
54. Modi AC, Quittner AL. Barriers to treatment adherence for children with cystic fibrosis and asthma: What gets in the way? *J Pediatr Psychol*. 2006;31(8):846–58.
55. Modi AC, Pai AL, Hommel KA, Hood KK, Cortina S, Hilliard ME, et al. Pediatric self-management: A framework for research, practice, and policy. *Pediatrics*. 2012;129.
56. Holbein CE, Carmody JK, Hommel KA. Topical review: Adherence interventions for youth on gluten-free diets. *J Pediatr Psychol*. 2018;43:392–401.
57. Hommel KA, Mackner LM, Denson LA, Crandall WV. Treatment regimen adherence in pediatric gastroenterology. *J Pediatr Gastroenterol Nutr*. 2008;47:526–43.
58. Severs M, Zuithoff PNPA, Mangen MJJ, Van Der Valk ME, Siersema PD, Fidder HH, et al. Assessing self-reported medication adherence in inflammatory bowel disease: A comparison of tools. *Inflamm Bowel Dis*. 2016;22(9):2158–64.
59. Simons LE, Blount RL. Identifying barriers to medication adherence in adolescent transplant recipients. *J Pediatr Psychol*. 2007;32(7):831–44.
60. Newton E, Schosheim A, Patel S, Chitkara DK, van Tilburg MA. The role of psychological factors in pediatric functional abdominal pain disorders. *Neurogastroenterol Motil*. 2019;31(6):e13538.
61. Blum RWM, Garell D, Hodgman CH, Jorissen TW, Okinow NA, Orr DP, et al. Transition from child-centered to adult health-care systems for adolescents with chronic conditions. *J Adolesc Health*. 1993;14(7):570–6.
62. Baldassano R, Ferry G, Griffiths A, Mack D, Markowitz J, Winter H. Medical position statement. 2002. Report No.: 1982;96:6734.
63. Maddux MH, Drovetta M, Hasenkamp R, Carpenter E, McCullough J, Goyal A, et al. Using a mixed-method approach to develop a transition program for young adults with inflammatory bowel disease. *J Pediatr Gastroenterol Nutr*. 2020;70(2):195–9.
64. McCartney S, Lindsay JO, Russell RK, Gaya DR, Shaw I, Murray CD, et al. Benefits of structured pediatric to adult transition in inflammatory bowel disease: The TRANSIT observational study. *J Pediatr Gastroenterol Nutr*. 2022;74(2):208.
65. Eros A, Soós A, Hegyi P, Szakács Z, Eross B, Párniczky A, et al. Spotlight on transition in patients with inflammatory bowel disease: A systematic review. *Inflamm Bowel Dis*. 2020;26:331–46.
66. Cole R, Ashok D, Razack A, Azaz A, Sebastian S. Evaluation of outcomes in adolescent inflammatory bowel disease patients following transfer from pediatric to adult health care services: Case for transition. *J Adolesc Health*. 2015;57:212–7.
67. Fishman LN, Kearney J, Degroote M, Liu E, Arnold J, Weir DC. Creation of experience-based celiac benchmarks: the first step in pretransition self-management assessment. *J Pediatr Gastroenterol Nutr*. 2018;67(1):e6–e10.
68. Philpott JR, Kurowski JA. Challenges in transitional care in inflammatory bowel disease: A review of the current literature in transition readiness and outcomes. *Inflamm Bowel Dis*. 2019;25:45–55.

69. Schmulson MJ, Saps M. Irritable bowel syndrome: From young to older age. *NeuroGastroLATAM Rev.* 2019;2(3):133–148.
70. Stollon N, Zhong Y, Ferris M, Bhansali S, Pitts B, Rak E, et al. Chronological age when healthcare transition skills are mastered in adolescents/young adults with inflammatory bowel disease. *World J Gastroenterol.* 2017;23:3349–55.
71. North American Society for Pediatric Gastroenterology Hepatology and Nutrition (NASfPGHa). Transitioning a patient with IBD from pediatric to adult care [Available from: www.naspghan.org /files/documents/pdfs/medical-resources/ibd/Checklist_PatientandHealthcareProdiver_Transitionf romPedtoAdult.pdf.
72. Schwartz L, Tuchman L, Hobbie W, Ginsberg J. A social-ecological model of readiness for transition to adult-oriented care for adolescents and young adults with chronic health conditions. *Child Care Health Dev.* 2011;37(6):883–95.
73. Gumidyala AP, Greenley RN, Plevinsky JM, Poulopoulos N, Cabrera J, Lerner D, et al. Moving on: Transition readiness in adolescents and young adults with IBD. *Inflamm Bowel Dis.* 2018;24(3):482–9.
74. Johnson LE, Lee MJ, Turner-Moore T, Grinsted Tate LR, Brooks AJ, Tattersall RS, et al. Systematic review of factors affecting transition readiness skills in patients with inflammatory bowel disease. *J Crohns Colitis.* 2021;15(6):1049–59.
75. Reilly NR, Hammer ML, Ludvigsson JF, Green PH. Frequency and predictors of successful transition of care for young adults with childhood celiac disease. *J Pediatr Gastroenterol Nutr.* 2020;70(2):190–4.
76. Bollegala N, Brill H, Marshall JK. Resource utilization during pediatric to adult transfer of care in IBD. *J Crohns Colitis.* 2013;7(2):e55–60.
77. Wood DL, Sawicki GS, David M, Smotherman C, Lukens-Bull K, Livingood WC, et al. The Transition Readiness Assessment Questionnaire (TRAQ): Its factor structure, reliability, and validity. 2014.
78. Ferris ME, Harward DH, Bickford K, Layton JB, Ferris MT, Hogan SL, et al. A clinical tool to measure the components of health-care transition from pediatric care to adult care: The UNC TRxANSITION scale. *Renal Failure.* 2012;34(6):744–53.
79. Parfeniuk S, Petrovic K, MacIsaac PL, Cook KA, Rempel GR. Transition readiness measures for adolescents and young adults with chronic health conditions: A systematic review. *J Transit Med.* 2020;2(1).
80. Vaz KKH, Carmody JK, Zhang Y, Denson LA, Hommel KA. Evaluation of a novel educational tool in adolescents with inflammatory bowel disease: The NEAT study. *J Pediatr Gastroenterol Nutr.* 2019;69(5):564–9.
81. Gray WN, Wagoner ST, Schaefer MR, Reed B, Morgan P, Holbrook E, et al. Transition to adult IBD care: A pilot multi-site, telehealth hybrid intervention. *J Pediatr Psychol.* 2021;46(1):1–11.
82. Huang JS, Terrones L, Tompane T, Dillon L, Pian M, Gottschalk M, et al. Preparing adolescents with chronic disease for transition to adult care: A technology program. *Pediatrics.* 2014;133(6).
83. Stark LJ, Hommel KA, Mackner LM, Janicke DM, Davis AM, Pfefferkorn M, et al. Randomized trial comparing two methods of increasing dietary calcium intake in children with inflammatory bowel disease. *J Pediatr Gastroenterol Nutr.* 2005;40(4):501–7.
84. Hommel KA, Herzer M, Ingerski LM, Hente E, Denson LA. Individually tailored treatment of medication nonadherence. *J Pediatr Gastroenterol Nutr.* 2011;53(4):435–9.

Chapter 21

Supervision and future challenges in pediatric psychogastroenterology

Bonney Reed, Simon R. Knowles, and Miranda A.L. van Tilburg

Chapter aims

Pediatric psychogastroenterology is a growing subspecialty dependent upon highly trained mental health professionals who apply psychological and behavioral principles to treat youth with gastrointestinal (GI) diseases through clinical practice and research. The subspecialty requires expertise in youth and family mental health as well as general knowledge on pediatric gastroenterology. As the current need for pediatric psychogastroenterology services far outweighs the available workforce of practitioners, there is a critical need to train mental health professionals in pediatric psychogastroenterology. The aim of this chapter is to provide a brief review relating to supervision and future challenges in pediatric psychogastroenterology.

Learning points

- Describe the goals of supervision in pediatric psychogastroenterology and detail training opportunities for early career trainees as well as licensed mental health professionals seeking further training.
- Describe survey results obtained from practicing pediatric GI mental health professionals regarding training and practice experiences.
- Understand the need to incorporate cultural differences in training, including training at national and regional levels, as well as include diversity and cultural sensitivity.
- Discuss future challenges in pediatric psychogastroenterology and opportunities for advancing the discipline.

The mental healthcare profession has a long history of teaching clinical skills through supervised sessions. Through the process of supervision, senior mental health professionals (i.e., supervisors) provide trainees or junior mental health professionals (supervisees) with instruction, modeling, and guidance on how to provide ethical and effective mental healthcare. Supervisors are responsible for evaluating the supervisee's work to ensure that treatment is appropriate, no harm is being done to the patient, and that the supervisee is advancing in skill acquisition. The field of pediatric psychogastroenterology is no exception to this supervisory model. High-quality supervision is a key component for subspecialty training, but training opportunities are currently limited. In this chapter, we will review aspects of supervision most relevant to the field of pediatric psychogastroenterology. For further information relating to supervision, including evidence-based supervision and supervisory models, see Bernard and Goodyear's *Fundamentals of Clinical Supervision* [1] and Chapter 21 of the adult psychogastroenterology book [2].

DOI: 10.4324/9781003308683-24

Pediatric psychogastroenterology supervision in clinical practice

For mental health professionals or trainees seeking training in pediatric psychogastroenterology, this subspecialty training should build on a foundation of training and experience in general youth and family mental healthcare. This training will prepare supervisees for subspecialty training. The practice of pediatric psychogastroenterology rests on and extrapolates from general evidence-based principles such as behavioral therapy, behavior modification, cognitive therapy, and interdisciplinary care.

The first task when training in pediatric psychogastroenterology is to build a supervisee's knowledge of the pediatric GI tract and its normative functioning as well as types of commonly presenting GI symptoms and conditions. Supervisees should also be introduced to the biopsychosocial model and how it informs care for GI youth. It is not uncommon to encounter trainees who still operate on the outdated model of separation of body and mind. Knowledge building can be done through lectures, readings, or shadowing of pediatric gastroenterologists.

Once the supervisee has developed a working knowledge of pediatric GI conditions and the biopsychosocial model, they should be exposed to a variety of training experiences to learn as many strategies and techniques as possible from their supervisor. It is important to note that some supervisors work in specific clinics seeing specific types of GI issues. For example, feeding clinics, inflammatory bowel disease (IBD) clinics, or disorders of gut–brain interaction (DGBI) clinics. A supervisee would not be exposed to all types of patients in GI when training in a specific clinic. Despite this specialization within a subspecialization, trainees should still be exposed to common presentations (e.g., functional abdominal pain (FAP) in a DGBI clinic) first and work toward more rare and complex cases (e.g., rumination disorder) as training continues. Some GI diagnoses, such as IBD or feeding disorders, would only be seen in tertiary care. Mental health clinicians expecting to work in general or primary care clinics are advised to receive training in common GI disorders such as FAP, functional constipation, and avoidant restrictive food intake disorder (ARFID).

Supervisees should also be trained in how to navigate a medical clinic, including communication with other clinicians in multidisciplinary care teams, as well as billing of mental healthcare for medical disorders. Given the fast-paced nature of medical settings, supervisees may have exposure to many training cases and diagnoses in a relatively short period of time. Training goals for each type of encounter should be established and monitored at regular intervals. It is especially important to establish training goals specific to psychogastroenterology that are above and beyond basic clinical skills, as these discipline-specific goals will be imperative for the supervisee's development as an independent GI mental health professional.

In a formal supervisory relationship, supervisors will be responsible for assessing the competence of supervisees and providing feedback, oftentimes both to the supervisee and to their formal training program. Methods of providing feedback and assessing competence should be discussed at the beginning of the supervisory relationship and agreed upon. This includes reviewing documentation that will be completed regarding the supervisee's performance. Supervisors should also establish dedicated opportunities for the supervisee to provide feedback on the process of supervision, both verbally and in written formats. It is important to emphasize that supervision is an iterative process that should be tailored to individual supervisee's needs and professional development goals. The use of a supervision contract outlining the expectations and roles within formal or informal supervision can be helpful for having a shared understanding of the supervisory relationship. In addition to hierarchical supervisory relationships, there will be instances in which mental health professionals seek consultation to develop expertise in pediatric psychogastroenterology. In these peer-to-peer consultation relationships, it is advisable to develop a shared understanding and expectations for the consulting arrangement. This may include frequency of meeting, duration of the consulting relationship, how the expert consultant will be able to provide feedback on clinical work, ethics surrounding the maintenance of patient confidentiality and privacy as cases are discussed, compensation to be paid to the expert consultant, and how knowledge and expertise gained will be measured.

Throughout training, supervisors should remain cognizant of helping supervisees meet their individual training goals while ensuring that youth receive appropriate care. Supervisors are responsible for helping supervisees establish and work toward professional development goals while also serving as gatekeepers to the profession. Ultimately, supervisors are responsible for ensuring that supervisees only progress after demonstrating mastery of training goals, with the ultimate goal of upholding the values of the profession.

Training opportunities in pediatric psychogastroenterology

Supervised training opportunities in pediatric psychogastroenterology are limited and in some countries non-existent. For clinical psychology doctoral trainees in the United States of America (USA), the Pediatric Gastroenterology-Special Interest Group (PG-SIG) of the Society of Pediatric Psychology maintains a current list of predoctoral internships and postdoctoral fellowships offering training in pediatric psychogastroenterology. These can be found on their website (www.pgsig.weebly.com/training--continuing-education.html). If no official supervised training positions are available in certain areas/countries, or if an established practicing mental healthcare provider cannot commit to full-time training spots, one can reach out to established clinicians for (remote) peer-to-peer supervision and training.

Workshops, continuing education, case conferences, and journal clubs are also available, mostly in the US. The website above provides access to specific training resources developed by the PG-SIG. In addition, the Rome Foundation Psychogastroenterology Group also offers regularly scheduled continuing education opportunities with pediatric-focused trainings. Opportunities can be accessed through their website (www.theromefoundation.org/rome-gastropsych/) as well as by joining their member listserv. These training opportunities are often virtual and available for clinicians across the world. Note that the training is usually given by the US, Canadian, or European professionals and their content/advice may or may not apply to other countries/cultures. This field needs more culturally sensitive practices and evidence.

Peer reflections regarding the methods and process of supervision

As part of writing up this chapter, a brief online survey was conducted involving mental health workers who were members of the Rome Foundation GiPSYCh listserv and the listserve of the Pediatric Gastroenterology-Special Interest Group (PG-SIG) of the Society of Pediatric Psychology. Twenty-four mental health professionals participated in the survey. The majority were fully licensed (*n*=21), with an average of 9 years (range: 2–20 years) working in psychogastroenterology. Almost all were psychologists (*n*=19, 79%), with the remainder physicians (e.g., psychiatrists, gastroenterologists; *n*=4, 17%), or a social worker (*n*=1, 4%). On average, practitioners reported that 52% of their patients had a DGBI, 18% had a feeding disorder, 26% had IBD, 9% had a motility condition, and 12% had another GI condition (e.g., celiac disease, diverticulitis). The most commonly reported treatment approaches were cognitive behavioral therapy (CBT; *n*=20, 83%), family-based behavior therapy (*n*=15, 63%), hypnosis (*n*=10, 42%), acceptance and commitment therapy (ACT; *n*=9, 38%), feeding therapy (*n*=5, 21%), interpersonal approaches (e.g., psychodynamic, psychoanalytic; *n*=3, 13%), mindfulness-based stress reduction (MBSR; *n*=4, 17%), and other approaches (e.g., behavior management training, medication, psychoeducation, and applied behavior analysis *n*=4, 17%). The following is a summary of feedback provided by this group in relation to their reflections on pediatric psychogastroenterology, including the provision of supervision in this area.

When you first started in psychogastroenterology, what kind of training did you get?

Less than 21% of participants (*n*=5) reported having had formal training via internships or postgraduate studies in a psychogastroenterology clinic. This reflects the fact that most general doctoral and clinical programs do not teach skills or knowledge in psychogastroenterology. Closest is training in pediatric psychology, which is training in child health psychology including developmental, emotional, and behavioral implications of a child experiencing a medical condition or injury. Although foundational to the practice of psychogastroenterology, general training in pediatric psychology leaves out specific skills needed for specific GI disorders. Twelve respondents (50%) reported being mostly self-taught (e.g., reading, online resources). We suspect this finding reflects a general lack of training resources in preceding decades when the field of pediatric psychogastroenterology was not widely developed. Many of these early trailblazers are authors in this book. Of those who reported receiving training, five had undertaken an internship or post-doc in a psychogastroenterology clinic (21%), eight reported receiving formal supervision by someone with expertise in psychogastroenterology (33%), and five received informal supervision by someone with expertise in psychogastroenterology (21%). Fourteen participants reported receiving training through workshops and/or continuing medical education (CME) events (58%).

What are the two to three most important skills that need to be developed in your supervisees?

Over 50% of those surveyed reported supervising students in pediatric psychogastroenterology (*n*=13, 54%), with an average duration of 6 years (range: 1–15). Besides traditional clinical child psychology skills, participants emphasized the importance of knowledge and skills specific to psychogastroenterology such as biopsychosocial case conceptualization, understanding of the pathophysiology of GI conditions, knowledge of gut-directed therapies, treatment protocols, and when to implement them. Other important skills included the ability to work within an integrated care team in gastroenterology, educating and working collaboratively with parents, developing behavior plans/reward systems, and implementing behavioral feeding strategies.

What are the two to three strategies/methods you found helpful in facilitating supervisee learning?

Participants highlighted live supervision, observation and collaborative case conceptualization, and report writing as beneficial. One respondent noted that the information, training, and treatment strategies associated with psychogastroenterology are harder and take longer to master than general psychology. This emphasizes the need for formal training and direct supervision. Yet, as discussed above, only a minority of mental healthcare providers in pediatric psychogastroenterology have access to (in)formal training/supervision. This is an important area for future development and should likely include collaboration with national professional organizations such as the American Psychological Association, the Australian Association of Psychologists Inc., the British Psychological Society, and other mental health training programs.

Participants also identified directed readings, educational videos, recorded presentations, and other learning materials as particularly useful components of supervision. The current book is developed specifically for such purposes: to provide guidance in training of pediatric psychogastroenterology.

What are the challenges associated with setting up a pediatric gastroenterology service?

Thirteen participants (54%) reported being involved in setting up a pediatric psychogastroenterology service (either in a hospital or in a private practice setting). Major challenges were identified such as getting "buy-in" from the GI team, lack of space and resources, time restraints, billing and insurance credentialing/coverage issues, as well as managing inherent differences in training between different subspecialties (e.g., GI and urology). These challenges are ubiquitous in hiring a mental healthcare provider in a pediatric GI clinic and leaves many patients without access to a mental healthcare provider.

Once a mental healthcare provider is hired, the participants offered advice and tips for those setting up a pediatric gastroenterology service. This included developing scripts for medical teams and providing psychoeducational handouts to patients/families, collaborating with medical providers where possible, and building relationships within interdisciplinary teams by appreciating other subspeciality's unique contributions. Participants also highlighted the importance of setting clear role expectations and providing online tools for helping patients (e.g., online CBT or hypnosis) to better manage the patient influx. Chapter 7 discusses in depth how to mitigate these challenges when developing a multidisciplinary clinic. The current survey results show the extent to which such specific advice is needed. One caveat: the advice is based on experiences within the US healthcare system. Although some challenges are ubiquitous, clinics in other countries may encounter other challenges and want to search for country/culture-specific solutions.

What are the future challenges in psychogastroenterology?

Participants emphasized the need for not only mental healthcare clinicians being trained in psychogastroenterology, but also physicians, for example, through integrating pediatric psychogastroenterology within fellowship training programs. For mental healthcare providers to deliver effective care to patients with GI diseases, physicians need to understand and value psychogastroenterology and know how to work with mental healthcare providers.

Some participants also highlighted the need to expand the workforce. Youth become adults and may miss adequate access to psychogastroenterology across the lifespan (i.e., pediatric to adult care). Some youth who have no access to adult clinics with expertise in psychogastroenterology may linger in pediatric care as young adults and eventually lose age-appropriate medical follow-up. Others who have no access to pediatric offices will prematurely (sometimes as young as age 12) be referred to an adult clinic with integrated pediatric psychogastroenterology. Neither is an ideal situation for obvious reasons.

Survey participants also emphasized that certain issues will remain challenges in the future. These are related to getting "buy-in" from administration and physicians, along with finding a financial model (e.g., value-based care) and billing structure that can be readily adopted. The reason why these issues have not yet been solved is likely due to the stigma of mental health, which reduces willingness of administrators/physicians to provide mental healthcare and for insurers to reimburse such care.

Cultural issues in pediatric psychogastroenterology

Pediatric psychogastroenterology is not practiced in a vacuum. Culture, healthcare systems, insurance, training and accreditation requirements, etc., vary from country to country and even within certain regions or certain cultural or ethnic groups. This variety impacts how pediatric psychogastroenterology is practiced. For example, children's toileting fears likely change with the type of toilet (pit latrine vs smart toilet), cultural stigma around defecation (can be discussed vs not), school toilets (private vs stalls without doors), parenting practices in toilet training, healthcare systems, etc. The rise of pediatric psychogastroenterology in the past few decades has been most notable in North America and in some European countries. This is reflective of our book authors – experts in their fields – who are predominantly from the US, with the addition of Canadian, Dutch, and Australian authors. As the editors, we tried hard to include culturally diverse international experts. We found that in some countries, particularly those in South America, Africa, and Asia, pediatric psychogastroenterology is in its infancy, and mental healthcare providers are rarely added to GI clinics.

It is important to recognize that the primary focus on practices in the US leads to a bias in the information presented in this book. Mental healthcare providers from other countries are advised to scrutinize recommended strategies, as they may or may not be valid for their patients. Even within the US, cultural and ethnic diversity can affect what are best practices. For example, parental beliefs about the appropriate age for toilet training vary by race, with Caucasian parents believing it should start after the child turns two, while Black parents believe it should start at 18 months of age [3]. A culturally competent mental healthcare provider will need to be aware of these cultural differences to work with diverse families.

Other areas that affect pediatric psychogastroenterology practices include how countries pay for visits (e.g., social medicine vs private insurance) and how school systems deal with medical issues (e.g., school nurses, formalized plans, special schooling). These may be a matter of access vs no access. For example, in the Netherlands, GI-focused hypnotherapy is now available to almost every child in the country, while in the US, access is limited and often concentrated in large (sub)urban areas. We hope this book will be an impetus for many to develop more culturally sensitive evidence-based practices, accreditation requirements, training guidelines, and increased insurance reimbursement for pediatric gastroenterology.

Future challenges in psychogastroenterology

As with any new and growing discipline, there are challenges for us to overcome collectively as pediatric psychogastroenterology health professionals and researchers. Similar to those who work with adults, the financial viability of pediatric psychogastroenterology within existing healthcare frameworks must be established. For pediatric psychogastroenterology to become mainstream as a critical treatment component for GI youth, financial models must be established to support the expertise, time, and space required to deliver psychogastroenterology treatment despite lower reimbursement rates compared to medical treatment.

To meet the clinical demands, pediatric psychogastroenterology must continue to be integrated into mainstream pediatric GI treatment, including access outside of major urban medical centers. Expanded opportunities for pediatric psychogastroenterology training experiences are also needed, both for early career trainees and for established mental health professionals seeking to develop expertise. A growing workforce of well-trained GI mental health professionals will allow the field to better meet clinical demands while increasing the visibility of the subspecialty as a critical component of holistic GI treatment. Existing evidence-based treatments need to be tested across the developmental spectrum to test effectiveness in different age groups and cultures.

Final comments

The initial idea of this book came after the original adult version *Psychogastroenterology for Adults* was published by Routledge in 2019. Mental health professionals, especially those working in psychogastroenterology, reported that the adult book was a valuable resource, and that a pediatric version is really needed. As the editors of this handbook, we are incredibly impressed and encouraged by the collective body of knowledge contributed by the authors of this volume. What began as a goal of developing a handbook to guide training for mental health professionals in pediatric psychogastroenterology developed into an exciting demonstration of the many areas of the subspecialty, with well-developed cross-disciplinary expertise and a growing evidence base. As the experience and expertise of these contributors attest, the future of pediatric psychogastroenterology is bright. For those entering the field, this handbook will serve as a collated guide to the conditions treated by GI mental health professionals, current evidence-based treatments, and clinical expertise to guide the "nuts and bolts" of practicing as a pediatric psychogastroenterologist. Ultimately, we envision this handbook increasing training accessibility to future GI mental health professionals and hopefully helping to develop a growing workforce of expert health professionals and scientists to meet growing and complex clinical demands.

References

1. Bernard JM, Goodyear RK. *Fundamentals of clinical supervision*: Boston: Allyn & Bacon; 2004.
2. Knowles SR, Keefer L, Mikocka-Walus AA. Supervision and future challenges in psychogastroenterology (Chapter 21). In: Knowles SR, Keefer, L, Mikocka-Walus, AA, editor. *Psychogastroenterology: A handbook for mental health professionals*. Oxon: Routledge Press; 2019. pp. 309–17.
3. Horn IB, Brenner R, Rao M, Cheng TL. Beliefs about the appropriate age for initiating toilet training: Are there racial and socioeconomic differences? *J Pediatr*. 2006;149(2):165–8.

Index

Page numbers in **bold reference tables.
**Page numbers in *italics* reference figures.

abdominal migraine 44
abdominal pain 189–190, 198; assessing 93; disorders of gut-brain interaction (DGBI)191–192; history of xxvii; non-pharmacologic management 194–195; organic GI disorders 192; pharmacologic management 194; treatment of 193, 201–204
abdominal X-ray 57–58
absorption of nutrients *13*
acceptance and commitment therapy (ACT): treatment of abdominal pain 204
ACEs *see* Adverse Childhood Experiences
acid 11, 18
ACT *see* acceptance and commitment therapy
acute pain 67
adaptive coping 104–107
ADHD *see* attention deficit hyperactivity disorder
adjustment to illness 240–241; evidence-based interventions **242–243**; promoting adherence 244–245
administrative leaders, recommended talking points with **96**
adolescents: adaptive coping 106–107; constipation 233; constipation and soiling 228–232; food refusal 148; nonadherence 244; promoting daily functioning 109; refractory symptoms 123; treatment adherence 104
Adverse Childhood Experiences (ACEs) 25
aerophagia 43–44
Aftertaste Challenge 173
ampulla of Vater 14–15
AN *see* anorexia nervosa
anatomy: of anorectal canal *17*; of GI tract *4*; of stomach *10*
anorectal malformations 38–39
anorectal manometry 60–61
anorectal/pelvic floor muscles 16–17
anorexia nervosa (AN)169–170
ANS *see* autonomic nervous system
antacids *37*
antecedent-based challenges, for feeding disorders 139
antibiotic refractory Clostridium difficile infections 18
antidepressants 194
antidiarrheal **37**
antihistamines 194
anti-inflammatory **37**
antinausea **37**
antiseizure medications 194
antispasmodics **37**, 194
antroduodenal manometry 60
anus 16
anxiety 105; brain-gut axis (BGA) 26; due to medical procedures 68; GI-related comorbidities 117–118; illness-specific anxiety 240; respiratory symptoms of 168
anxiety comorbidity 179
ARFID *see* avoidant/restrictive food intake disorder
ASD *see* autism spectrum disorder
aspiration 7–8
assessing: abdominal pain 193, 201; constipation 221, 229; fear 68, **70**, 170; pain 68, **70**; youth with nausea and vomiting disorders (NVD)179–181
assessment best practices: behavioral observations 81; clinical interviews 78–80; medical examination 78; validated measures and screeners 81–83
assessment findings, implications of 83–84
assessment questions/comments, regarding food refusal *149*
attention deficit hyperactivity disorder (ADHD) 117

autism spectrum disorder (ASD): constipation 233; food selectivity 159
autonomic nervous system (ANS) 25
avoidance: fears of aversive consequences 168; school avoidance 179, 193
avoidant/restrictive food intake disorder (ARFID) 132–133, 136–137, 169–170; history of *134*

behavioral assessment of constipation 222–223
behavioral intervention: of cyclic vomiting syndrome (CVS)183–184; of rumination 185–186
behavioral modification for constipation 224–225
behavioral observations 81
behavioral rigidity 117
behavioral strategies, of constipation 231–232
behavioral treatment, of constipation 223
belching 36
BGA *see* brain-gut axis
bile 3, 14–15
biofeedback 234
biologics 194
biomedical model xxviii, 23
biopsychosocial model xxviii, 77–78, 87; brain-gut axis (BGA) 22–23
bite-size fading *146*
blood supply 6
blood tests 54–55
body image 241
bowel management 231
bowel urgency, GI-related comorbidities 115–116
brain-gut axis (BGA) 7, 22–25; anxiety 26; biopsychosocial model 22–23; catastrophizing 26–27; depression 27; environmental factors 27–28; gut microbiota 28; influence of stress 25–26; influencing psychological factors during therapy 28–30; metaphors to explain **29**; post-traumatic stress disorder (PTSD) 27; somatization 27; trauma/PTSD 27
breath tests 56–57
brief screen for tobacco, alcohol and drugs (BSTAD) 180
burping *see* belching

C. difficile infection 18
capsule endoscopy 62–63
caregiver education 71
caregivers 101; catastrophizing 105; collaborating with 102–103, 125–126; constipated children 232–233; education of 102; evidence-based collaboration to promote adaptive coping 105–107; helping promote adaptive coping 104–105; helping promote adherence 103; overprotection 107–108; promoting daily functioning 107–109; supporting 109–110; training in food refusal 147
case conceptualization 81–82; biopsychosocial model 77–78
catastrophizing: brain-gut axis (BGA) 26–27; caregivers 105; psychosocial aspects of pain 199
CBT *see* cognitive behavioral therapy (CBT)
CD *see* Crohn's disease
celiac disease 41, 219; treatment adherence 103
central nervous system (CNS) 23; pain 190
cephalic phase 7; gastric secretion 11–12
challenges for psychogastroenterology in the future 256–258
chemical digestion 11
chief cells 11
child mental health professionals **92**
children: adaptive coping 106; constipation and soiling 228–232; treatment adherence 103–104
children's libido xxvii
cholesterol 15
chronic abdominal pain 192–193; *see also* abdominal pain
chronic GI conditions: psychosocial functioning with 239–241; self-management of 241–244; transitioning to adult care 245
chronic GI symptoms 35; metaphors to explain **29**
chronic pain 67; acceptance and commitment therapy (ACT)204; *see also* pain
classical conditioning 7
clinical interviews 78–80
clinical practice, supervision of 253–254
CNS *see* central nervous system
coaches, collaborating with 124–125
codes for pediatric feeding disorder (PFD) 136
cognitions: catastrophizing 199; hurt *vs.* harm 199–200
cognitive behavioral therapy (CBT) xxviii, 101, 182, 241; food refusal 148; treatment of abdominal pain 201–202
cognitive restructuring, treatment of abdominal pain 202
colic 193
colitis xxvii
collaborating with: caregivers 125–126; multidisciplinary teams 125; schools/coaches 124–125
colon (large intestine) 16
colonic manometry 60
colonoscopy 63
common characteristics of, complex cases 114
common GI conditions **36**
communication: with caregivers 102; family-provider communication 109; in multidisciplinary care **93**; strategies for **92**
community-based treatment, of food refusal 143
comorbidities: anxiety disorders 117–118; obsessive-compulsive disorders (OCDs) 117–118; *see also* GI-related comorbidities

complex cases: common characteristics of 114; difficulties in therapeutic alliance and misconceptions about treatment 120–122; GI-related comorbidities *see* GI-related comorbidities; social determinants of health (SDOH) 119–120
compliance training, punishment and 231
constipation 219, 228; assessing 221, 229; autism spectrum disorder (ASD)233; behavioral assessment 222–223; behavioral modification 224–225; behavioral strategies 231–232; behavioral treatment 223; bowel management 231; cycle of 220; education of 223–224, 230–231; functional constipation 46, 229; history of xxvii; interventions for 233–234; psychogenic constipation xxvii; psychosocial assessments 230; toilet training 223; treatment adherence 224; treatment of abdominal pain 221–222
consultations for feeding disorders 138
coping kit 106
coping strategies for medical procedures 68–70
Crohn's disease (CD) 19, 40
cultural issues in psychogastroenterology 257
CVS *see* cyclic vomiting syndrome
cycle: of constipation *220*; of somatic avoidance resulting from fear generalization *167*
cyclic vomiting syndrome (CVS) 45–46, **178**, 179; sleep disruptions 180; treatment of 183–184

D-cells 11
deep enteroscopy 63
deglutition *see* swallowing
depression, brain-gut axis (BGA) 27
desensitization, strategies to address food refusal 146
diagnostic comorbidity 114–115; anxiety disorders 117–118; GI-related comorbidities 115–117; obsessive-compulsive disorders (OCDs) 117–118
diarrhea 36, 55
diet, microbiome 18
difficulty swallowing 169
disability, pain and 192–193
disorders of gut-brain interaction (DGBI) xxvi, xxviii, 7, 19, 23, 41–43; abdominal migraine 44; abdominal pain 191–192; aerophagia 43–44; cyclic vomiting syndrome (CVS) 45–46; functional abdominal pain (FAP) 45; functional constipation 46, 219; functional dyspepsia (FD) 43; functional nausea 45; irritable bowel syndrome (IBS) 44; nonretentive fecal incontinence 47; pain 190; rumination syndrome 43
distraction: coping strategies for medical procedures 72–73; treatment of abdominal pain 203–204
duodenum 15
Dutch protocol, hypnotherapy 215
dysautonomia 116
dysphagia 36, 169

EA *see* esophageal atresia
early childhood, promoting daily functioning 108
eating away from home, food selectivity 159
eating disturbance 136
education of, constipation 223–224, 230–231
emotional and behavioral functioning 239–240
emotional distress, psychosocial aspects of pain 199
endoluminal functional lumen imaging probe (EndoFLIP) 61–62
endoscopy 62–63
enemas 222
enhanced toilet training (ETT)233–234
enteric nervous system (ENS) 6, 23; pain 190
enterochromaffin-like cells 11
environmental control, strategies to address food refusal 145
environmental factors, brain-gut axis (BGA) 27–28
enzymes 3, 14
eosinophilic esophagitis (EoE) 39–40
escape extinction, strategies to address food refusal 147
esophageal atresia (EA) 36–37
esophageal manometry 59–60
esophageal phase, of GI tract 8
esophagus 3, 7–8
ETT *see* enhanced toilet training
exposure therapy, treatment of abdominal pain 204

fading, strategies to address food refusal 146
family involvement 182
family-provider communication 109
FAP *see* functional abdominal pain
FAPDs *see* functional abdominal pain disorders
FD *see* functional dyspepsia
fear: assessing 68, **70**; cycle of somatic avoidance resulting from fear generalization *167*; helping youth manage medical procedures 68; of stooling 224–225; of toileting 222–223
fear-learning model 170–171
fear network, emergence of (feeding difficulties)165–169
fears of aversive consequences (FOAC) 164–165; diagnosis of 169–170; emergence of maladaptive fear network 165–169; integrating treatment approaches 170–171; strategies for addressing 171–173
fecal alpha-1 antitrypsin test 56
fecal fat test 56
fecal microbiota transplantation (FMT) 18

feeding behaviors, positive reinforcement 145–146
feeding difficulties 131–133; avoidant/restrictive food intake disorder (ARFID) 136–137; best practices for 137–139; fears of aversive consequences *see* fears of aversive consequences; food refusal *see* food refusal; food selectivity *see* food selectivity; pediatric feeding disorder (PFD) 133–136; *see also* nausea; vomiting
feeding skill assessment 132
feeding skill dysfunction, pediatric feeding disorder (PFD) 133
feeding strategies 147–148
feeding treatment providers, state of practice 137
feeling and body investigators (FBI agents) 171
FGIDs *see* functional gastrointestinal disorders
fight or flight response 25
FMT *see* fecal microbiota transplantation
FN *see* functional nausea
FOAC *see* fears of aversive consequences
food hierarchies 157
food refusal 142–143; assessment questions/comments *149*; community-based treatment 143; contributing factors of *144*; strategies to address 145–147
food-related concerns, GI-related comorbidities 116
food rewards 157
food selectivity 152; autism spectrum disorder (ASD) 159; creating food hierarchies 157; interventions 152, 154; maintaining progress 159; parent and family factors 154; parent-child feeding interaction *155*; parent training (PT) 154; reinforcement 154–155, 157; selective attention 154–155, 157; strategies to increase appropriate mealtime behaviors 154, 157; tasting time 158; treatment planning 154
food sensitivities 116
functional abdominal pain (FAP) xxvi, 45, 101
functional abdominal pain disorders (FAPDs) 191–192, 198
functional constipation 46, 219; clinical presentation of 229; *see also* constipation
functional disability **178**, 181
functional dyspepsia (FD) 43
functional gastrointestinal disorders (FGIDs) 198
functional nausea (FN) 45, **178**; treatment of 182–183
functional vomiting (FV) **178**; treatment of 183
functioning, promoting daily functioning 107–109
FV *see* functional vomiting

gagging 173; *see also* vomiting
gallbladder 3, 14–16
gastric belching 8
gastric emptying 12
gastric emptying studies 59
gastric juices 11
gastric phase, gastric secretion 12
gastric relaxer **37**
gastric secretion 11–12
gastroesophageal reflux disease (GERD) 8, 36, 39
gate control theory of pain 26
G-cells 11
general anesthesia 73–74
GERD *see* gastroesophageal reflux disease
GI conditions: common in youth **36**; disorders of gut-brain interaction (DGBI) 41–47; inflammatory GI conditions 39–41; structural conditions 36–39
GI immune system 19
GI mental health professionals 71–72, **92**; assessment phase 91; case conceptualization 81–82; clinical interviews 80; role of 68–70; validated measures and screeners 82–83
GI-related comorbidities 115–117; trauma/PTSD 119
GI tract 3; anorectal/pelvic floor muscles 16–17; basic structure and function of 3–5; blood supply 6; gallbladder 14–16; gut microbiota 18; immune system 19; large intestine (colon) 16; layers of 5–6; liver 14–16; nervous system 6–7; pancreas 14; signs 19; small intestine 12–13; stomach 8–12; swallowing 7–8; symptoms 19
glucagon 14
guide to food refusal 147–148
gut-directed hypnotherapy 215; stages of hypnosis **212**; *see also* hypnotherapy
gut microbiota 18, 28, 191

H. pylori (*Helicobacter pylori*) 55–57
H&B CPT codes 80
harms of overtesting 63–64
health-related quality of life (HRQoL) 240
helping youth manage medical procedures: acute and chronic pain 67; coping strategies for medical procedures 68–70; pharmacological strategies 73–74; physical strategies for 72; procedural pain and fear 68; process and preparatory strategies 71–72; psychological strategies 72–73
Hirschsprung disease 38, 219
histamine 11
history of: avoidant/restrictive food intake disorder (ARFID) *134*; pediatric feeding disorder (PFD) *134*; of psychogastroenterology xxvii–xxviii
HPA *see* hypothalamic-pituitary-adrenal axis
HRQoL *see* health-related quality of life
hurt *vs.* harm 199–200

hypnosis, coping strategies for medical procedures 73
hypnotherapy 211–215; challenges associated with 216; discussing with parents/youth 215; individual versus home-based treatment 215–216
hypothalamic-pituitary-adrenal axis (HPA) 25

IBD *see* inflammatory bowel disease
IBS *see* irritable bowel syndrome
imaging 57; abdominal X-ray 57–58; gastric emptying studies 59; upper GI X-ray 58–59
immune system 19
immunomodulator **37**
incontinence, nonretentive fecal incontinence 47
infants/toddlers: adaptive coping 106; constipation 221–222; constipation and soiling 220–226; eating disorders 139; pain 193; treatment adherence 103
inflammatory bowel disease (IBD) xxvi, 40–41, 101, 192; body image 241; history of xxvii
interdisciplinary care 91–93
intestinal phase, gastric secretion 12
intrinsic factor, stomach 11
irritable bowel syndrome (IBS) 7, 19, 44, 103, 115, 191

laboratory testing, common indications for **55**; *see also* medical procedures/testing
language adaptations, by age and development level **79**
large intestine (colon) 16
laxatives 222, 229
layers of GI tract 5–6
LES *see* lower esophageal sphincter
limbic circuit 168
liver 3, 14–16
lower esophageal sphincter (LES) 8, *10*

maladaptive fear gradient *166*
meal schedules, strategies to address food refusal 145
mealtime behaviors, strategies for increasing 154, 157
mealtime structure 138
medical assessment of constipation 229
medical dysfunction, pediatric feeding disorder (PFD) 133
medical examination 78
medical procedures/testing: blood tests 54 55; breath tests 56–57; endoscopy 62–63; harms of over-testing 63–64; imaging 57–59; motility and pH testing 59–62; stool tests 55–56; *see also* helping youth manage medical procedures
medications for GI conditions **37**; rumination syndrome 43
memory reframing, coping strategies for medical procedures 73
metaphors to explain, brain-gut connection, nervous system hypersensitivity and chronic GI symptoms **29**
middle childhood, promoting daily functioning 108–109
mind-body skills 182
misaligned treatment goals 122–123
miscarried helping 107
miscommunication 122
misconceptions about treatments 120–122
modeling, social influences on GI pain 200–201
motility 59–62; anorectal manometry 60–61; antroduodenal manometry 60; colonic manometry 60; common testing indications **62**; EndoFLIP (endoluminal functional lumen imaging probe) 61–62; esophageal manometry 59–60
mouth 7–8
mucosa 5
mucus cells 11
multidisciplinary assessment, for feeding disorders 132
multidisciplinary teams, collaborating with 125
multidisciplinary treatment: determining starting state 95–98; identifying the ideal state 87–93; moving toward the ideal state 98; selecting your team 94–95
muscle tensions, coping strategies for medical procedures 72
muscular layer, of GI tract 5–6

nausea 177; GI-related comorbidities 115–116; *see also* functional nausea
nausea and vomiting disorders (NVD)177, **178**; assessing 179–181; treatment primer 181–182
nausea severity scale 180
nervous system 6–7
nervous system hypersensitivity, metaphors to explain **29**
neuropathic pain 189
NFI *see* nonretentive fecal incontinence
nociceptive pain 189
nonadherence 244
non-pharmacologic management, of abdominal pain 194–195
nonretentive fecal incontinence (NFI) 47, 234
nurses 89
nutritional assessments 132
nutritional deficiencies, autism spectrum disorder (ASD) 159

treatment: of abdominal pain 193, 201–204; of constipation 221–222; of cyclic vomiting syndrome (CVS)183–184; of functional nausea 182–183; of functional vomiting (FV)183; misaligned treatment goals 122–123; of rumination 184–185
treatment adherence 103; adjustment to illness 244–245; adolescents 104; children 103–104; for constipation 224; infants/toddlers 103
treatment nonadherence, troubleshooting 124–125
treatment planning, food selectivity 154
treatment primer, on nausea and vomiting disorders (NVDs)181–182
treatments, misconceptions about 120–122
troubleshooting treatment nonadherence 124–125
tube weaning 173

ulcerative colitis (UC) 40, 192
upper GI X-ray 58–59

validated measures and screeners 81–83
visceral hypersensitivity 190–191
visceral pain 189
vomiting 173, 177; GI-related comorbidities 115–116; *see also* functional vomiting

X-ray: abdominal 57–58; upper GI X-ray 58–59